MW00446863

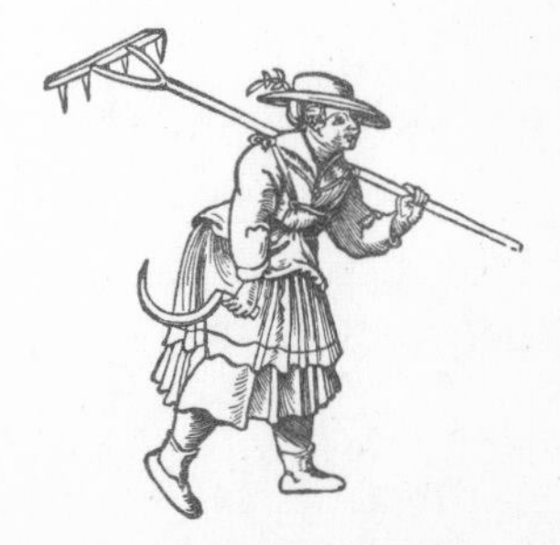

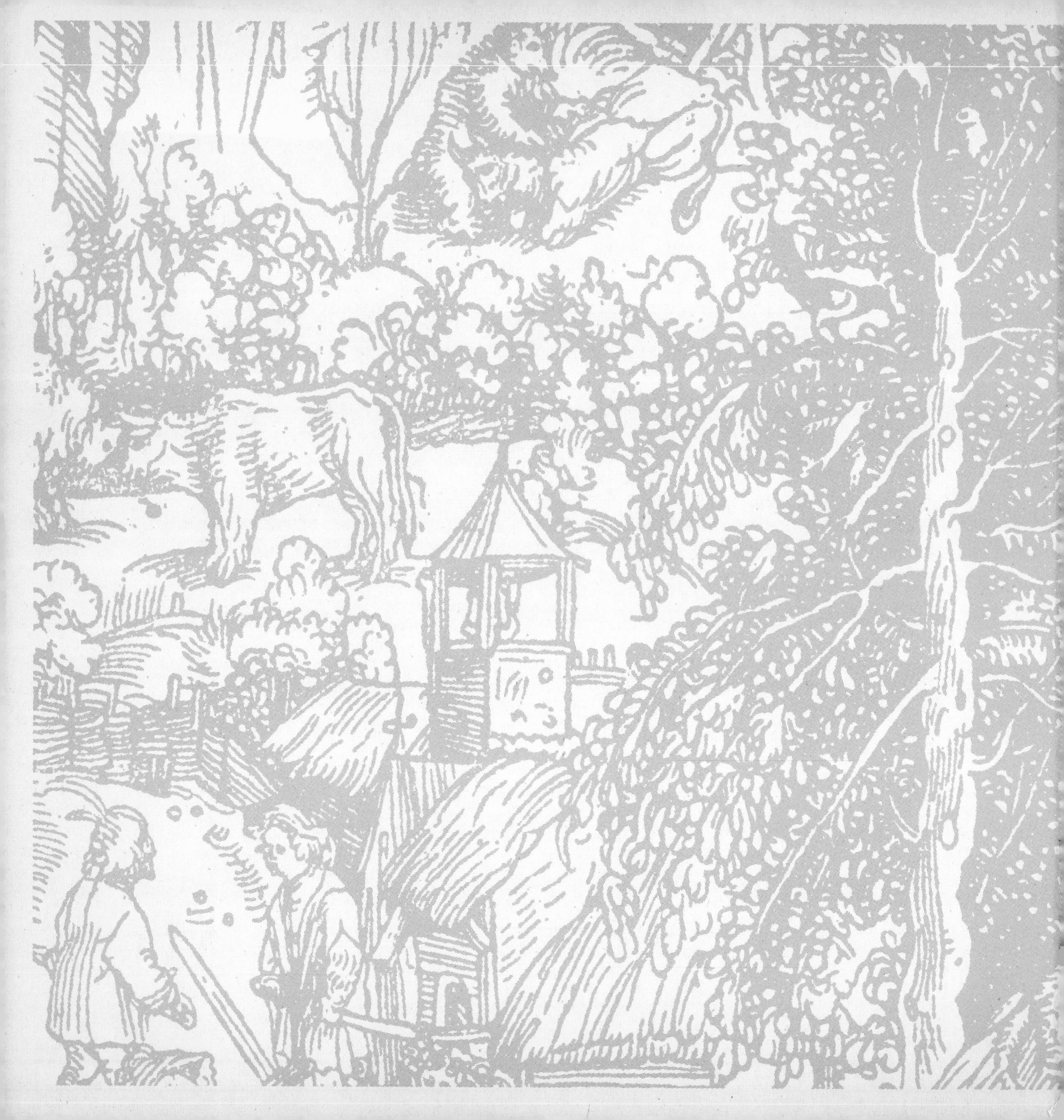

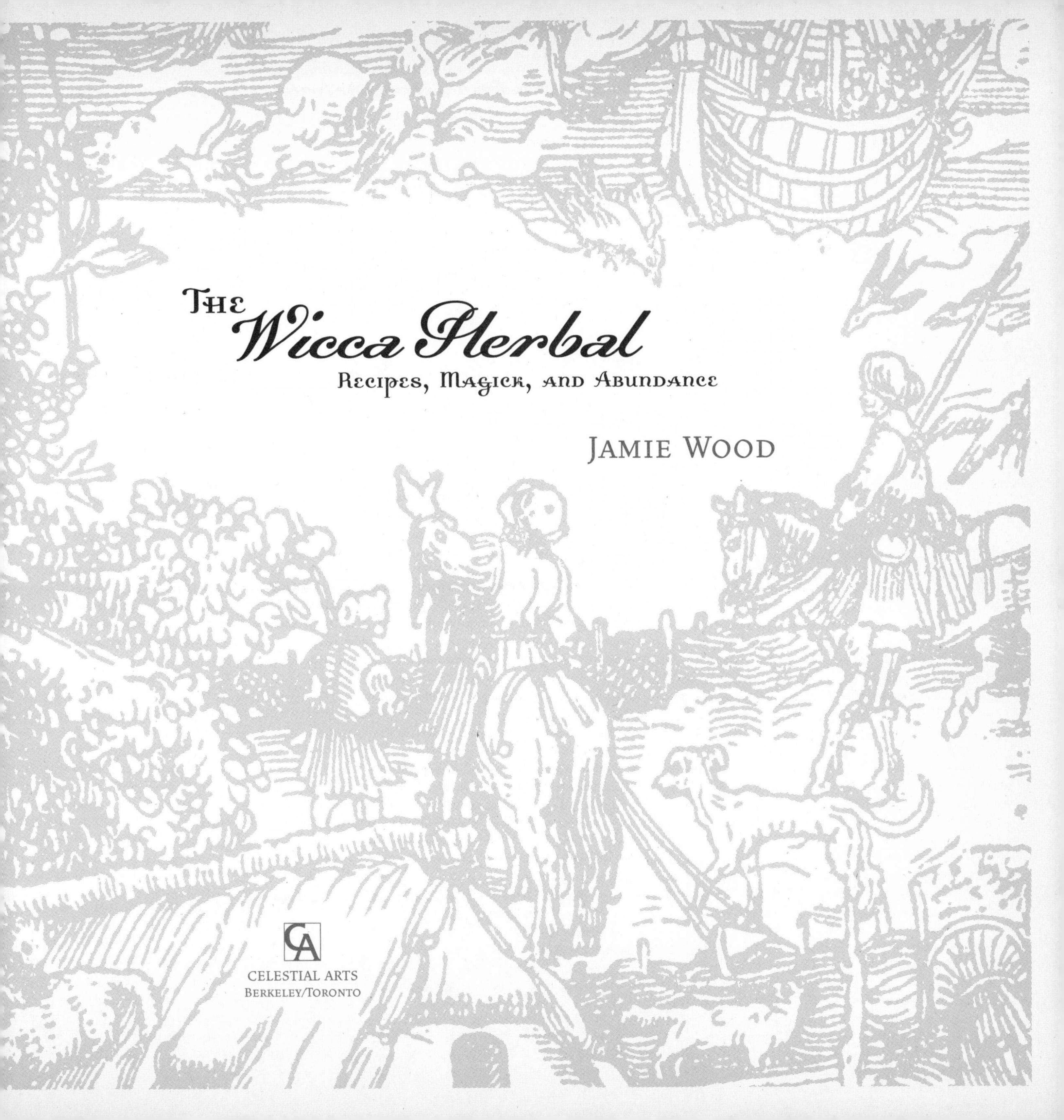

The Wicca Herbal

Recipes, Magick, and Abundance

Jamie Wood

CA
CELESTIAL ARTS
BERKELEY/TORONTO

I dedicate this book to the faeries and offer energy to the continuing relationship between their world and ours.

A Kirsty Melville Book

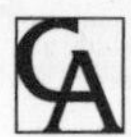

Celestial Arts
P.O. Box 7123
Berkeley, California 94707
www.tenspeed.com

Distributed in Australia by Simon and Schuster Australia, in Canada by Ten Speed Press Canada, in New Zealand by Southern Publishers Group, in South Africa by Real Books, and in the United Kingdom and Europe by Airlift Book Company.

Cover and text design by Jeff Puda

The information contained in this book is based on the experience and research of the author. It is not intended as a substitute for consulting with your physician or other health-care provider. Any attempt to diagnose and treat an illness should be done under the direction of a health-care professional. The publisher and author are not responsible for any adverse effects or consequences resulting from the use of any of the suggestions, preparations, or procedures discussed in this book.

Library of Congress Cataloging-in-Publication Data
Wood, Jamie.
The Wicca Herbal: recipes, magick, and abundance/Jamie Wood.
p. cm.
"A Kirsty Melville book"—T.p. verso.
Includes bibliographical references (p.) and index.
ISBN 1-58761-169-4 (paper)
1. Witchcraft. 2.Herbs—Miscellanea. 3. Magic. I. Title.

BF1572.P43W662003
133.4'3—dc21

2003048452

First printing, 2003
Printed in Canada

1 2 3 4 5 6 7 8 9 10 — 07 06 05 04 03

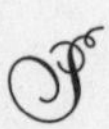

Yes,

I

Am

Wiccan

Yearning breaths slips through the cracks of my being

Everything stills to the sound of the question: who am I

Suspended in the downy void of existence I recall

I echo in my soul the eternity of woman and her grace through adversity

Armored in her resolution and cloaked in her compassion for all things

Maiden. Temptress, Mother, Crone—many faces, yet, one soul

Wondering in awe of my connection to all that came before and all that shall be

Intricacies that Mother and Father Nature placed before me as gifts to be unwrapped

Cradled in the magic and mischief that surrounds my tenuous existence

Compassion that bleeds forth from a place of my remembering

Aroused with the suspicion that I am but a guest upon this sphere

Never forgetting to love myself, my fellowman, flora, fauna, and the future . . .

—Cheryl Martel Hardin

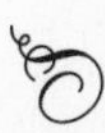

Contents

1

Wicca & Mother Earth

2

Magickal Herbs & Plants

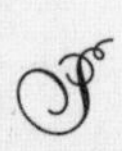

Acknowledgments

I offer my thanks to three wonderful people who helped shape and encourage *The Wicca Herbal*: my magickal midwives Connie, James, and Michael. Without your support and encouragement, I would have been lost. Thank you for the guidance, presence, and peace of mind you offered. Thank you Jacquie for your wise wimmin advice; big, fat, wet faery kiss to Rue for listening to my ramblings; and lots of thanks to Sara for checking my culinary dishes. I truly appreciate my advocates: Windy Ferges, an awesome editor and even more incredible woman; Julie Castiglia, a fantastic agent, lovely lady, and true friend; and Lisa Regul, my patient cornerstone, with whom I enjoy sharpening the tools of my wit. Much appreciation to Jeff Puda for the beautiful design of this book, as well as the other books in my Wicca series.

I am also very grateful, to the tips of my glittering wings, to those who lovingly contributed recipes, rituals, and information or assistance. They are: Cheryl, Cindy, Crimson Dragon entourage, Dawn Marie, Deborah, Elise, Jeannine, Jeff, Jenny, Jimi, Johanna, Julie, Kristen, Melinda, Robynn, Sharon, and Tara. Lots of squishy, faery hugs for the warm and caring support and friendship from Babsikins, Barbara, Chrystie, Crystal, Julia, Lisa, Megan, Rocky, Tammy, and Victoria. Big kisses to my family: Kevin, Alethia, Skyler, Kobe, and Buck. It's time to play with the faeries. Let's create Findhorn wherever we are! The Goddess is back.

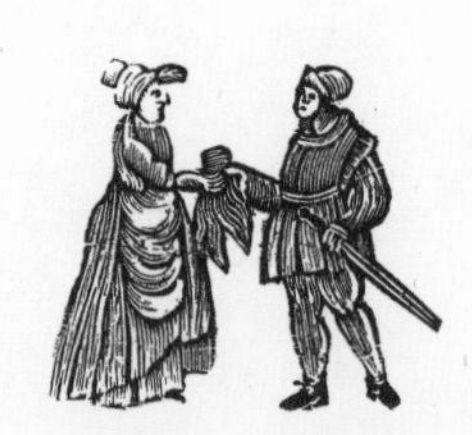

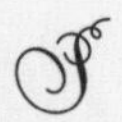

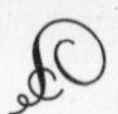

Preface

Wicca is a way of life that asks you to attune yourself with nature's ebb and flow. I believe Wicca is a guide for living with a strong spiritual emphasis, though not every follower adheres to this. You must find your own path. It requires great responsibility and a personal connection to Spirit; no one person should be your sole source of information. Books help, but primarily you need to be in nature. The God and Goddess are attributes of the Creator, and help you focus or invoke their divine essence, but it is not necessary to know all the pantheons.

Magick is the manifestation of our thoughts and desires. The word comes from an ancient term meaning "to be able." In Wicca, it is spelled *magick* to distinguish it from the more general term *magic*. The "k" in *magick* balances the energy of the word; the "k" reaches for heaven while the "g" roots down to earth. Spells are cast on very special occasions. They serve as tools to remind us of our ability to manifest even without the right herb or a candle of the right color. Wicca reminds us of our divine nature by pointing to the fact that the Divine is within. The ceremonies remind us of our part in the connection with nature and All That Is.

Witches heal. We lead, by example, a life at one with the cycles and rhythms of nature. Throughout time, until today, witches have sought to bring healing by using the gift of herbs. The herbs I have selected for this book are those most often used by Wiccan healers to maintain harmony and good health, clear blocks from abundance and joy, and actualize dreams and desires.

If you are interested in Wicca and witchcraft, your interest is all that is necessary. You cannot become a witch by casting spells or buying lots of incense and oils. Rather, observe a bird's flight—the way he lets go and allows the wind to carry him—and apply it to your life; watch how nature grows quiet in the winter and allow for the same rest and introspection in your life.

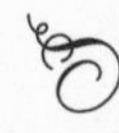

1

Wicca & Mother Earth

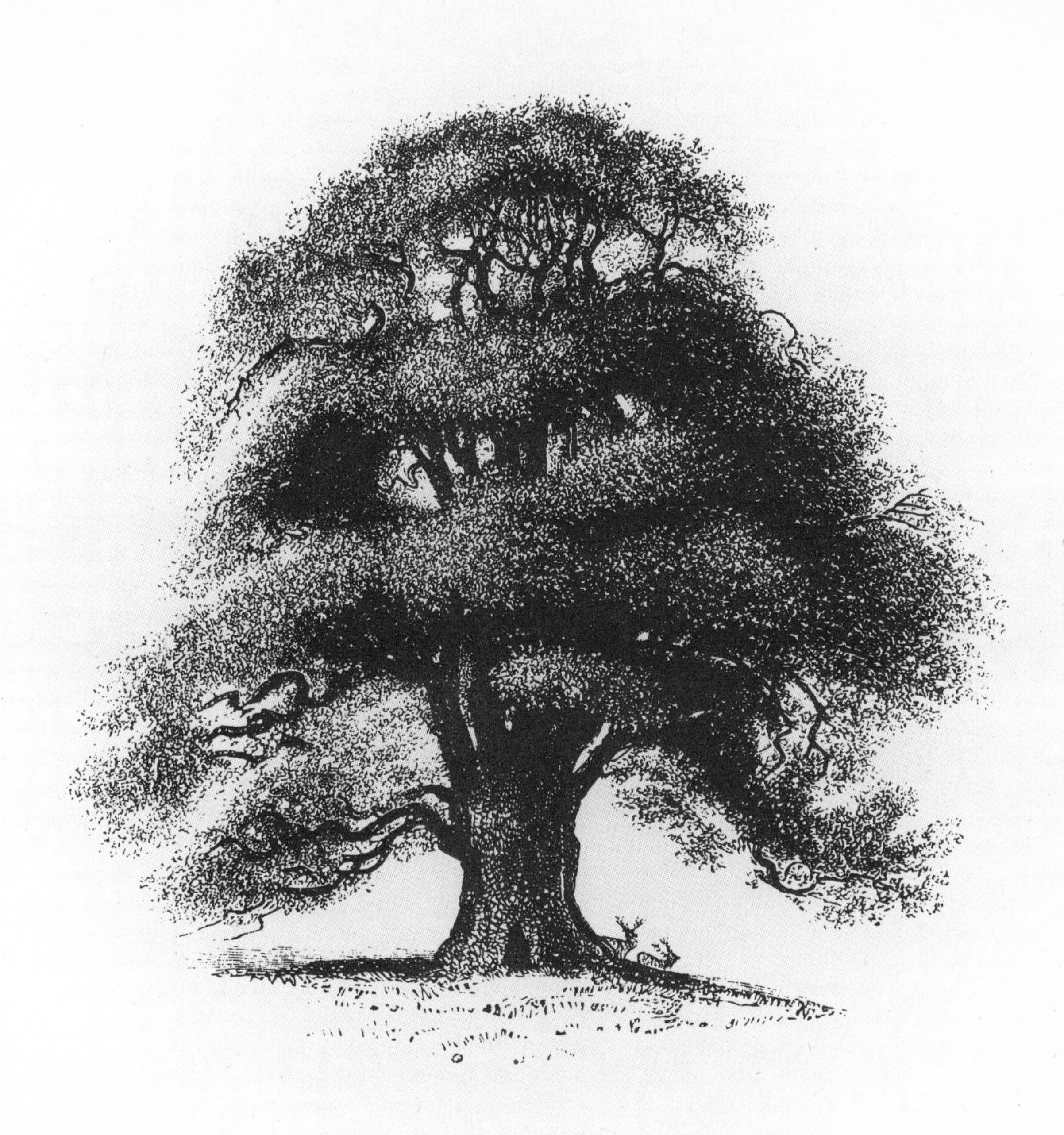

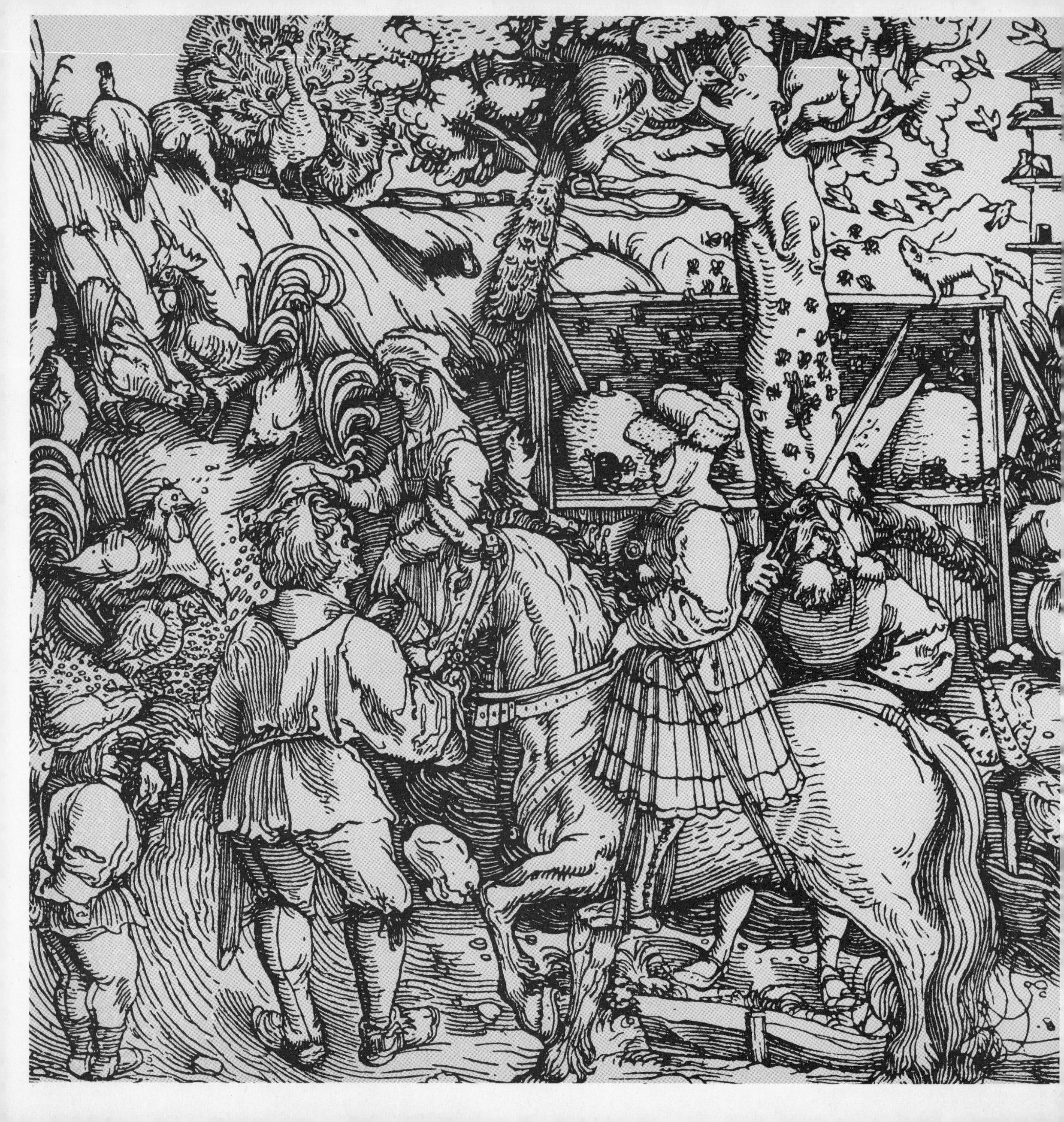

Introduction

CENTURIES BEFORE CHEMISTS concocted potent drugs and manufactured beauty supplies in high-tech laboratories, people went to Mother Earth in search of ingredients for healing, ritual, and beauty. The earth's rich supply of herbs and plants comforted the people, allowing and inviting them to recognize the abundance and security the Mother provided. From the dawn of time, Mother Earth has offered ready remedies to meet the physical, spiritual, and emotional needs of her children. It matters not if the need is for serenity, soothed with chamomile on a quiet desert night, or relief from depression, to be found in St. John's wort (as well as in looking at a rainbow). The living, breathing Mother Earth—often known as Gaia in the Wiccan faith—is quite literally supportive; we drink her waters, walk upon her, breathe oxygen from her trees, and find our needs met through using the curative power of herbs.

Although our collective connection with nature has been challenged for many years, the popularity of herbs is enjoying a renaissance. Digging into the earth and allowing the Mother's rich soil to sift through our fingers as we gar-

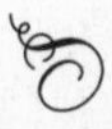

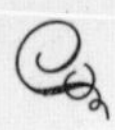

den grounds us with a sense of well-being. We take comfort in knowing that we are always protected and our needs provided. When we take the time to care for a garden and make our own therapeutic remedies, we are affirming that we want health, beauty, and happiness. Cultivating an ongoing relationship with nature and Mother Gaia connects us with a higher order of intelligence and a rhythm not often perceptible by our limited human minds. We tap into this wisdom when we grow and use herbs. Herbs teach us balance between resting and blooming, the need and value of our dependency, and the universe's perfect harmonic timing.

Rub the leaves of the aromatic rosemary or chew on the sweet licorice-tasting seeds of anise, and a world opens up to you. Every seed contains the knowledge it needs to grow. An acorn doesn't wonder if it will become a mighty oak, for it already is. All of nature's wisdom and self-actualization is available to you. Follow Mother Earth's pattern, and you will find an impeccable design of divine beingness.

Tuning in to nature and herbs can help bring the spiritual to the mundane, heaven to earth. We align ourselves with the vibration of the plants as we tend a garden of herbs, or as we use them medicinally, magickally, for body care, or in cooking. There is an energy force within each plant. Focusing on the properties of a plant increases its ability to heal and enhances its flavor. When we turn our attention to anything, it becomes manifest on the physical plane. Our focus alone makes it so.

Utilize herbs at their seasonal peak, and you will reap more of their medicinal and magickal properties. The more you use, the more they increase their availability. This symbiotic relationship honors the gift and the giver. The ebb and flow of abundance and dormancy provide guidance for our lives. We can maximize our potential by harmonizing with the cycles of the seasons, allowing parts of ourselves to die during the fall months, going inward for introspection during the winter months, birthing a new self during the spring months, and dancing in every ray of sunlight we can during the summer months.

Plants and humans draw from the same life force. We are "children of the universe, no less than the trees or the stars," in the words of the "Desiderata." Within the Wiccan belief system, it is not appropriate to force our will on another, including our sister and brother plants. So how does our focus on a plant raise its vibration and curative abilities? Plants respond to our energy by their own will.

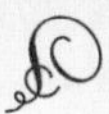

The same thing happens when you pay attention to other people. When you really look at them, acknowledge them, accept them as your equal, and love them, the natural response is to want to give back.

To bring the knowingness of our connection to Mother Earth to the everyday state of existence, it is helpful to satisfy the linear-thinking mind by explaining how the plants work. In this way, the left side—or logical part—of our brain can rest at ease, and the right side—the cyclical or spiritual part—can explore the ethereal realms where magick and healing take place.

Within each medicinal plant is a unique combination of active chemical ingredients that point to the mystery of their healing potential. Herbs and other plants contain varied curative powers of healing. Bitters, found in the roots and leaves, are detected on the taste buds, and activate the brain's response to release the hormone gastrin, which stimulates gastric acids, bile flow, and digestive juices. Herbalists recommend beginning each meal with a bitter to aid the digestive system, which is why we eat salads at the start of a meal. Some herbs that contain bitters are angelica, dandelion, hop, and burdock.

Flavonoids are found in flowers, leaves, stems, fruits, and roots. They are the reason some plants are bright yellow to rich orange, colors that attract birds and insects to pollinate as well as drawing animals to eat them. Flavonoids strengthen blood vessel walls, which guards against oxidation, and they relieve water retention, inflammation, and muscle spasm. Herbs that contain flavonoids include dandelion, elder, and passionflower.

Volatile oils are located in leaves, bark, flowers, and fruit. The volatile oils are responsible for a plant's signature scents, as in mint, lavender, ginger, and rosemary. These aromas are believed to repel predators, protect against disease, and attract pollinators. They are also associated with stress relief, stimulating circulation, easing water retention, and enhancing appetite.

Alkaloids are found in roots, seeds, and leaves. Some herbalists attribute to alkoloids the regulation of plant growth and a powerful life force that repels predators. These compounds also fight fungal and bacterial infections. Tobacco, poppy, and goldenseal all contain alkaloids.

Gums and resins are located in branches and trunks of shrubs and trees. Gums and resins are forms of sap that work as the blood sending the life force from the roots out to the branches; they are the plant or tree's circulatory system. Early in

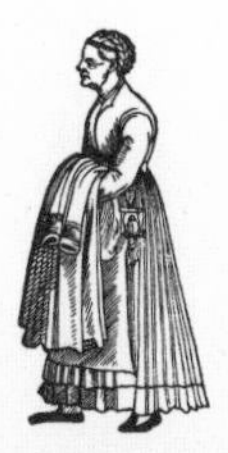

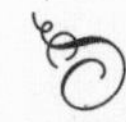

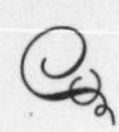

spring, you can hold a stethoscope to a tree and hear the pumping of the sap. Many gums and resins contain antibacterial properties. Myrrh and pine contain gums and resin.

Mucilage, found in the inner bark, roots, and seeds, is a water-retaining agent that helps germination. Its uses for people are to aid constipation and soothe irritated mucous membranes. Flax and slippery elm are rich in mucilage.

Saponins are located in the leaves and roots. Botanists theorize that the soap-like taste attributed to saponins repels predators. Possible benefits associated with these chemicals include strengthening blood vessels, counteracting stress, and regulating hormones. Mullein and black haw contain saponins.

Tannins are found in the roots, leaves, and bark. Tannins have an astringent action that protects and heals mucous membranes and skin. Oak bark is full of tannins.

Interacting with all the elements of herbs and plants can be a luscious experience of third-dimensional living—in the awareness of the earth-plane existence. If you are attracted to a particular tree or other plant, follow your feelings and reach out to it with willing openness. Physical contact with a plant will help balance your body's energy, and as you stand or sit with a tree you might receive some insights and inspirational thoughts. When you have made a deep bond with a plant or tree and are ready to end that connection, move slowly out of it and visualize sending some love and light around the tree or offer water. It has been proved that the plant world is greatly enhanced by this offering. An attitude of thanks and gratitude for nature's gifts is a sure way of opening up the channels of communication with trees and plants.

In this fast-paced society, we need to take time to discover the power and joy of living in the present moment. Satisfy your desire to connect with nature by tuning in and appreciating her bounty; the result is nothing short of magickal.

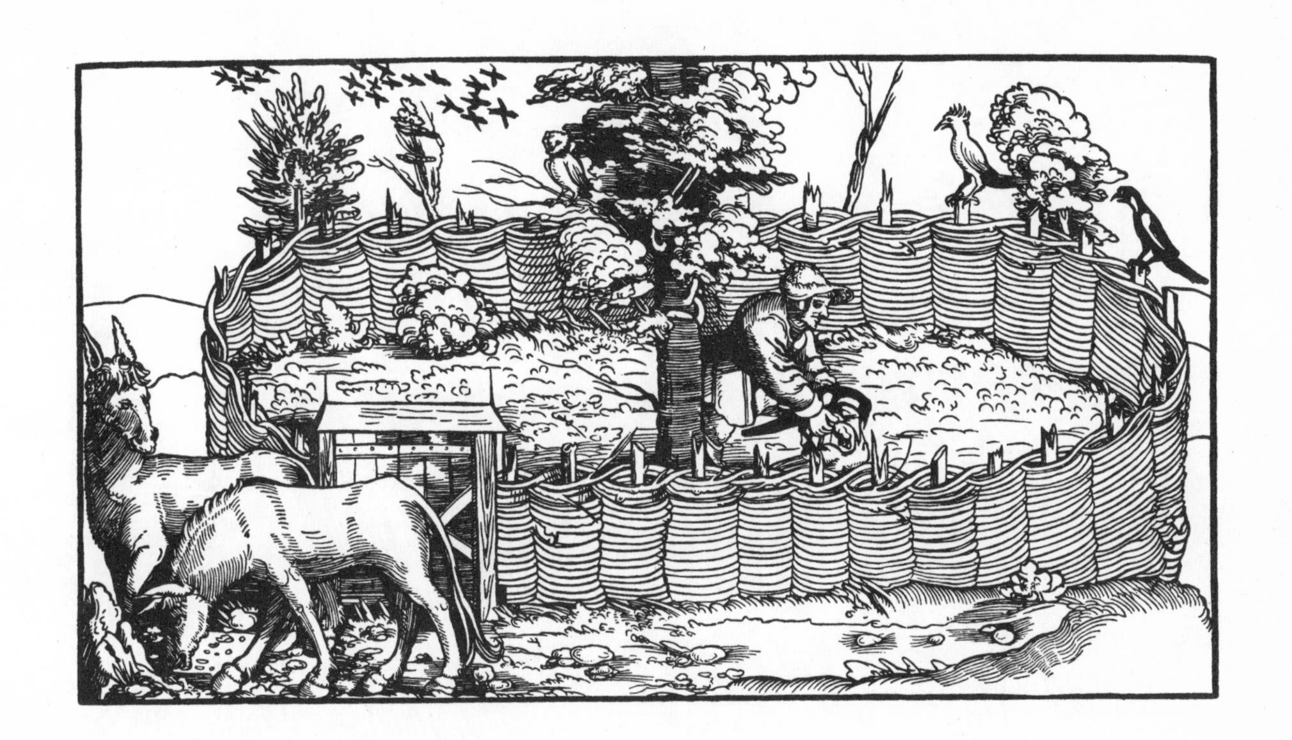

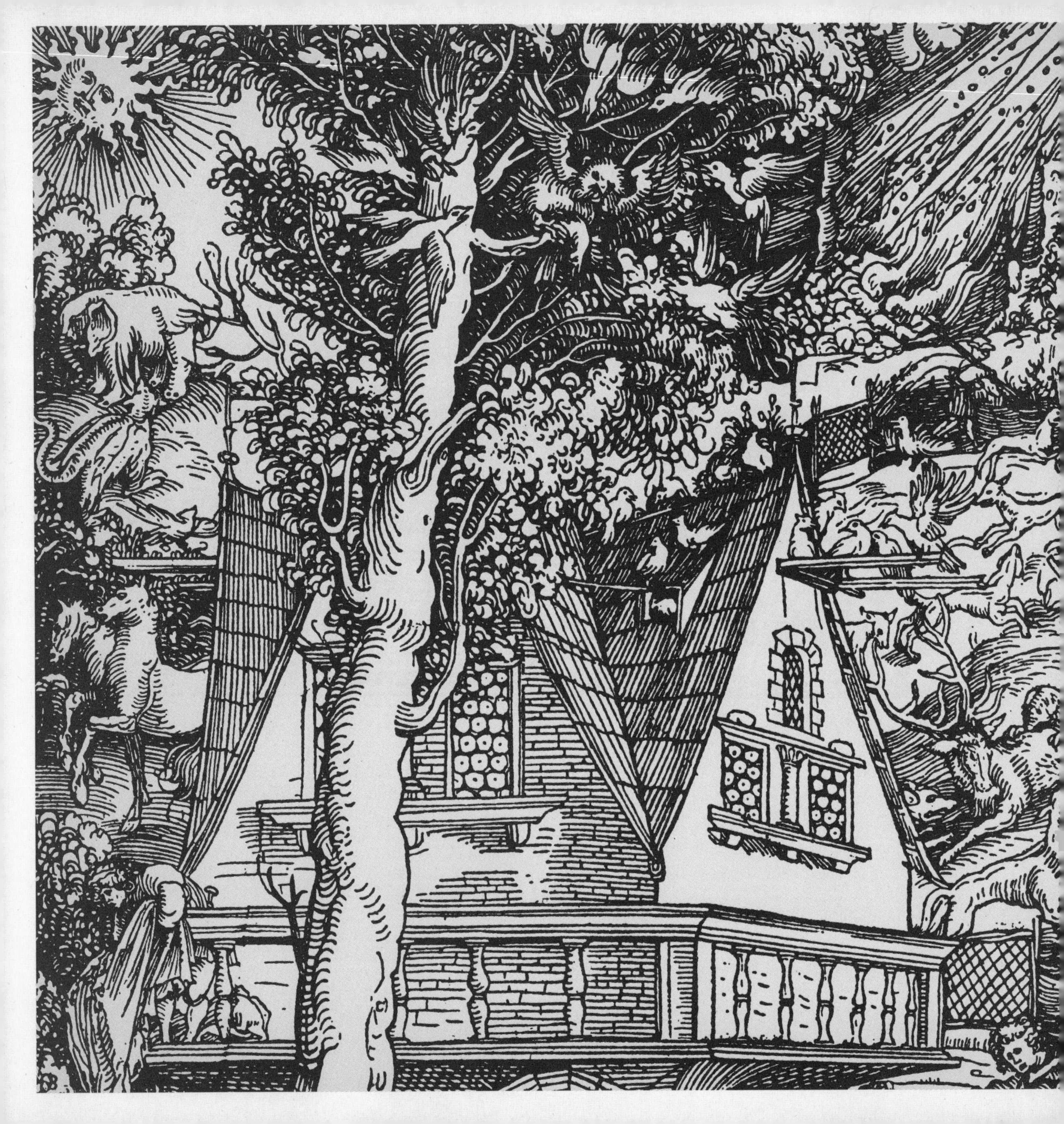

The Wiccan Tradition

WICCA IS A BEAUTIFUL spirituality encompassing gentleness, awareness, and responsibility. Wicca—sometimes called witchcraft or the Craft—follows the wise woman ways of tending Mother Earth. We look to nature for guidance, observing the natural world to find a teacher powerful and true. We approach our work with reverence for all things alive and sacred. Each moment and all people are holy. We nurture and manifest for ourselves, love others, and create our destiny from a courageous and peaceable sustenance known as Goddess and God.

Many believe the word *wicca* derives from the Old English *wicce,* (pronounced "weecha"), meaning "wise" or "to bend or shape unseen forces." Others say it is properly spelled *wica,* meaning "one born into the craft." People in all walks of life have used herbals, or books of herbs, for centuries; they are of particular importance to those practicing witchcraft, Wicca, and other earth-based spiritualities.

Wicca draws from many different traditions, which span divergent civilizations across the breadth of land and time. Central to all Wiccan beliefs is a spirituality that calls on

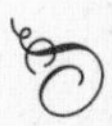

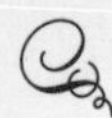

one to attune to the rhythms of nature and reach an individual connection with Spirit.

Throughout history, followers who agree about theory, philosophy, or lore have formed traditions and customs specific to their desires and needs. They have organized themselves to support one another politically, emotionally, and mentally—to inspire conversations that would explore their spirituality.

Historical and archeological evidence indicate that in earlier millennia of human history, the feminine Divine worked harmoniously with her male counterpart, in a theology that paid reverence to mysticism. With the move into the Piscean Age, the pendulum swung and the focus shifted to a patriarchal society in which the linear mind, an aggressive nature, and a purely male god commanded the masses. Since before the time of Christ we have lived in this epoch of leaders and followers. In this worldview, arbitrarily straight lines were placed around and through the infinite and ever-evolving entity known as our relationship with the Divine. Still, for the most part, many commoners and noblemen alike continued to believe in the sanctity of aligning everyday life with nature. It may be this patriarchal focus occurred so that as a human tribe we could bring forth great mental works of mathematics and science, giving birth to the Industrial Age. During this era, some practiced spellcasting publicly as herbal healers, but others took their spirituality underground for preservation.

In the Aquarian Age, which began in the late twentieth century, the emphasis shifted to autonomous experience and a self-governing people. Heightened awareness of karma, of every action causing a reaction, has propelled people toward taking responsibility for their actions. The shift has begun, and many now seek and follow their own inner spiritual guidance. At its worst, this process can be painful and incomprehensibly lonely; at best, it is liberating and feels like a homecoming.

In the context of this era of individuality, Wiccan beliefs and styles of participation vary. Some manifest the rhythms of nature in their everyday lives but do not possess the desire to buck modern society and label themselves with touchy words such as witch or Wiccan. Others may find beauty in varied forms of worship (as in my eclectic personal combination of the Faerie Tradition of Wicca, mystic Christianity, Buddhism, and Native American spirituality). Some practice alone because they cannot find one group to satisfy all their pleas for connection with the Divine. Still others appreciate Wiccan spirituality but have no interest in

organized systems, especially when it comes to religion, mythology, or spellcasting. Whatever your preference, your choices are authentic because you are honoring your unique understanding of what Spirit means to you. You do not need to have three generations of witches in your broom closet, know every god and goddess in all pantheons, or have appreciation for every Wiccan holiday to practice some form of this nature-based spirituality. Finding your way within Wicca is a matter of making peace with, and congruency between, your soul and ego, your higher self and your personality, your ideals and practicality.

Spellcasting

Wicca gives us an opportunity to practice and explore our ability to manifest the life we want through spellcasting. And yet, this is one of the most misunderstood aspects of Wicca. Spellcasting is an appendage of the religion: not all Wiccans cast spells; it is not a requirement.

A spell is a focused prayer or wish. Spells are used as a last resort after the practitioner has assessed four major questions: Is what I'm asking for a need or a want? Have I done everything humanly possible on the mundane level to bring about the desire? Will it harm? Does it serve the highest good of all concerned?

Spellcasting draws on the divine energy, reminding us that in every moment, we are creating our lives. Instead of being a mixed-up bundle of wants and needs, we slow down, savor each desire individually, and concentrate. Spells help us focus on one emotion or need, giving it recognition and a full day in the sunlight of our awareness. After all, each desire is a full universe of one facet of our expression. Spells and rituals remind us how to manifest our thoughts to make them appear on the physical plane. When we remember to recognize ourselves as creators, we can choose whether we want to keep the door open for an experience, feeling, or thought to pass through again. Our mundane life is a dream state full of illusions. In this state, first we forget our limitless ability, and then slowly, step by step, we regain our awareness of our divine, immeasurable, and boundless self, which is fully unaffected by the trials that we pretend are so important while we are visiting earth in this incarnation.

A ceremony, spellwork, or ritual combines the three modalities of learning—kinesthetic, auditory, and visual—as a means of redirecting the course of your life.

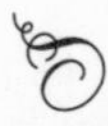

Physical movement locks in the sensation of power you feel during the meditative state of a magickal space. The rhymes, symbols, and chanting used in ritual bypass the doubts, worries, and complications focused on by the left brain. The scene of a circle in balance, with appropriate symbols and colors, communicates with people who learn from visual stimuli.

Spells create an intention that moves through time and space, breaking through the linear boundaries of ordinary life. They create doorways to new perspectives, transforming all subsequent or dependent effects.

The most essential tool in any ritual or spell is your will or intent. You can envision the center of your will as being in your mind, your solar plexus, your heart, or—when your need is a fervent one—in all three. Other tools of the trade, such as wands, athames (ritual knives or daggers), pentagrams, and chalices, pale in comparison to the importance of your intent and the power of your will. A wand symbolizes air, athames represent fire and the ability to draw and define magick circles, pentagrams represents the element of earth and the harmony of four directions and spirit working together, and a chalice epitomizes water and the Mother's receptivity; but it is your intent when you use them and your assessment of their importance that make them effective. If you need to, you can change a black candle to a white candle. If you change from street clothing to a cloak or put on a special necklace with intent, you can transport yourself to a magickal realm. Ask yourself if you could cast the spell on a deserted island; if so, then you will know how strong your intent is.

Elements of a Ritual

Within this book, you will find magickal rituals or spells. When possible, cast a full circle before using these. Doing so helps you to concentrate, clear a doorway connecting the mundane and the Divine, and hold a protective space. You can follow the general description below or make up your own process. When there is neither the time nor the place to cast a circle, you will want to at least center and ground yourself. Centering is an internal process of calming the mind and bringing the whole body to the present moment. Concentrate on your breathing. Relax your muscles, and focus on the space between your eyebrows. Let all thoughts pass

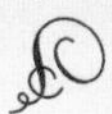

without getting caught up in them. Grounding is an external process in which you connect with the divine source. Visualize sending an energy cord from the energy center known as your root chakra, located at the perennial floor, to the center of Mother Earth. When you feel balanced like a tree, firmly rooted to the earth, begin the ritual.

Many magickal rituals contain similar elements. These are:

— cleansing and blessing the area
— laying or casting the circle
— putting quarters up and calling on the guardians
— raising the cone of power or raising the energy
— calling Goddess and God
— the work
— sharing cakes and ale (optional; you can also offer a chalice and snack)
— bidding farewell to Goddess and God
— taking down the cone of power or grounding the energy
— bidding farewell to quarters and guardians
— closing the circle

Cleansing and Casting a Circle

Walk in a clockwise direction around the area you have designated for your circle, holding a smoldering bundle of dried sage, or your choice of appropriate incense. Before each person enters your circle, direct the sage smoke or incense over her or his body (this procedure is called smudging). Anoint and bless her or his third eye (the center of the forehead) with oil in a pentagram or just draw a small line if that works best for you. Invite your guests to gather in a circle around the altar. Next have the participants center and ground by using the method described above.

Hold hands around the circle, right palms up, left palms down. Visualize a ball of light energy descending from the heavens to rest above your altar. Watch as an individual spoke grows from the ball and enters your solar plexus. Allow the light to envelop you. Pass the light clockwise around the circle, forming a wheel, then push the energy outward to encompass the room. Say,

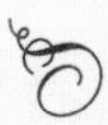

As we are connected to the Wheel of Life
We hold our place between here and the Divine
Blessed Be!

This wheel of energy symbolizes your relation to one another as individual yet unified creators of life. Open your eyes and drop hands.

Point your athame fingers (index and middle fingers together) toward the east with your arm fully extended. Go around the circle clockwise, pointing, and say,

I conjure thee, O Circle of Power
That you may serve as a barrier this very hour
Between the outside world and we, I create a sacred place
Outside of the realm of time and space
By my will, so mote it be

Calling the Guardians

When you reach the east again, ask everyone to face in that direction. Hold your hands up, palms facing the east—guardian of the element of air—and say,

All hail ye guardians of the eastern quadrant
I ask for your protection upon this ritual
I call upon the blessings of Archangel Raphael
I invoke the guidance of the hawk and eagle
I welcome the spirit of the Sylphs
Bestow inspiration, creativity, and openness to new beginnings
If anyone has a symbol, name, word, or animal that represents this direction to you, call it out now!
By my will, so mote it be.

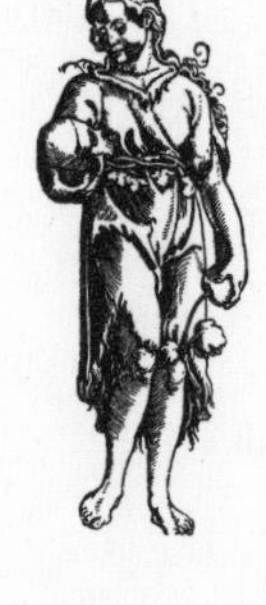

Turn to the south, and ask the rest to follow. Hold your hands up, palms facing the south—guardian of the element of fire—and say,

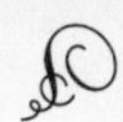

All hail ye guardians of the southern quadrant

I ask for your protection upon this ritual

I call upon the blessings of Archangel Michael

I invoke the guidance of dragon, horse, and lion

I welcome the spirit of the Salamanders

Bestow energy, passion, and healing

If anyone has a symbol, name, word, or animal that represents this direction to you, call it out now!

By my will, so mote it be.

Turn to the west, and ask the rest to follow. Hold your hands up, palms facing the west—guardian of the element of water—and say,

All hail ye guardians of the western quadrant

I ask for your protection upon this ritual

I call upon the blessings of Archangel Gabriel

I invoke the guidance of dolphin and whale

I welcome the spirit of the Undines

Bestow safety with emotions, expression, and feelings

If anyone has a symbol, name, word, or animal that represents this direction to you, call it out now!

By my will, so mote it be.

Turn to the north, and ask the rest to follow. Hold your hands up, palms facing the north—guardian of the element of earth—and say,

All hail ye guardians of the northern quadrant

I ask for your protection upon this ritual

I call upon the blessings of Archangel Uriel

I invoke the guidance of stag and snake

I welcome the spirit of the Gnomes and Dryads

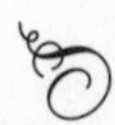

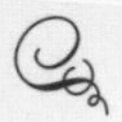

> Bestow grounding and the wisdom of the ancestors
>
> If anyone has a symbol, name, word, or animal that represents this direction to you, call it out now!
>
> By my will, so mote it be.

Last but not least, walk from the north back to the east, and nod your head once to the east, thus completing your quarter calls.

Raising the Cone of Power

Raising the cone of power creates a place that stands outside the boundaries of time and space, a place in which the participants can perform magick. Ask everyone to join hands, right hands up, left hands down. Invite them to visualize their roots growing downward from their solar plexus, spiraling in a clockwise direction, through the many layers of Mother Earth. A short distance away glows the molten crystal core of the Mother. On the count of three, wrap your roots around her core. Raise the Mother's white light up to your body, spiraling up in a clockwise direction through her many layers. Feel the energy enter your feet; pass through your legs, hips, stomach, and heart. Now imagine a circular doorway opening at the crown of your head. See above you a brilliant star. Focus your awareness or attention in a clockwise direction and send it spiraling toward that star, rising higher and higher into the heavens. On the count of three, wrap your energy around the brilliant star. Watch the white-golden light spiral down to enter the top of your head, traveling down through your throat to your heart. Send the light around your circle, securing your sacred space. When you are ready, drop hands. You have now created a cone of power that no outside force can penetrate, and each person is now a channel or conduit for Love's power.

Calling God and Goddess

We call in God first so that he may open the door from the Divine to the mundane for the Goddess. This door remains open during the duration of your work so that you may receive divine inspiration. At the altar, sprinkle cornmeal or grain around a candle that represents the God (if you are outside, sprinkle it around the circle). Light the candle. Say,

O God, our divine father

He whom we have called upon since the beginning of time

Come to us now

Grant us the security of your golden light and
divine confidence

Blessed Be!

At the altar either pour wine (into a small glass) or sprinkle rose petals around a candle that represents the Goddess (if you are outside, sprinkle around the circle). Light the candle. Say,

O Goddess, our divine mother

She whom we have called upon since the beginning
of time

Come to us now

Grant us the protection of your luminescent light
and divine nurturing

Blessed Be!

Work

Now is the time to perform your magick within the safe confines of the circle and under the protection of Goddess, God, and the guardians. If you are working solo, now is the time to cast your spell. When you have finished it, if you had cakes and ale designated for this ceremony, now would be the time to bless them and eat. "Cakes and ale" are symbolic food and drink you have selected. Cakes and ale mean different things in different Wiccan traditions. To some, they are a symbolic connection to the Divine (similar to the body and blood of Jesus Christ in Communion); to others, they are a symbol of the interconnectedness of the Divine and the earthly; to others, they are simply a way to guide participants from the realm of the spiritual back to the mundane. Choose what you want the cakes and ale to mean for your ritual or invite each participant to feel their own connection. If you are conducting a healing ritual, it is better to eat after the circle has been closed.

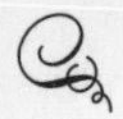

Ending the Ritual

First bid farewell to Goddess as the doorway is open, and then God will close it behind them. Say,

> Dear Goddess, our divine mother
> Thank you for your guidance
> Stay if you will, go if you must
> Hail and farewell
> Blessed Be!

Extinguish the Goddess candle. Say,

> Dear God, our divine father
> Thank you for your guidance
> Stay if you will, go if you must
> Hail and farewell
> Blessed Be!

Extinguish the God candle. Hold hands around the circle. Visualize your sacred space, and let the energy circle up through the roof or trees, back up the star to which you have linked your power; on the count of three unlock your energy from the star. Watch the energy spiral downward in a counterclockwise direction. See it move through the heavens, down through the trees or rooftop, through the top of your head. As the energy spirals down through your body, keep what you need and let go of the rest. The energy continues to spiral down through your feet and through the earth. The roots that once kept you tied to Mother Earth begin to dissolve. On the count of three, imagine those roots disengaging from the Mother's core. Open your eyes.

Walk to the east, again nod your head in that direction, and walk counterclockwise to the north.

Face the direction of the north, ask everyone to do the same, and say,

> Dear guardians Archangel Uriel, stag, snake, and the spirit of the Gnomes and Dryads

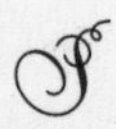

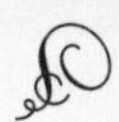

Thank you for your protection, blessings, and guidance
Stay if you will, go if you must
Hail and farewell
Blessed Be!

Walk to the direction of the west, ask everyone to turn the same way, and say,

Dear guardians Archangel Gabriel, dolphin, and whale, and the spirit of the Undines
Thank you for your protection, blessings, and guidance
Stay if you will, go if you must
Hail and farewell
Blessed Be!

Walk to the direction of the south, ask everyone to turn the same way, and say,

Dear guardians, Archangel Michael, dragon, horse, lion, and the spirit of the Salamanders
Thank you for your protection, blessings, and guidance
Stay if you will, go if you must
Hail and farewell
Blessed Be!

Walk to the direction of the east, ask everyone to turn the same way, and say,

Dear guardians, Archangel Raphael, hawk, eagle, and the spirit of the Sylphs
Thank you for your protection, blessings, and guidance
Stay if you will, go if you must
Hail and farewell
Blessed Be!

Point your athame fingers with your arm extended toward the east. Release the circle in a counterclockwise direction as you say,

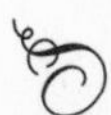

I erase thee, O circle of power
That you no longer exist as a barrier
Between the outside world of man, and this sacred place
As my will, so mote it be!

Hold hands around the circle and say,

I send this energy out to the universe to do my bidding
The circle is now open but not broken
Merry meet, merry part, and merry meet again.

Do not be nervous or worry if you mess up a word or two. The most important thing to remember in any ritual is your intent—not your perfection. Magick is fun, not a test.

A Final Word on Spells

Magickal work is often done in a group, whereas an actual spell is most often cast individually or by a group of three. Spells create a space for the caster to make a declaration of intention. Etymology says that one origin of the word *spell* is a term that connotes "to speak a tale." The spells created in this book are means to affirm your will; they are not to be used as a form of manipulation. Suggestions are given for the appropriate phase of the moon or day of the week to do your working, appropriate colors to use, and so on. These guidelines help the worker to draw on the energy represented by the time or symbol, but in a time of need it is not absolutely necessary to follow each recommendation.

You cannot determine the specific manifestation of a spell, so don't get attached to a predetermined outcome. Spirit is omnipotent, possessing a knowledge and range of possibilities that our mind does not even know exist. Here on earth, we are just one facet of the light, and we are not often in possession of the whole truth.

A spell or ritual manifests in a way and at a time that fulfills our destiny. The met desire is always right and good for one's higher self. The seed of our destination was long ago placed in our hearts. That destination is coming home to our

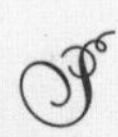

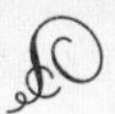

divine state of being. From this state of actualization, we can do great things. Only when our hearts find solace and joy with an idea should we cast a spell.

If you listen to your heart, you will not need to prove anything by casting many spells, one after another. Give rituals and spells time to work. If you don't wait, then the intents and desires stack up against one another like a traffic jam: some can collide or combine. Often once a spell comes to fruition, other needs are answered or no longer exist.

You may wonder if each and every one of the incantations and recipes in this book has been tried. The truth is that they have all been tried, though not always on the physical level. Every spell I write is something I need to know. Teachers teach that which they need to learn. I also know that I represent only one facet of Spirit's diamond, so to present as many beings and thought forms as possible, I have included contributions from other people. This is important to do because it presents a wider range of needs, questions, and desires and provides a stronger foundation for this representation of Spirit.

The new millennium brings with it a call for balance between mystic spirituality and earthly needs. We are corporal yet unfathomable—a perfect light trying to shine forth from a flawed casement. The craft of Wicca helps us find harmony between these seemingly opposing forms. Nature is our best guide, for here we can truly see the face of God and Goddess. When we follow the sabbats and honor nature's cycles, we find harmony.

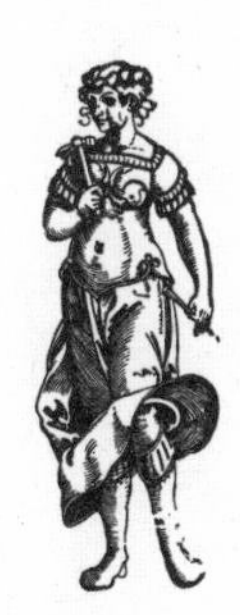

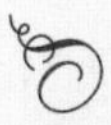

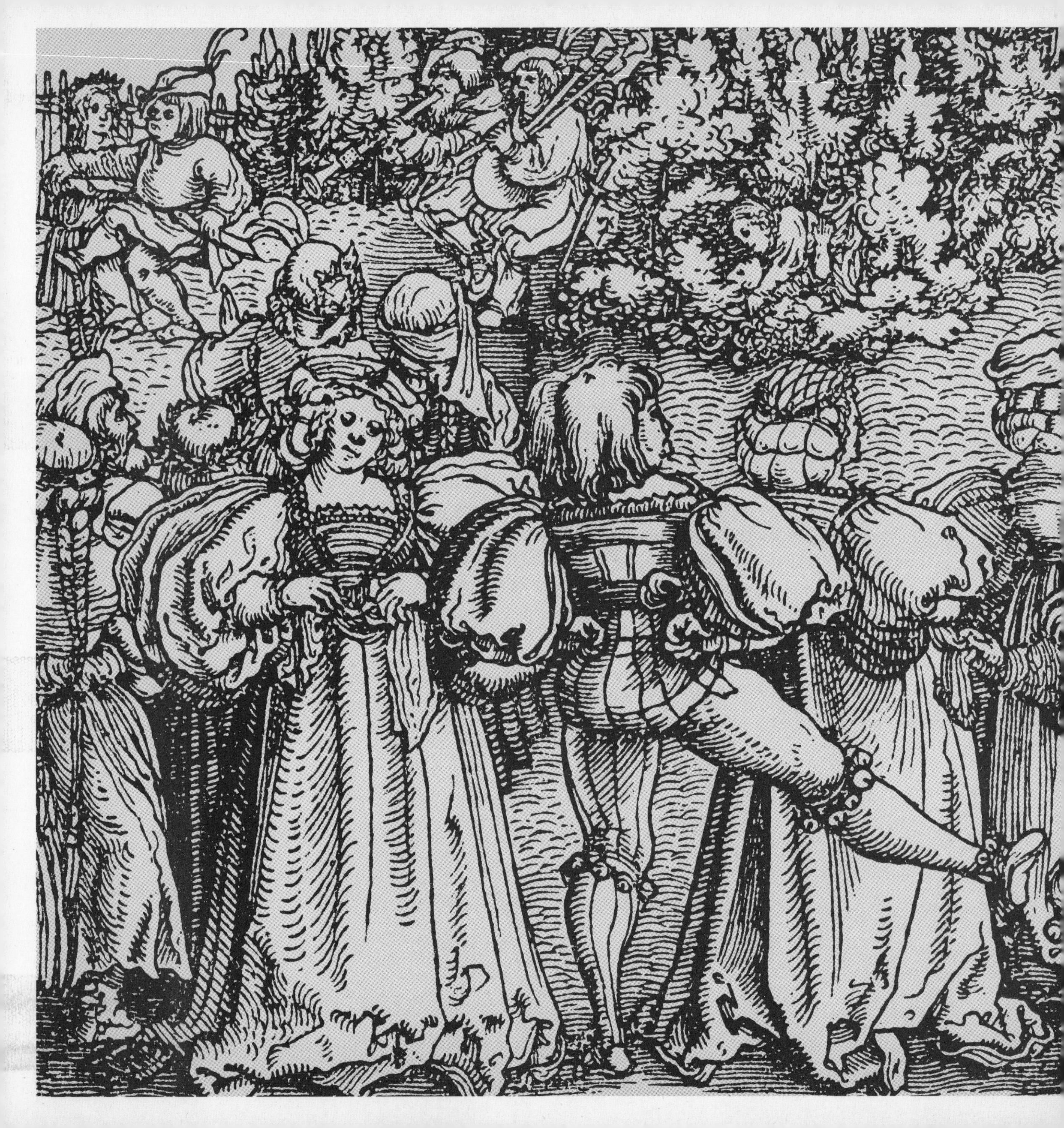

The Sabbats

WITHIN THE WICCAN TRADITION, there are eight holidays (holy days) known as sabbats that are celebrated during the year. Each one can be observed in various ways, depending on your liking, your coven's preference, or the high priestess or priest orchestrating the sabbat ritual. The one common theme is that each of the sabbats honors a season. Four are based on the movement of the sun, marking the solstices and the equinoxes; these are often referred to as the minor sabbats. The other four mark traditional northern European planting and harvesting cycles, and are known as the major sabbats. Together they make up what is known as the Wheel of the Year or the Mandala of Nature. You can choose to literally ride the seasons, finding comfort in following the rhythm of nature's ebb and flow. The holidays offer a connection to the best teacher Spirit offers us—nature.

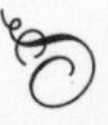

Samhain

Celebrated on October 31, Halloween (known as Samhain) is the Witches' New Year's Eve and third harvest. It is a time to play with our shadow selves and sit in the woods between the worlds of light and darkness, knowing all things are possible. Nature is recessing into the quiet barrenness of winter. It is a season to acknowledge that both light and darkness are necessary to our growth. Remember departed loved ones and their gifts, harvest strength, trust the mirror reflecting your light, salute health, believe in enchantment, and tell stories as the veil between the mundane and magickal worlds is at its thinnest. Symbols of the holiday are pumpkins, skeletons, marigolds, fall leaves, pomegranates, and witch hats. Herbs and other plants associated with this sabbat include apple, broom, milk thistle, mint, mullein, nutmeg, oak, sage, and wormwood.

Yule

Celebrated between December 20 and 22, Yule or winter solstice is a time to recognize that the wheel of nature and of life will continue no matter what. Life is an ever-evolving spiral. It is a season to join friends and family and appreciate them. This holiday marks the longest night of the year and the rebirth of the sun. Days will be longer from this point on. Bring in the light and joy in your life as your divine right; trust in life and celebrate all its forms, trust your faith, open doors, and ask for great things. Symbols of the holiday are wreaths, holly, yule logs, and lights. Herbs and other plants associated with this sabbat include ash, bay, chamomile, frankincense, hazel, holly, juniper, milk thistle, mistletoe, oak, pine, rosemary, sage, sandalwood, and walnut.

Imbolc

Celebrated on February 1 or 2, Imbolc or Brigid's Day marks midwinter. Animals begin to come out of hibernation and ewes begin lactating; light is returning. This is a time to acknowledge our individual gifts and feed our talents with supportive action. Imbolc is connected to the powerful new life awakening in the depths of the earth and thus also represents the rebirth and upsurge of personal power. Now

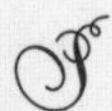

we can plant seeds of inspiration, acknowledge the returning light, invoke patience, find virtue in perseverance, and inspire others. Symbols of the holiday are seeds, wells, and fire. Herbs and other plants for this sabbat include angelica, basil, bay, cinnamon, frankincense, myrrh, nettle, orris root, rosemary, rowan, and saffron.

Ostara

Celebrated between March 20 and 22, Ostara or spring equinox is one of the two times of the year when night and day are of equal duration; it is a holiday of balance. Ostara is a time to rebirth our new selves, clear away the clutter in our minds, and wipe the slate clean in our lives. See life in nonextreme terms—neither too terrible nor too fantastic. In nature, flowers are blooming and the world is abuzz with new life. Ostara rejoices in the beauty of our unique selves and in playing with impish delight. Find balance, plant individual expression, believe in abundance and fertility, face fears, cry, and allow for all emotions. This sabbat represents dawn on the Wheel of the Year, so if the night owls in your group do not object, celebrate the holiday at sunrise. But remember, ritual is a celebration, not drudgery, and it does not need to be a test of your endurance. Symbols of the holiday are eggs, rabbits, and flowers, including violets. Herbs and other plants associated with this sabbat include broom, cinquefoil, jasmine, lavender, lily, rose, sage, and willow.

Beltane

Celebrated April 30 and May 1, Beltane (or May Eve and May Day) is a time to revel in life's absurdities and have fun. The sun is gaining strength and thought to hold the characteristics of youth—playful and mischievous. Flowers abound, waiting for you to enjoy the beauty of life's physical pleasures. Smell the flowers or dance in a secluded part of overgrown wilderness, as you relish the light and laughter of faeries and children. Traditionally, the holiday represents the marriage of the divine masculine and divine feminine, as seen in the maypole dance. Weave together the magick of the male and female aspects of yourself. Honor the collaboration and patchwork that is you. Respect the soul's journey, and always

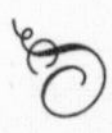

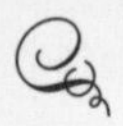

remember to take the ride of life lightly—it is only a dream, after all. Symbols are the maypole, strawberries, faeries, and flowers such as the daisy. Herbs and other plants associated with this sabbat include angelica, apple, ash, calendula, cinquefoil, red clover, frankincense, hawthorn, honeysuckle, red clover, rose, rowan, St. John's wort, and woodruff.

Litha

Celebrated around June 20 or 21, Litha, summer solstice, or midsummer is a time to spread warmth, and enjoy the sun's energy. The sun is at its highest point in the sky. This is the longest day of the year. Everywhere you look nature shows her bounty; praise the opulence and abundance available to you for the asking. This is a day to celebrate your gifts of healing, whether they are intuitive or use plants. Make peace with the impermanence of life and changing relationships, knowing that you are always guided and watched over. Bloom where you are planted. Respect male energy, honor your light, hug yourself. You are one with the infinite sun. Symbols are the sun, and all things yellow or orange or round. Herbs and other plants associated with this sabbat include basil, chamomile, cinquefoil, elder, fennel, frankincense, lavender, lily, mistletoe, mugwort, oak, pine, rose, St. John's wort, thyme, vervain, and yarrow.

Lughnasadh

Celebrated August 1 or 2, Lammas or Lughnasadh is the first harvest of the year. Corn and grains are gathered with reverence and gratitude. Now is a time to harvest your resources, assess your needs, and use your gifts wisely, releasing any burdens and grudges. Soon you will move into the darkness of winter; sacrifice the unwanted from your life by throwing symbols of them into the sabbat fire. Harvest fruits from your garden with your family. Bless the tools of your trade in order to bring a richer harvest next year. Share your harvest with others who are less fortunate, for after Lammas you will begin to make contact with the darkness again, recognizing that nothing lasts. Every feeling and event passes through your awareness like clouds across a sky. Zero in on your truth. Make a commitment to honor your strengths and many skills. Find the beauty in the muggles (non-magickal

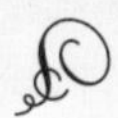

people) and mundane. Symbols are corn, grains, and breads. Herbs and other plants associated with this sabbat include acacia, calendula, frankincense, mistletoe, oak, rose, and sandalwood.

Mabon

Celebrated between September 20 and 22, Mabon or autumn equinox is the second day when daylight and darkness are equal, creating a mirror for you to look into as you seek balance and acceptance, weighing the bounty of your own personal harvest gained through life's experience. It is a time to honor and separate your truth from your physical experience. This acknowledgment sanctifies the people, events, and experiences impacting your being and your journey, without getting caught up in how life should look. It is a time once again to balance the light and the dark. Mabon is the second harvest of the year and the witches' day of giving thanks. Simplify your life and rid yourself of unnecessary activity and clutter, in preparation for the silence of the darker months. Donate what you don't need. Clear the disorder of your mind and learn to sit with the quiet of the soul. Without rushing around, you will need to make peace with your shadow, which will help you release a bit more of the mask you show to the outer world and reliance on appearances. Give thanks and harvest what is helpful. Symbols of the season are leaves and cornucopias. Herbs and other plants associated with this sabbat include apple, balm of Gilead, calendula, cypress, milk thistle, mugwort, myrrh, oak, orrisroot, passionflower, pine, rose, and sage.

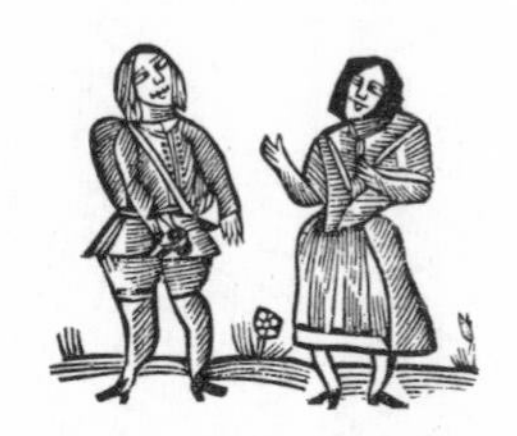

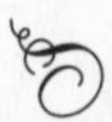

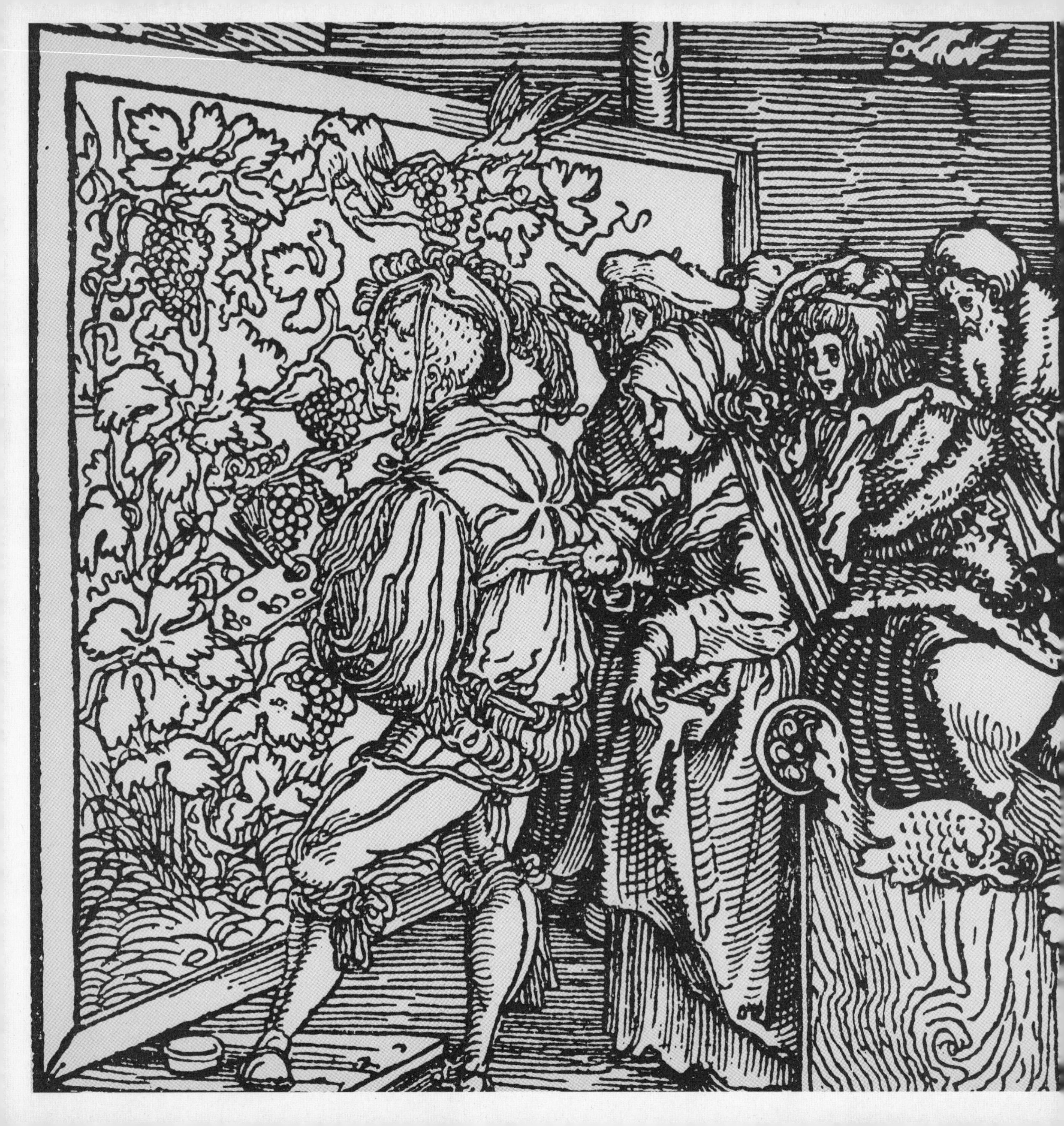

Medieval Herbalogy

HUMAN BEINGS HAVE PRACTICED herbal medicine for thousands of years. Anthropologists and archeologists confirm that human societies everywhere have utilized plants as medicine throughout history. During the medieval period, when professional physicians in the modern sense did not yet exist, herbs and other plants offered the only medical relief available. Plants also provided dyes, cosmetics, and food.

In medieval northern Europe, extensive information about the properties and uses of plants was common knowledge. The responsible wife and mother learned to find and use plants to heal her family and animals. Welsh herbalists showed particular skill in using plants. In fact, members of one Welsh family handed down their herbal skills for one thousand years in unbroken tradition. Like their predecessors, medieval healers may not have understood technical matters, such as that some plants had astringent properties while others had soothing properties, but they could observe the results of the treatments. Throughout history and during the Middle Ages, healers ascribed the effects of

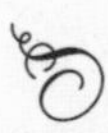

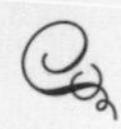

plants and herbs to a combination of physical properties and spiritual reinforcement. Gods, goddesses, and spirits were enlisted to aid healers in their work. This system of belief continued well into the Christian era.

Medieval healers brewed infusions and mixed herbs in lard poultices; they burned dried herbs to make a healing smoke to inhale. Healers sought out the uses of plants, often testing plants' effects on themselves and carefully observing effects on others through repeated use. Among the most commonly used plants were garlic, lily roots, and horehound. Most people found the plants they needed growing wild, including some Mediterranean plants that immigrated to northern Europe with the Romans.

Particularly reliable places for obtaining various plants would be noted and the plants carefully harvested, leaving enough to regenerate the supply for the next year.

Monasteries took this process further by creating herb gardens within their walls. In these gardens, more refined varieties of wild herbs and other plants were cultivated. Skilled monks often extended their healing practice to the local population, reinforcing bonds of community between monks and villagers. Medieval people, along with their more ancient predecessors, handed down herbal lore as part of the everyday education of the young. The teachings were mostly oral and hands-on, allowing young people to test and find the herbs themselves. The ancient ones believed one must seek out the plants, watch them grow, hold them, and love them. Only then could one ask permission to take from these living beings, thereby showing respect for the life that dwells within. This way, the plant's spirit would go with the healer and help treat the sick. Practicing this ongoing give-and-take ensured the survival of plants and people alike. Although most people knew something about using herbs, commonly it would be an older woman in a village who provided healing wisdom along with potions and such for magickal purposes.

Magick and herbal knowledge went hand in hand as medieval people sought to understand and control their world. Medieval people gathered specific plants at particular times of the month and year depending on the use they had for them. Often people avoided letting the plants touch iron, as it was thought that metal would draw the plants' powers to itself, leaving them useless. Plants became associated with particular characteristics, including astrological signs, planets, or masculine or feminine traits. Herbs particularly associated with magickal properties

included cumin, elder, and periwinkle to encourage fidelity; catnip, lavender, marjoram, and St. John's wort to promote happiness; basil, chamomile, mint, and cowslip for wealth; or dill, peppermint, thyme, violet, and yarrow for love.

Plants provided a wide range of dyes used for different purposes. Woad, a dye well known to the ancient Britons before Roman times and later to the Saxons, produced a blue dye through a process of fermentation and combination with limewater (an alkaline solution). Weld produced yellow, blue, or green, depending on how it was mixed. Saffron produced a yellow dye for coloring food—especially favored by upper-class folk. It was also good for dyeing clothing, but its cost put it out of reach for all but the wealthiest. Walnuts and the roots of the water lily supplied various brown dyes. Lichens produced dyes ranging from browns to reds, oranges, and yellows. Madder, found mostly in the Netherlands, gave good red and brown dyes—and could even be used as a hair dye. More exotic dyes could be imported from countries far away along the active trade routes of the Middle Ages.

The medieval housewife used plants for virtually every aspect of housework. As most people lived in houses with stone or dirt floors, plant material would be strewn on the floor to provide warmth, comfort—and a place for waste to fall! More well-to-do households would use rushes for this purpose. Often sweet-smelling herbs such as woodruff were mixed with rushes to mask the odor of wastes. Fleas plagued even the best of homes, so the conscientious housewife mixed flea repellents such as pennyroyal and fleabane into the rushes. Other favorite plants to mix in included sweet flag, rue, tansy, marjoram, and juniper. The use of rushes and herbs on floor continued well into the eighteenth century, when permanent flooring became available to the general populace.

As monasteries extended herbal knowledge and created cultivated versions of useful plants, herbal wisdom became not only the province of the common people, but also scholars. The first European herbal treatises that have survived were written in the early Middle Ages, and many of them were amongst the first books to be printed in the late fifteenth century. Modern knowledge of the uses of herbs derives from these ancient traditions. Western society has once again begun to recognize and value the use of herbs as humans did in the distant past. Wiccan traditions seek to reclaim this understanding of the natural world and the human's place in it. Learning herbal wisdom and utilizing it in our own lives can help us find our place.

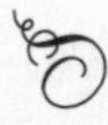

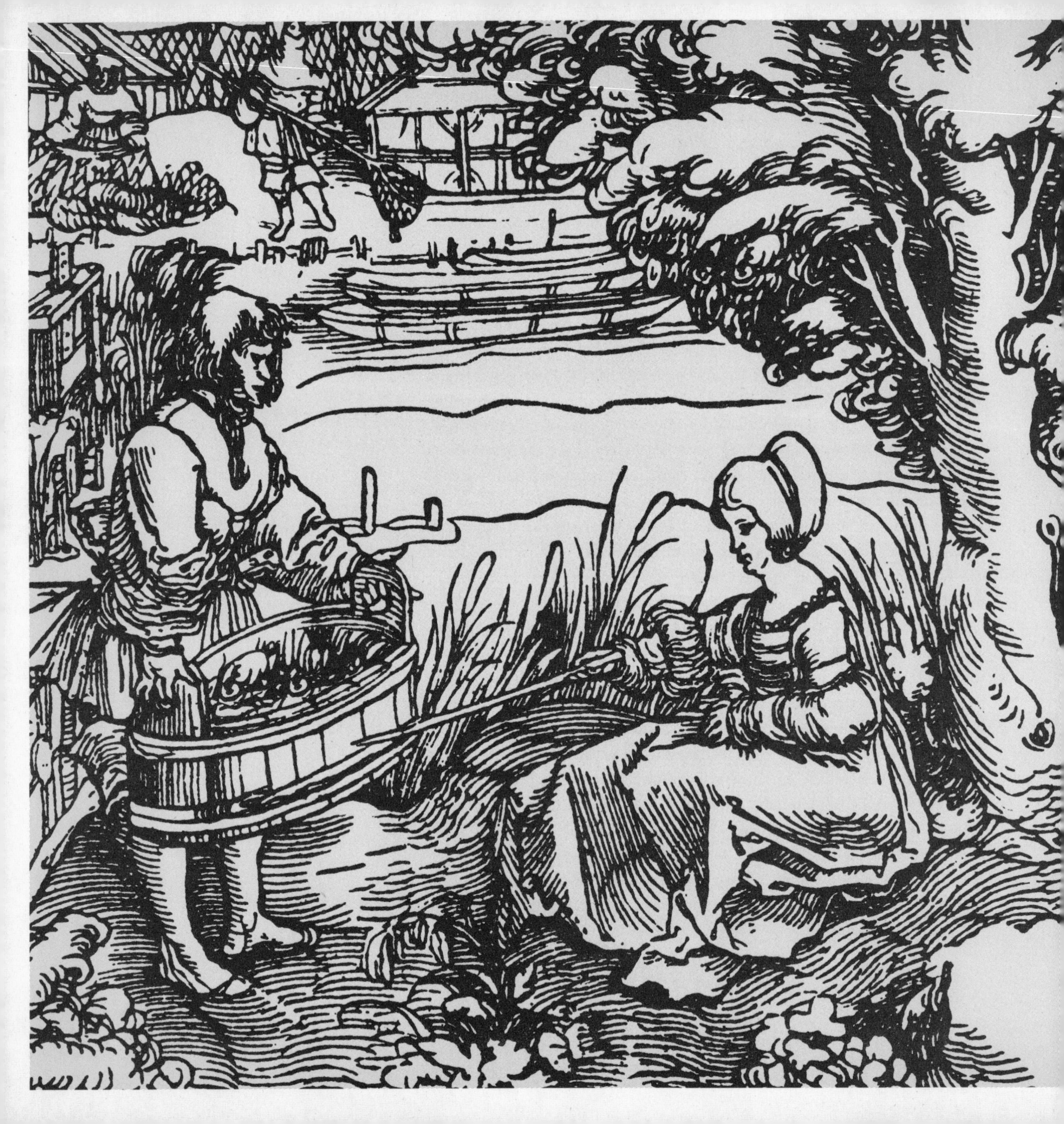

Wise Woman Ways

GROWING, USING, AND PLAYING with herbs can be as complicated or as simple as you like. There are scientifically precise methods that follow medical indications and counterindications, meaning what the herb can do for your physical body; and there are wise woman, folkloric ways. The wise woman method takes into account the herbs' vibratory effects on our emotional and spiritual bodies, based on the magickal intentions you attach to the plant's flavor, aroma, or appearance. Similarly, there are ceremonial magick ways of doing ritual and providing healing, and there are green or earth magick ways, which are guided more by intuition, inspiration, and accumulated experience. (Ceremonial magick is a formal magickal practice that grew out of the study of occult traditions in Europe and the Middle East and bases its concepts on ancient philosophical ideas. Earth magick draws from the folk traditions of medieval Europe discussed in the previous chapter.)

In the wise woman practice, it is important to make a connection with the herb you are using. As you peruse these pages, you will notice that many

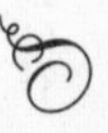

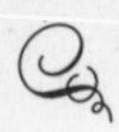

different herbs are said to produce similar results, such as reducing stress and fatigue or eliminating toxins. The reason I include overlap is that everyone's body is unique, and herbs must harmonize with a particular person in order to be effective. Incorporating herbs is quite a personal process, as some but not others will fit your individual needs.

There are many ways to test the relationship between you and an herb. Begin with tasting or smelling it. If the aroma or taste appeals to you, the chances are it will have a positive effect.

Next, you can try muscle testing. Lie down and hold the herb against your solar plexus (this can also work standing). Located under your diaphragm, the solar plexus is the center of your power. Extend your dominant arm straight out in front of you. Ask a friend to apply pressure to your wrist or hand, while you attempt to resist. If your resistance is weak, then the herb most likely will prove ineffective for you. If your resistance is strong, then the herb will work for you.

You can also do muscle testing alone. Place your middle finger over your index finger. With your other hand, hold the herb against your solar plexus. Apply pressure with your middle finger while resisting with your index finger.

Another method of testing is the pendulum. Before you begin, ask the pendulum to show you which directions are yes and no. (The answers can vary from person to person.) Then ask the pendulum if the plant will work for you. Meditation with live plants is also effective.

Begin with the mildest herbs before going for the most potent ones. For example, if you are having difficulty sleeping, begin with chamomile tea. If that doesn't work, try hops. If you are still experiencing difficulties, go with valerian. And, cycle your herbal use, alternating periods when you use them with periods without. You can choose to cycle by days (for instance, five days on, two days off), or by weeks (two on, one off), or by months. When substituting dried herbs for fresh, halve the amount you use.

Once you have found an herb or herbs that work well with you, make a healing pouch out of chamois leather. Start by cutting a circle three inches in diameter. Using a hole punch, make holes all the way round the edge. Thread a strip of leather or strong thread through the holes for pulling the pouch closed. Place the herb (or herbs) in your pouch and wear it around your neck, next to your skin if possible.

Last, connect with herb consciousness. Ask yourself, what does the herb do? What do I need? What can I give back to the herb? Tobacco, for example, is often used as an offering. A blessing ritual for tobacco used in offerings and prayer work is found in my description of that plant in the "Magickal Herbs & Plants" section. A good watering or a gift of crystals work, too.

The following is a list of common categories of ailments and the herbs most likely able to help because of their healing properties.

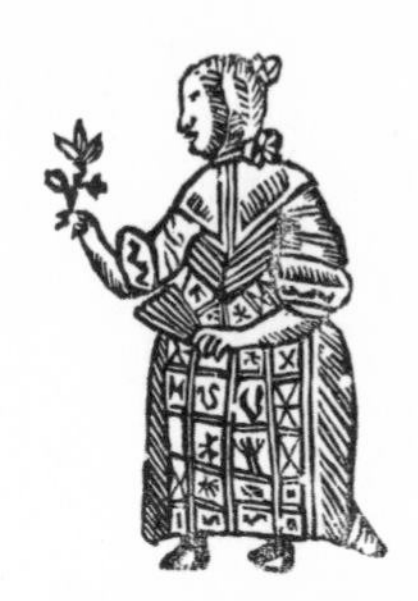

Sleep — chamomile, skullcap, hop, valerian

Stress — lavender, St. John's wort

Digestion — peppermint, ginger, fennel, anise

Immune system — echinacea

Women's issues — evening primrose

Heart System — hawthorn, motherwort

Blood Purification — dandelion, burdock root, echinacea

Balance — geranium, bergamot

The following is a list of the most common subjects for spells and the herbs most likely to help because of their magickal intent and vibration.

Stress — sage, frankincense, dragon's blood

Love — orrisroot, apple, rose

Prosperity — calendula, cinquefoil

Clairvoyance — mugwort, wormwood

Protection — angelica, rue, rosemary

Communication — bay, cinnamon, vanilla

Women's issues — vervain, motherwort, peppermint

Success — cinnamon, high John the conqueror, rowan

Balance — geranium, angelica

Harmony — basil, lavender, chamomile

Lust — clove, patchouli, ylang-ylang, sandalwood

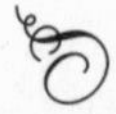

There are basic preparations used for treating both medical conditions and the emotional and spiritual issues listed above. These are infusions (or teas), decoctions (oil-based), poultices, washes, and ointments. The most widely used is the herbal tea. Begin with a small dose of a weaker tea to test for side effects. If need be, slowly increase the strength. For a weak infusion, steep half an ounce of herbs in one pint of water for fifteen minutes. For a medium strength infusion, steep two-thirds of an ounce of herb in one pint of water for twenty minutes. For a strong or medicinal infusion, steep one ounce of herb in one pint of water for twenty minutes. Teas made with magickal intent will vary depending on the degree of need, but usually they do not have to be strong to be effective. If a tea is to be drunk for medicinal purposes, always consult a healing practitioner.

Ancient ways of healing are included in this book. There is no way to contain all of the knowledge about healing herbs in one book, but know that the prominent qualities of these herbs have been included to the best of my ability. When you use any healing remedy of the wise woman ways, it is important to have a "healthing" intent. Focus on your health, not on the sickness. These remedies are not intended as an alternative to the care of a healing practitioner. Consult your healing practitioner or doctor before applying these methods.

When you decide to apply herbs in your life, take into consideration your own intuition. Focus on the curative or magickal properties you need for a particular situation, including the planetary and deity associations. For example, vanilla is associated with Venus—both the planet and the Goddess. You may choose to call upon the Goddess of Love or the planet ruling love; whichever works for you is the right one.

There may be some recipes in this book that call for ingredients with which you are not familiar. A list of where to find these ingredients is located on page 260. When recipes call for plant oils, keep in mind that essential oils should be used for any internal use, such as culinary dishes, while perfume oils and essential oils can be used interchangeably for external applications, such as lotions or potions.

The herbs have been organized in an alphabetical format for easy reference. Magickal and mundane information for each herb includes the plant's botanical and folk names, parts used, medicinal applications, magickal powers, gardening tips, and examples of culinary, beauty, healing, and ritual recipes.

This book combines the expertise of Wiccan and magickal herbalism with aromatherapy, natural medicine, and organic gardening. It is a dance, illustrating the art of working with herbs as a way of striving for balance, and it is a catalyst for creating harmony in your life. Wicca is a religion that asks you to take responsibility for making your connection to Spirit. No one book or person can spell out which essence of an herb is the only one for you to use, because no one can be an intermediate between you and Spirit. You must practice by doing magick. Magick cannot be defined in terms of the mental, linear, or word form. Strengthen, tone, and trust your intuition, and you will find magick all around you.

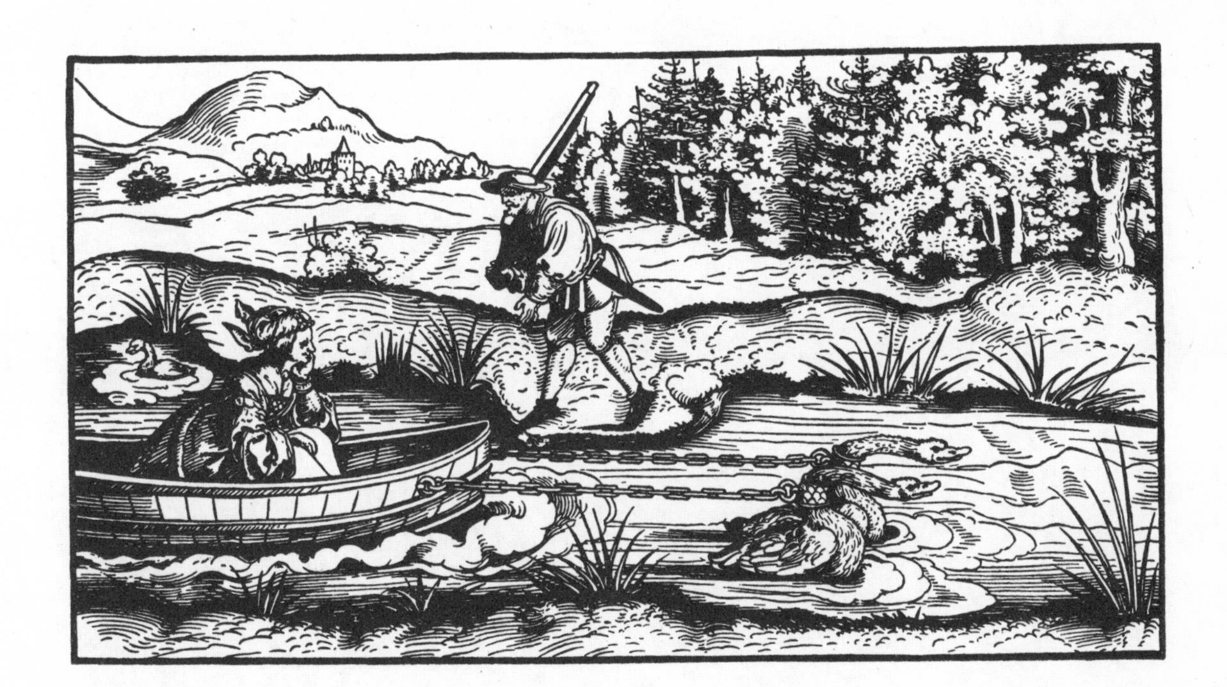

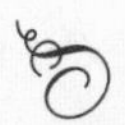

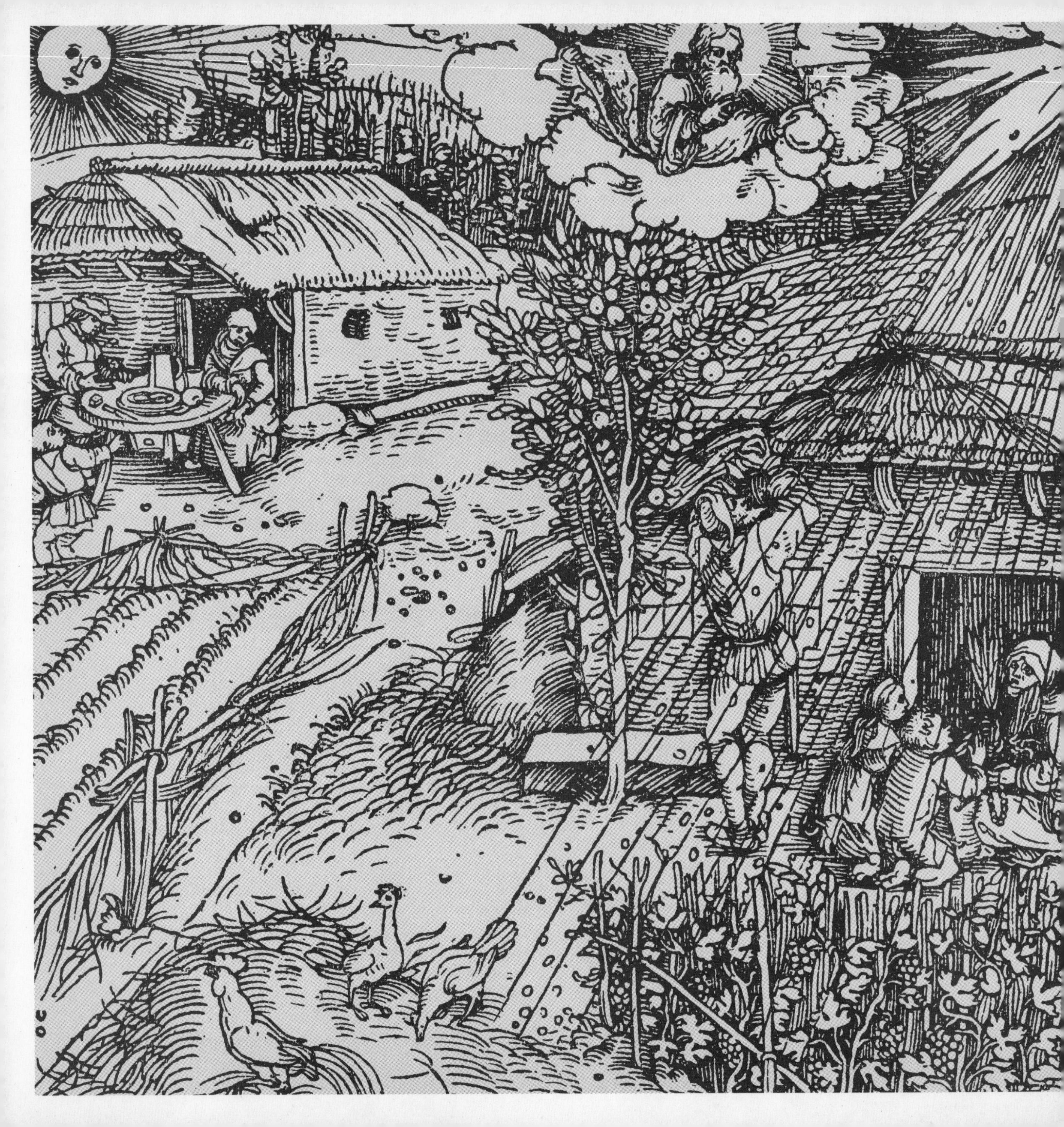

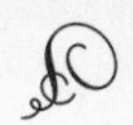

Natural Gardening

WORKING WITH MOTHER EARTH as you garden seems an obvious thing to do, but as we have "progressed" further away from living with the land, the rhythms of nature do not come easily to our minds. There are three types of natural gardening that will help us attune to nature: lunar gardening, biodynamic gardening, and composting.

Lunar gardening is not a new practice. The Muslims of the Middle Ages studied lunar gardening extensively. Western European manuscripts dating back to the 1600s list the advantages of planting by the moon. According to the principles of lunar gardening, the moon influences the growth of plants in two areas: phases and astrological signs. As the moon waxes (increases) and wanes (decreases), it pulls on the ocean, causing changes in the tides; in the same way, it is thought to pull moisture in the soil to rise to the surface or retreat into the depths, depending on its phase.

There are four phases of the moon that correspond to distinct gardening patterns. During the new or dark moon is the time to plant and transplant

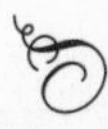

above-ground annuals that produce seeds outside the fruit, as well as fast-germinating and extra-slow-germinating seeds. During this time, leaf and root growth are balanced. As the moon waxes, it is in its second quarter. Now is the time to mow lawns for increased growth, harvest root crops, and plant and transplant above-ground annuals that form seeds inside the fruit. (Incidentally, it's also a good time to cut your hair for good growth.) When the moon is full, roots experience the most growth. Plant slow-germinating (two weeks) seeds, as well as bulbs, biennials, perennials, and root crops. Mow lawns (or cut your hair) to slow growth. Take indoor plants outside to bathe in the full moonlight. As the moon wanes, it enters the resting period of the fourth quarter. Harvest plants for storage and drying, prune, cultivate, and weed. During this phase, control pests using the least-invasive method, so you do not harm beneficial insects. Sow plants that require strong root systems. Begin compost piles.

The second way the moon influences growth has to do with the astrological sign through which the moon is passing. Consult a lunar calendar, as the phase changes every few days. Generally speaking, earth signs are good for root crops, flowers do well when planted during the moon's transit of air signs, most plants enjoy the fertile water-sign periods, and harvesting, cultivating, and weeding are done during the transit of the fire signs. Plants sown with a favorable combination of phase and astrological sign produce larger harvests and do not go to seed as fast.

Of course, between all these great plans and intentions, life happens. You may decide to integrate either the phase of the moon or the sign's influence into your gardening, or choose one over the other based on time constraints. Both techniques work best when using organic matter and composting.

The earth has a spirit. Its vitality is the focus of *biodynamic gardening*. In our modern age of science-driven agriculture, we have lost touch with the energy of the earth, and in doing so, we have caused the earth's energy to wane, resulting in the decline in health of our plants, animals, and water. We have even lost touch with the most basic principle of our existence as children of the earth, causing a drying out of our own souls. With a little awareness, this problem becomes all too apparent. Biodynamic gardening is the search for this original vitality and once we find it, channeling its immense energy to heal our food, plants, and planet.

Biodynamics is a science of life forces, a recognition of the basic principles at work in nature, and an approach to agriculture that takes these principles into

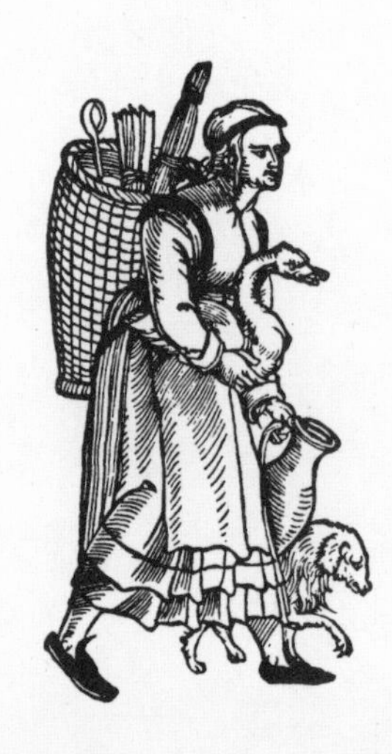

account to bring about balance and healing. Observation is the key to biodynamic gardening principles. With careful focus on natural phenomena, clear thought, and the ever-present awareness of the earth's spirit, we can attune ourselves again with the natural rhythms and the life force guiding us. With this focus, we become aware of the subtle balances necessary to heal our ailing planet.

Biodynamics is a continuous path of knowledge, as opposed to predetermined methods and techniques. The theories are based on the ideas of Rudolf Steiner, a philosopher, educator, agricultural expert, and clairvoyant. Steiner was born in the Austro-Hungarian Empire in 1861. He lived in a strange balance between the old peasant way of life in the mountains of Austria and the rapidly changing world of the nascent Industrial Age. With his childhood bound up in the intimate relationships peasants maintain with the earth's natural rhythm and his adulthood lived in the rapidly advancing industrialization of society, Steiner found himself interested in bridging the gap between these two worlds. He gave more than six thousand lectures and wrote dozens of books on the subject of balancing a spiritual connection with the earth and the new science and technology, a school of thought he called anthroposophy. It is this work that led to the basic principles of biodynamic gardening.

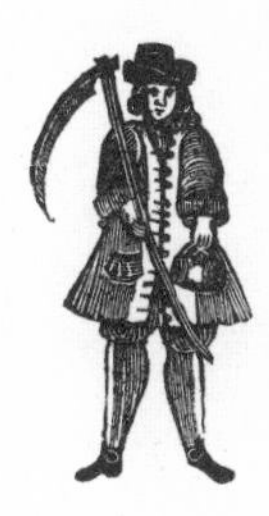

Biodynamic gardening is truly a never-ending path of learning, as the Mother continues to evolve. Through observing nature, we gain understanding of all that affects plants and their growth. Unlike the modern belief that with access to soluble compounds of nitrogen, potassium, and phosphorous, plants will grow, biodynamic gardening takes into account all things that influence or manipulate plant health and development. This technique considers the movement of the stars, weather patterns, animal reactions—all things from the heavens to the depths of the earth. According to Sherry Wildfeuer, author of *Stella Natura*, we can rely on our ability to "read the book of nature."

Nature reveals itself on its own accord, and it offers more knowledge than can be readily understood. Through continual observation and study of various changing environments and conditions, we begin to grasp what is essential for each individual plant. Herbs require varying levels of sun, water, and attention. As Wildfeuer says, we must observe nature in "shade, as well as full sun, in wet and dry areas, and on different soils." Only by paying close attention can we hope to understand the language of the elements, hear the voice of nature, and regain

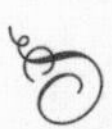

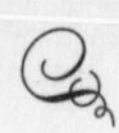

ancient wisdom. As we fall into the rhythms of the seasons, we can create balance and harmony in our solidarity with nature.

Seasons come and go. Life seemingly comes from nothing in the spring, and then we see it fade away in the fall. With an understanding of these cycles and their effects on individual crops, we can time our gardening efforts. Food and herbs grown in harmony with the eternal rhythm of the earth's energy are richer and full of the essential positive vibrations necessary for a healthy life. Steiner believed that food grown this way was full of energy, whereas food grown without the proper attention lacked essential vitality. The more this energy is within us, the easier it becomes to be in tune with the natural flow of the earth itself (or Gaia herself).

There has been a major shift in food consciousness in the late twentieth century. For the past forty or fifty years, food supplies in the United States and other industrialized countries have grown primarily on what we could call the chemical revolution. After World War II and the proliferation of chemical pesticides and fertilizers, commercial agriculture turned away from traditional farming practices. Unfortunately, many growers lost the instinctive knowledge of tradtional methods and adopted synthetic dependency. The revered chemicals began to hide and distort the ancient heartbeat of the Mother, until the farmers could no longer hear the spirit of the earth. It has been said that farmers of old were able to walk through their fields and feel the energy of the soil radiating everywhere. They sensed any lack of energy or disharmony in the soil, and were able to balance it with composting and reenergizing methods.

This deep connection to the earth as a living, breathing macrocosm is very similar to the principles that the famous experiment at Findhorn was based on. In 1962, three lovely people moved to the western tip of Scotland, where they built a garden on impossible sandy, dry land. Eileen received guidance from Spirit or God, Dorothy received guidance from the deva, or spirit, of the plants, and Peter translated their visions into action. With careful attention to the cycles of the seasons and the individual needs of each plant, they reaped forty-pound squash and eight-foot-tall foxgloves.

Biodynamic gardening principles can be applied at any time in a plant's life. You will find secrets of the earth hidden within you. Think of how much information you possess that cannot be put into words. The knowledge of the earth is like this: it is an ever-evolving book that can never be read, but rather only felt. Through

careful observation, the broadening of our perspectives to see and believe in the connection between ourselves and each plant, and our gradual attunement to the natural rhythms of the earth, we return to an ancient way of living. Listen to the gentle lessons the Mother has to teach, and you will promote the healing of our planet and the hearts of human population.

Soil, like the earth itself, is a living, breathing organism with a complex, interdependent cyclical system of growth, fruition, death, decay, and renewal. When your soil is in balance and healthy, it consists of chemical breakdown and realignment of air, water, and nutrient absorption, retention, and release. When it is not, it can become so acidic or alkaline that almost nothing will grow in it. It can retain so much moisture that oxygen is depleted and plants drown and rot away; or conversely, it can shed water so quickly that plants wither and die of thirst. It can even become so finely compacted that almost no amount of water can seep in, and roots can barely penetrate even a few inches. Ultimately, when the wind blows, the fine surface of it will simply blow away, leaving behind a hard concrete-like layer that seems as if it is well on its way to becoming solid rock.

Fortunately, there is another solution to all but the most extreme soil conditions, and that is composting. From a Wiccan or other earth-based religion's point of view, composting just makes sense. It is recycling on a biological level, the way the Goddess intended. Also, Wiccans are taught as part of our Code of Hospitality that a gift deserves a gift, and in return for all the fruit, flowers, vegetables, and herbs that your garden gives you, you are honor-bound to return the favor. Now, it may not seem to you that your kitchen garbage, dead cut flowers, and yard trimmings are a very fair trade, but they are just what the soil needs to replenish itself. In particular, the nutrients that a plant takes from the soil and utilizes to grow are largely still present in the decaying material of that plant after death. So by returning the stems, peels, tops, spent flowers, dead leaves, or even chopped-up pruned branches back to the soil, you give those nutrients the opportunity to return to a usable state and nourish a new generation of growth.

Composting can be as simple or as elaborate as you wish to make it. If you have the space, you can build one or more large bins. The simplest method of composting is "sheet composting," the best and most detailed explanation of which is found in *The Ruth Stout No Work Garden Book*. It is by far the easiest composting method, and the one intended to mimic most closely the processes of

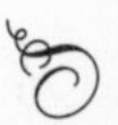

the Mother herself. First the garden soil is turned once, to loosen it. (This step can actually be omitted, but it slows down the results to do so.) Then a thick layer (about six inches or so) of organic mulch is spread over the entire loosened area. On top of that, dump all of your (or even all your neighbors') nondiseased yard waste, vegetable scraps, hair and nail clippings, ashes from the fireplace, eggshells, nut shells, and coffee grounds. The mulch will shrink down in time as decomposition proceeds. Straw is an ideal organic mulch, and one of the most universally available. When using straw, it is important to keep in mind that it contains seed, and the layer must be kept thick enough to keep them from sprouting. Other mulches, mostly the by-products of agriculture, can work as well. Some people even use newspaper now that the ink is soy-based, but I personally find this unsightly.

The composting process will vary, depending on your waste. Soil can be added each time you add green or kitchen waste. Otherwise, straw or dry leaves or grass clippings can go on top, just to keep the flies away. Compost should be kept moist but not wet, kind of like a cake. The amount of watering will depend on the quantity of compost, the weather, and the amount of ventilation. Sometimes you don't need to water at all, especially if you have a lot of green material. Turning is necessary if you have a huge compost pile, or to speed up the process. Green material and watering both do approximately the same thing—add moisture. Water is always available; green material is available only sporadically, so watering becomes the way that you adjust the moisture content when there is no green material to add. If the pile becomes too wet, add dry material or turn it to dry it out.

If weeds should appear in whatever mulch you are using, simply bury them under more mulch. When you have kitchen scraps or yard trimmings to add, scoop or rake some of the mulch away from an area, spread out your would-be compost, and replace the mulch topping. The mulch will continuously decompose wherever it comes in contact with the soil surface and will need to be replenished with a new layer periodically. This is much like the natural cycle of litter and decay found on the floor of a forest or meadow. Once the process gets going, you will never have to till the soil again. Weeds become much less of a bother, as long as your mulch stays thick enough, and your topsoil will gradually grow richer, softer, and deeper.

Don't be surprised if a tomato plant sprouts in your compost pile. Ideally, the center of a compost pile will rise to a temperature of well over a hundred degrees Fahrenheit. This is why well-composted material is often almost black and

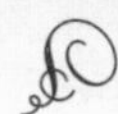

charred-looking. It has been cooking slowly to the consistency of crumbly charcoal, breaking down the complex chemicals found in plant materials and rendering them soluble again. Ordinarily, this heat is enough to kill almost anything, including most plant diseases and insects. Beneficial insects and earthworms will be found only in the much cooler, bottom few inches of the pile. Tomato seeds, however, can readily withstand the heat of virtually any compost pile. In fact, research has shown that the heat may actually increase the likelihood and percentage of germination. The germination of most other seeds in your compost, however, is a good indication that it is not "cooking" enough and probably needs to be either watered more often or fed more green material, or possibly even have a little compost starter added to get it going again.

Another possibility is a composting tumbler; there are many varieties on the market. They hold a reasonable amount of material for a small garden, are easy to use, and cost anywhere from fifty to a few hundred dollars, depending on size, style, and where you buy it.

Many people cultivate specific plants to add to their compost. The thinking behind this practice is that these species have the ability to absorb certain types of nutrients and minerals from the soil, or even the air, that other plants cannot touch because these nutrients are chemically bound up in such a way that most plants cannot absorb them. These are some of the plants and the nutrients they supply:

- Clover, vetches, peas, and beans supply nitrogen by taking it right from the air. Nitrogen is essential for growth. Clover in particular will send down deep roots, which can help break heavy clay soils and bring up to the surface nutrients that other plants' roots can't reach.

- Dandelion and chickweed add copper to your compost. Dandelion and groundsel will also add soluble iron to the soil. In alkaline soils, iron is often present but chemically bound up and inaccessible to plants, causing chlorosis. The conventional solution is to add chemical acidifiers or iron chelates containing sulfur, but these can actually compound the problem in the long run. A gentler solution is to compost your dandelions and throw in your coffee grounds and teabags.

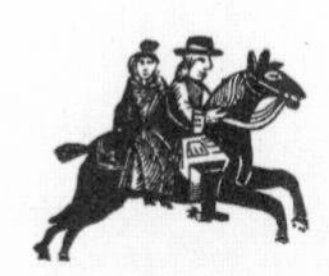

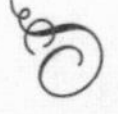

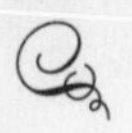

— Yarrow gives copper, phosphates, and potash to the soil. The first is essential for green growth, the last two for flowering and fruit.

— Roman chamomile provides calcium.

— Dead nettles are rich in quite a number of trace minerals.

— Mexican marigold and tobacco are sometimes added to the compost for their insect-repellent properties. The marigold will actually kill harmful species of nematodes, and tobacco is said to kill cutworms. If you are sheet composting, you can put a bit of the appropriate herb under the mulch next to the most susceptible plants.

— Eucalyptus leaves, if you have them, can be added as well—but sparingly, as they actually inhibit plant growth as well as deterring insects.

— Comfrey leaves are high in minerals and quite effective in compost piles.

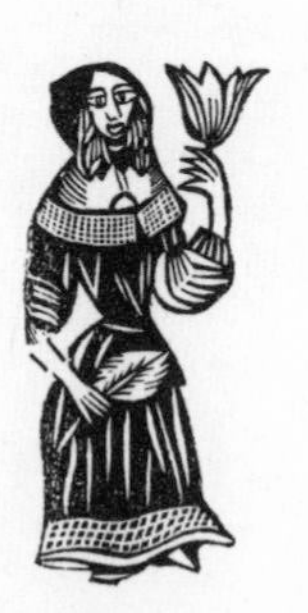

If want to speed up the decomposition of the various materials in your compost, add horse, sheep, or poultry manure from the local stable or barnyard, or exotic (and expensive) organic and inorganic ingredients such as greensand, cottonseed meal, or rock phosphate. Manure is also an excellent source of nutrients for the soil. But not all manures are created equal, so to speak. Commercially available steer manure is so high in salts that it will burn most plants. By the time the salts have been leached out, so have the majority of the nutrients. It is also of questionable merit to people who prefer more organic methods because of the large amounts of hormones and antibiotics fed to both beef and dairy cattle. A far superior alternative is horse manure. Most horses are treated as prized and well-loved pets, well fed and exercised, and given medicines only when necessary. This is a far cry from the factorylike treatment many cattle and poultry receive. The extra chemicals given to animals to stimulate growth or milk or egg production pass right through their systems and end up in their manure—and ultimately, in your herbs, fruits, and vegetables. Some of these chemicals break down; some don't. Some individuals feel that there is a moral or spiritual issue involved as well.

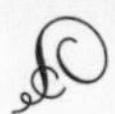

Though not exactly vegetarians, they won't consume food from these "animal factories" and don't wish to use the manure from them either.

Another advantage to horse manure is that it is often free; but the downside is that it doesn't come in handy bags from the store. You usually have to go to a stable and shovel it yourself. This is not as bad as it may seem. Horse people are a friendly lot and are often willing to help in some way just to get rid of the stuff. (They always seem to have plenty of it, you see.) Usually it has been piled up someplace and is semicomposted already, from just sitting around waiting for you to haul it away.

If all this is highly distasteful to you, there is still an alternative, but it's going to cost you. Bat and bird guano, mostly imported from South America, can be purchased in some of the high-end nurseries or even ordered by mail. It is composted, bagged, and a very high-quality manure. It is also rather expensive, and very chic among gardeners. (That is, if manure can be chic. Personally, I don't mind using the shovel, and you definitely know where the stuff comes from that way.)

Here are some other additions that you might make to the compost, or even directly to your soil.

Dolomitic limestone can make your soil less acidic and increase the amount of available calcium. Fish emulsion is rich in both nitrogen and phosphorus. It is rather odorific, however. Cottonseed meal will help acidify soil that is too alkaline, and it is a good source of nitrogen. Blood meal has both nitrogen and phosphorus, but as it is the product of commercial slaughterhouses, some shun it for reasons delineated above. Bone meal is high in phosphorus and calcium, but it has the same stigma as blood meal for some. Kelp (seaweed) is a good overall product for trace minerals, but it is often expensive. Greensand is rich in potash. Other products that may be available only regionally, such as ground peanut shells, cocoa palm, or bagasse, can be excellent sources of nutrients at low cost in areas where they are plentiful.

For much more detailed information on this topic, I recommend Rodale Press's *Encyclopedia of Organic Gardening*. And remember, when you compost, you are not just saving money, recycling waste, improving the quality of your garden, or giving back to the earth, you are doing *all* of these things. What is more, you are confirming the interconnectedness of all things and participating in the magickal ritual of renewal which Mother Earth performs every day.

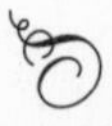

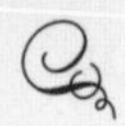

Tips for Gathering, Storing, and Preserving Fresh Herbs

Harvesting or gathering herbs with attention and the greatest care ensures their quality and infuses further love and healing potential into the plants. As you gather, ask the plant's permission to take, and seek guidance for which leaf, flower, or fruit to cut. Never take more than one-quarter of any particular plant, and try to remember to give an offering, such as a pinch of tobacco, food, crytals, water, or heartfelt thanks.

To glean the highest life force from the herbs, harvest after the roots have developed fully, during the peak of their growth, and in the morning after the dew has evaporated. Harvest the fresh young leaves below the flowers.

Different parts of the plant need to be gathered in different ways and at different times. Flowers and leaves should usually be collected in the spring and early summer. For a plant with useful leaves, you can pinch back the flowers so the energy does not leave the leaves and diminish their flavor. When drying leaves or flowers, snip off long stalks. Harvest leaves when they are young for the most concentrated medicinal and magickal powers. Do not use insect-bitten, yellowed, or blotched leaves or insect-bitten or wilting flowers. Gather flowers soon after they open, before insects have frequented them. Pick off seeds after they have had ample time to ripen on the plant: yellowed leaves are a great indicator that the seeds are ready. The best time to harvest root crops is in the early spring, when the sap rises, or in autumn, though you can also gather after the plant sheds its leaves in the late fall or early winter. When gathering the bark, take from the fallen branches and only from the bigger ones. If a lot of bark is required, you may need to saw off a branch first. Gather bark in early spring or autumn.

To increase growth in woody perennials such as rosemary, harvest at the point that the new branches leave the central stem. Some gardeners prefer to harvest annuals to the ground, while others like to leave one or two plants in their bed to reseed and return earlier next year. With woody perennials such as sage or rosemary, harvest no more than one-third of each plant.

Preserving and storing herbs properly will ensure their quality for up to two years after collection. Submerge fresh herbs in clean water. You may choose to add about two tablespoons of salt per sinkful to rid the leaves of insects. Blot gently

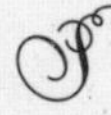

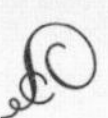

with a cloth or paper towel to dry. Hang upside down in a cool, dry place with a good flow of air for three weeks. Leave seeds and fruits attached to the plant during the drying process. Another method is to dry the leaves flat between thin, soft sheets of paper. You can dry culinary perennials such as sage and thyme in the refrigerator. Loosely stack clean, dry herbs in a covered container and separate layers with parchment paper. Seal tightly. You can experiment with freezing some herbs, such as thyme, rosemary, and sage, for up to four months. The freezing method preserves the flavor but dissipates the medicinal value. A dehydrator works well, leaving color, taste, and scent intact.

You can choose to separate the dried leaves from the stems and put them in dark glass jars. To remove tiny leaves or flowers, hold the stem at the top and run your fingers down the stem in a shredding motion, severing leaves from the stem. Tiny leaves such as thyme or marjoram can be used as they are; larger leaves such as basil or rosemary should be chopped or torn. Pack lightly in the jars. Or leave the flowers, leaves, or seeds on the plant and store in brown paper bags with the stems protruding and the bags securely tied around the stems.

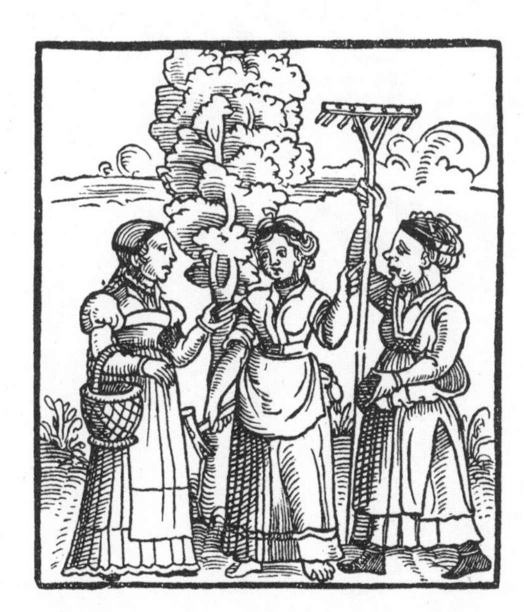

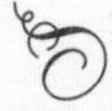

2

Magickal Herbs & Plants

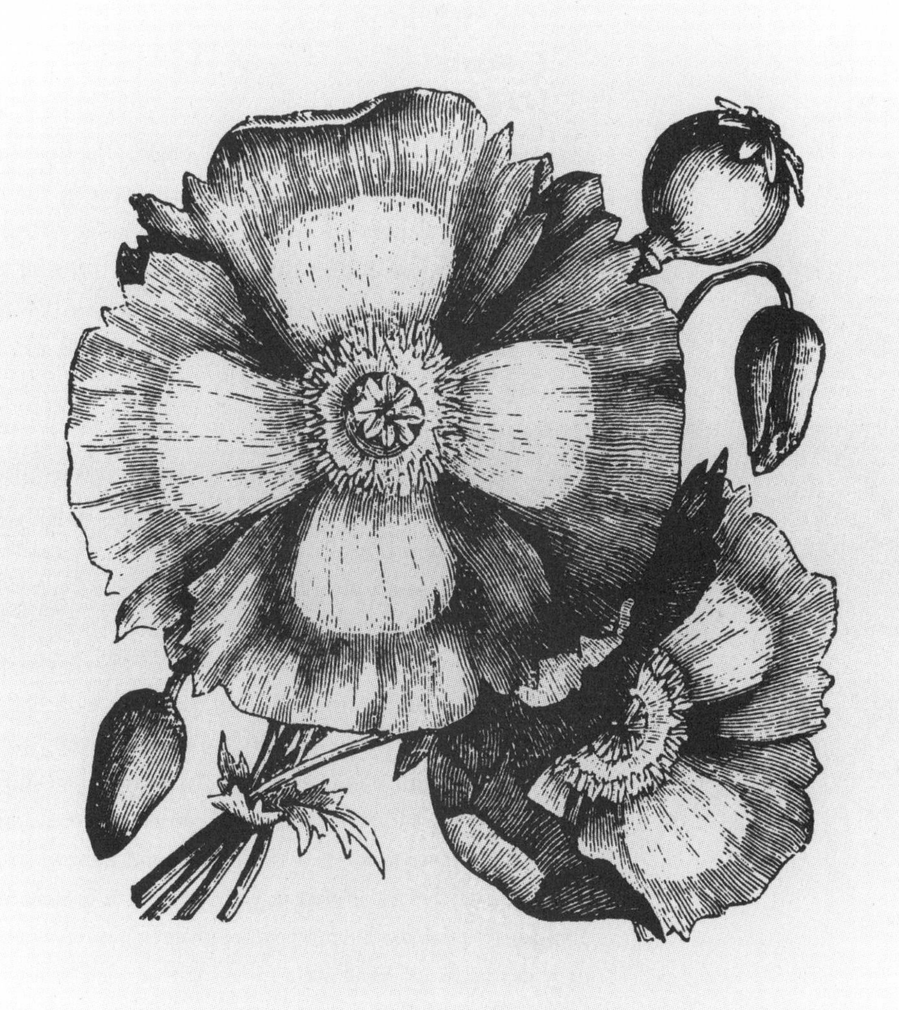

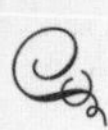

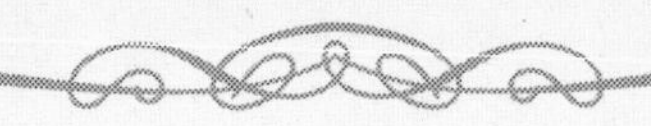

Acacia

Acacia Senegal

CAPE GUM, GUM ARABIC TREE, EGYPTIAN THORN

Parts Used: twigs, root

Acacia comes in many varieties, but *Acacia Senegal* is the source of true gum arabic, used in inks, pharmaceuticals, and candies. Many of the leaves are feathery, and most of the flowers are cream, yellow, or orange. Acacia aids meditation and the development of psychic powers. It is used to anoint altars as it possesses high spiritual vibrations, protection powers, corresponds to the element of air, and is associated with the planet and god Mars.

Akashic Authenticity

The Akashic Records register the memories of each person's heart as the soul moves through various incarnations. When we reclaim the seed of our destination, which was already planted in our hearts, we can begin to awaken to the delight of being. Acacia attunes you to the highest spiritual vibrations, the place where the Akashic Records are accessed.

This meditation can be incorporated into an Ostara ritual or any new moon ritual. It honors your authenticity, the way you work with light and magick; it affirms that whatever method you employ is valid as long as you have positive intent. It helps you release self-scrutiny and allow it to die, and lets you surrender to the fate that is your divine manifestation: a perfect and complete expression of Spirit.

Burn acacia incense for this meditation and perform it on the day of the new moon or the day before or after it. Cast a circle, or ground and center yourself.

Imagine that you are in your favorite place in nature, whether it be a beach, mountain, or desert. Relax. Visualize a mirror surrounded by a white glowing light. Walk toward that mirror. You are undertaking a journey you have long desired.

Now you are in a forest glen. Everywhere you look there are trees. Hear the pitter-patter of drops from an earlier rain falling from drenched branches. A great stag steps

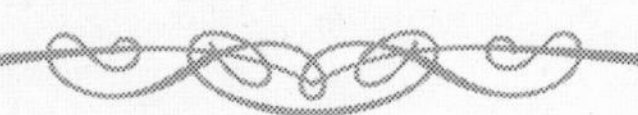

into the clearing. He beckons you to follow him. Instinctively you follow. Soon you notice that you are climbing up a steep mountain. The pinnacle is pointed and sharp. After much hiking, your body feels very heavy. You feel a great weight upon your back. Just at the point that it becomes nearly unbearable, you reach the top.

On the plateau stands a magnificent woman, Lady Luna. She is draped in winter white, ice blue, and indigo. Around her neck are a strand of garnet and a garland of acacia flowers. She asks, "What do you seek, my child?" You reply, "I seek peace. I want to release these burdens." "Give me your pain," says Lady Luna. "I will transform it." You see that Moon Mother is another aspect of Spirit, which means she is part of you. You search through your being for all hurt and sad feelings and then send this negative energy streaming toward her open hands. When all the energy has left your body, it forms a gray, murky ball. Lady Luna throws the ball up in the air, and it transforms into doves of peace.

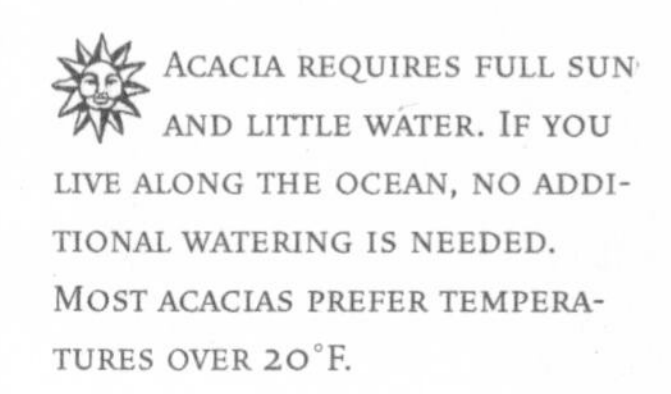

Acacia requires full sun and little water. If you live along the ocean, no additional watering is needed. Most acacias prefer temperatures over 20°F.

"Look at this drop of dew on a spider web," she says. "There are worlds within worlds. Surrender the stories that keep you weighted down. You do not need a ballast to float. See for yourself." A pond appears before you. You wade in to where the water is deep and cool. As you swim you feel calm and contented. Your reflection reveals compassion, a state of the freedom, and acceptance. After some time you come out of the pool feeling clean and refreshed. "What is it that you desire?" Lady Luna asks. Pour out your desires from your heart center. Their energy forms a crystal ball into which the doves of peace swirl. Place your hands on the sides of the ball. Guide the ball into your solar plexus, and push the energy down your legs to your feet, so that they will know the path to walk upon. Lady Luna walks toward you and melts into your being. The stag, king of the four-legged, reappears. His antlers grow from his forehead near the third eye, which represents his inner knowledge. He allows you to ride upon him for the journey back to the forest glen. When you are once again surrounded by the glen's trees, the stag says, "I give you unconditional love and support for your intentions and desires." Then he too melts into you. You are whole and complete with both male and female aspects. You step through the mirror and are back in your favorite place. Rest there for a bit. Concentrate on your feet; they will help you walk toward your intention and destiny. On the count of three you will come back to the earthly plane. Release the circle, if you have cast one.

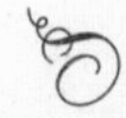

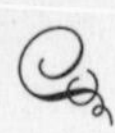

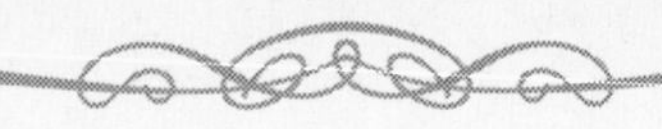

Alder

Alnus (various species)

FEVER BUSH

Parts Used: leaves, bark

GIVE AMPLE WATER OR GROW BESIDE A CREEK. ALDER GROWS WELL IN SUN OR SHADE. ALDER IS NATIVE TO EUROPE, ASIA, NORTH AFRICA, AND NORTH AMERICA.

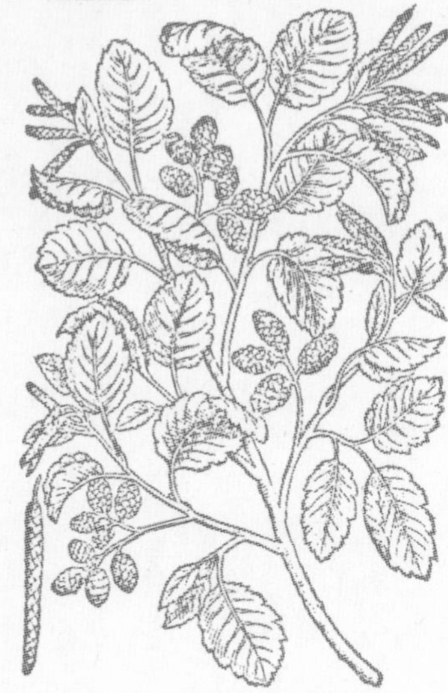

The presence of alder indicates that water is nearby. Alders grow as shrubs or thick-trunked trees in swamps and along riverbanks. Alder trees have shiny oval leaves and catkinlike flowers. Alder is an astringent and long ago was used to alleviate gangrene. An infusion of aged alder bark is used for stomachaches, as a blood purifier, and to facilitate childbirth. Dry rot from the tree has been traditionally mixed with powdered willow bark as a poultice for burns. Native Americans placed leaves in their moccasins to relieve tired, aching, and hot feet and made flutes and whistles from its branches. In magick, alder is used for strength, protection, emotions, and to attune with the element of water. Alder is associated with the planet and goddess Venus and the astrological signs Cancer and Pisces.

Alder Poultice

This poultice can be used to reduce and relieve most swelling, including swollen or inflamed breasts.

1 cup fresh alder leaves
1 tablespoon warm milk

Grind the alder leaves to a pulp. Add the milk. Place the mixture in a cheesecloth bag and lay directly on the inflamed area until the poultice grows quite warm, about 10 minutes.

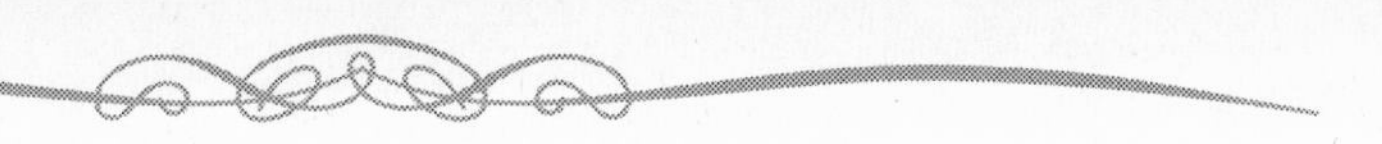

Aloe

Aloe vera

ALOES, ALOE VERA, BURN PLANT, MEDICINE PLANT

Part Used: leaves

Aloe leaves grow tall and wandlike, with spines along the sides to protect them from grazing animals. According to legend, aloe is the only plant to come directly from the Garden of Eden. Aloe is usually found in dry, sandy, and rocky regions. It is used to treat gastrointestinal ailments, boost the immune system, and relieve pain. Aloe can be taken as a laxative in small doses; do not overuse. For a diuretic, mix a little of the fresh juice from the leaf with fruit juice and drink it before meals. Aloe juice is exported all over the world as an effective blood cleanser and laxative. Aloe's magickal properties include healing, luck, the gift of life, and protection. Planetary and deity associations for aloe are Mars and Venus.

ALOE LIKES FULL SUN OR LIGHT SHADE INLAND. WATER DEEPLY BUT INFREQUENTLY. GROW IN LOOSE, DRY, WELL-DRAINED SOIL RICH IN HUMUS IN REASONABLY FROST-FREE AREAS. TO PROPAGATE, SEPARATE AND REPOT THE ROOTED SUCKERS AT THE PLANT'S BASE. ALOE IS NATIVE TO EASTERN AND SOUTHERN AFRICA.

DO NOT USE ALOE INTERNALLY IF YOU ARE PREGNANT.

Aloe Gel

While not a panacea, aloe can alleviate the sting and speed healing from cuts, burns, ulcers in the mouth, insect bites, and mild skin irritations. This gel will keep in the refrigerator for two months and is useful to have around for emergencies, especially if there are small children in your household.

- 1 large outer aloe leaf
- contents of 1 500 mg powdered vitamin C capsule
- 20 drops lavender essential oil

Peel the leaf with a peeler or paring knife and place in a blender or food processor. (If you do not own a blender or food processor, you can use a mortar and pestle.) Blend thoroughly. Measure ⅓ cup aloe puree; reserve any remaining puree for another use. Place the measured puree and all remaining ingredients in the blender and blend thoroughly. Store in a clean glass jar with a tight-fitting lid.

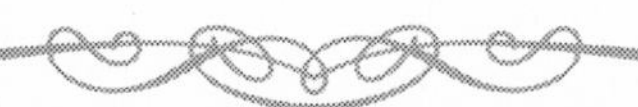

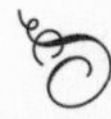

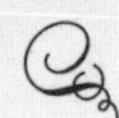

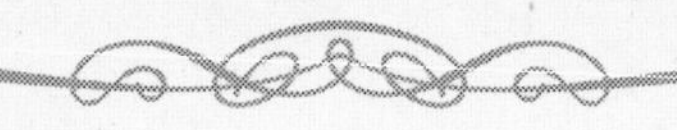

Angelica

Angelica archangelica

ARCHANGEL, GARDEN ANGELICA, HERB OF THE ANGEL, MASTERWORT, ROOT OF THE HOLY GHOST, SINGER'S HERB

Parts Used: root, leaves

Angelica is cultivated in gardens and found in woodlands and damp places. The plant has fragrant umbrella-shaped heads of greenish yellow flowers and divided, toothed leaves. Angelica possesses a wide range of benefits. In 1555, a Benedictine monk prayed for guidance to provide a treatment for the plague; angelica was his answer. The bitter chemicals in angelica trigger the digestive system and help to alleviate gas and stomach cramps, colic, and heartburn; to stimulate appetite; and to promote elimination. Candied angelica stalks are a popular sweetmeat in Spain and France, valued for their fertility properties. Angelica can also be used to flavor wines. Suck on the root to relieve a sore throat. Planetary and deity associations for angelica include Atlantis, archangel Michael, Venus, the sun, and the astrological sign of Leo. Angelica resonates with the element of fire, which also coordinates to the direction of the south, the cornerstone for passion. In magick, angelica is used for protection and to reach the astral plane.

IF YOU ARE PREGNANT, YOU SHOULD NOT USE ANGELICA.
ANGELICA CONTAINS KNOWN CARCINOGENS AND SHOULD BE USED SPARINGLY.
ANGELICA RESEMBLES WILD PLANTS IN THE CARROT FAMILY THAT ARE POISONOUS, SO DO NOT ATTEMPT TO HARVEST IT IN THE WILD.

Passion-Enhancing Elixir

In a patriarchal society, even before young women reach puberty they are taught to cover up and cast aside the enchantress side of their nature. Before a young woman has a chance to honor the power of her sexuality, she is shamed or exploited. She can feel the power of her sex appeal but often cannot enjoy it.

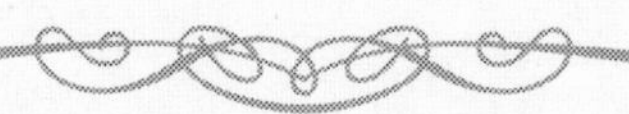

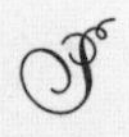

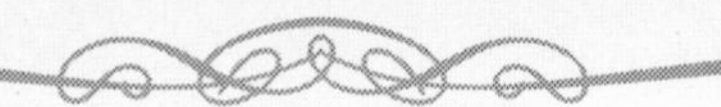

Some ancient societies honored the women who had the gift of a passionate nature. They created sacred spaces for women such as Cleopatra and let them loose, so to speak. Women's sexual passion is an integral part of our divinity. You know that it feels good! Join the resurgence today: honor and respect the sacred slut within.

Make this elixir during a waxing moon, preferably after the crescent or pubescent phase has passed. In this recipe, the moon phase reflects the space between the maiden phase and the mother phase of her life, when a young woman feels the power and possibilities of fertility.

ANGELICA ENJOYS PARTIAL SHADE. GROW IN MOIST, RICH, SLIGHTLY ACIDIC SOIL. TO PROLONG THE PLANT'S LIFE, CUT BACK THE FLOWERS BEFORE THE BUDS OPEN. ANGELICA PREFERS TEMPERATE REGIONS, AND IS COMMON IN WESTERN EUROPE.

1 red candle

1 teaspoon angelica tincture (see page 261)

1 cup passion fruit juice or apple juice

Light the candle and combine the tincture with the juice (the juice symbolizes the Goddess and her divine nature, with special attention given to building and strengthening the temptress within). Hold your hands over the drink and say,

Dear Goddess of sex, fire, and love
I call upon my passion from above
To honor as sacred my sexual face
As one with you in a divine space.

Drink the juice and reflect on your sacred sexuality.

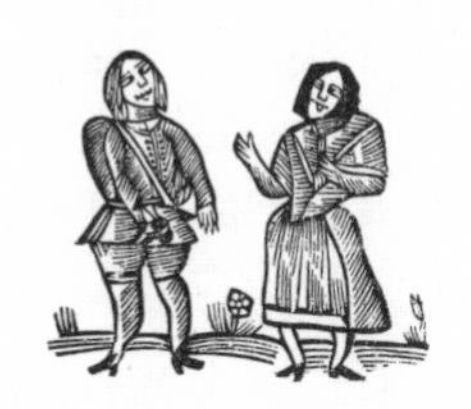

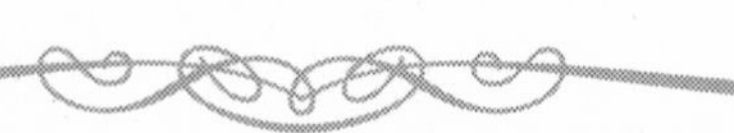

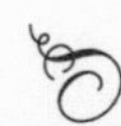

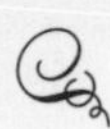

Anise

Pimpinella anisum

ANNEYS, ANISEED

Part Used: seeds

Anise is recognized by its feathery, moss-green leaves and umbrellas of cream-colored flowers, which form yellow seeds that smell distinctly like black licorice. It has naturalized in the United States and can be found in fields and hedgerows, and on rocky hillsides. The seeds, which usually mature in August, can be chewed as a breath freshener or to settle an upset stomach; anise is known as a terrific digestive aid. The seeds are useful for dental purposes, and can be added to toothpaste or infused as a tea to fight cavities. Cookie confectioners are known to use the seeds to flavor their baked goods. Planetary and deity associations for anise are the moon, ruling emotions; Jupiter, the Romans' supreme god; Apollo, who rules with the Sun in honor of fertility, light, truth, medicine, poetry, fine arts, and eloquence; and Mercury, who rules over communication and travel.

Pan de los Muertos

MAKES 1 LOAF

Anise is used in protection and purification rituals, often during the dark phase of the moon. The herb is believed to allay nightmares, attract luck, and cleanse spaces. During the Dias de los Muertos celebrations traditional in Mexico, it is widely used to flavor sweets and cooked in breads to entice the deceased to visit. Julie Boyer, a good friend whose life journey has her wandering between northern and southern California, brought this yummy bread to a Dia de los Muertos celebration. It sweetened the palates of our honored guests—both living and dead.

¼ cup milk

4 tablespoons (½ stick) chilled unsalted butter, cut into 8 pieces

¼ cup plus 2 teaspoons sugar

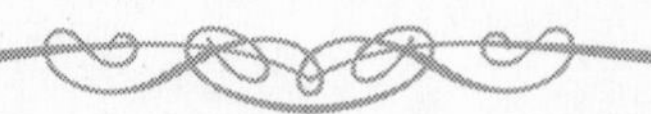

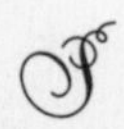

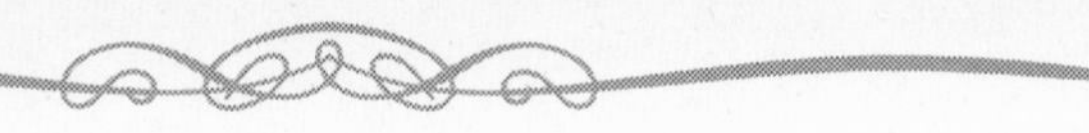

½ teaspoon salt
1 package active dry yeast
¼ cup very warm water
2 large eggs
3 cups all-purpose flour, unsifted
½ teaspoon anise seed
¼ teaspoon ground cinnamon

In a saucepan, bring the milk to a boil and remove from the heat. Stir in the butter, ¼ cup of the sugar, and the salt. In a large bowl, mix the yeast with the warm water until dissolved; let stand 5 minutes. Add the milk mixture. Separate the yolk and white of 1 egg. Add the yolk to the yeast mixture; place the white in a bowl and reserve. Add the flour to the yeast and remaining egg. Stirring with a spoon, blend well until a dough ball is formed. Flour a pastry board or work surface and place the dough in the center. Knead until smooth. Return the mixture to the large bowl and cover with a dish towel. Let rise in a warm place for 1½ hours.

Grease a baking sheet and preheat the oven to 350°F. Knead the dough again on the floured surface. Divide into fourths, setting 1 piece aside. Roll the remaining 3 pieces into ropes. On the greased baking sheet, pinch 1 end of the ropes together and braid. Finish by pinching the ends together on the opposite side. Divide the remaining dough piece in half and shape into 2 bones. Lay them atop the braided loaf, forming an X shape. Cover the loaf with a dish towel and let rise 30 minutes. Meanwhile, in a bowl, mix anise seed, cinnamon, and the remaining 2 teaspoons sugar. Beat the egg white lightly. After the 30 minutes has passed, brush the top of the bread with the egg white and sprinkle with the anise seed mixture, avoiding the crossbones. Bake for 35 minutes, or until the bread springs back to the touch.

Grow in full sun and light soil. Sow the seeds in warm ground. Anise does not transplant easily. Anise enhances the growth of coriander when planted nearby, but harms carrots. Anise is native to north Africa, western Asia, and the eastern Mediterranean.

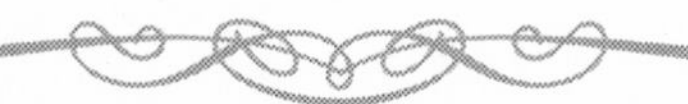

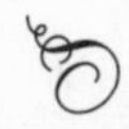

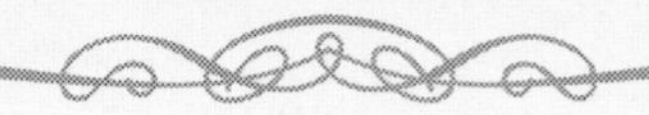

Apple

Malus pumila

FRUIT OF THE UNDERWORLD, SILVER BRANCH, SILVER BOUGH, TREE OF LOVE

Parts Used: fruit, blossoms, branches

Apples are the Goddess's sacred fruit, used in love and healing arts, and are strongly associated with the Samhain, Mabon, and Beltane sabbats. Their powers to invoke love were once believed so powerful that the flowers were used in all bridal bouquets. Apple pies are often the center of love spells; the latticework atop the pie symbolizes the containment of the maker's love. In the ancient ogham alphabet of the British Isles, the letter *q* is called *quert*, which is the word for "apple." Apple wands are often employed as an aid to Otherworld journeying. Apple is associated with many deities including Aphrodite, Apollo, Athena, Diana, Dionysus, Hera, Hercules, and Venus.

Applesauce Muffins

MAKES 1 DOZEN MUFFINS

Apples represent our immortality. The timelessness of apples points to both the vibrancy of youth and the flame of Spirit that continues to burn forever. We are children of earth, children of Spirit. As children, our life force pulsates with fire. Even as we cross to other planes of existence, our light continues to shine. The impressions and relationships we create during our lives will also live a deathless existence. Like all things, they will transmute and grow. Be conscious of what you create and be aware that at every moment you are inventing your world. What will you send out? Infuse your intent to make space for a world of light. Be mindful of the timelessness of life and your participation in it.

Nonstick vegetable oil spray
¾ cup unsweetened applesauce
1 tablespoon vanilla extract

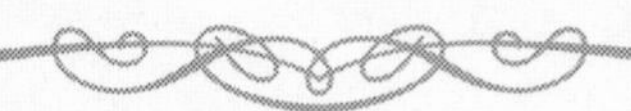

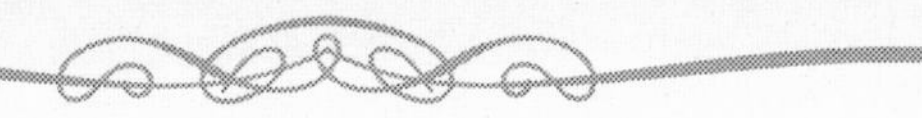

1 cup milk
1 large egg
2 cups whole wheat flour
1 teaspoon ground cinnamon
1 tablespoon baking powder

Preheat oven to 400°F.

Spray 12 standard muffin cups (⅔-cup capacity) with nonstick spray. In a bowl, mix together the applesauce, vanilla, milk, and egg. In a small bowl, mix the wheat flour, cinnamon, and baking powder. Add the dry ingredients to the applesauce mixture; stir until just combined. Fill the muffin cups ¾ full. Bake 17 to 20 minutes, or until the muffins spring back into place when touched. Let the muffins cool 5 minutes, then turn onto wire racks to cool completely.

Apple trees prefer full sun and frequent watering, especially during long dry periods. All apples require pollination. Most apples need approximately forty days of temperature below 45°F to grow and blossom properly.

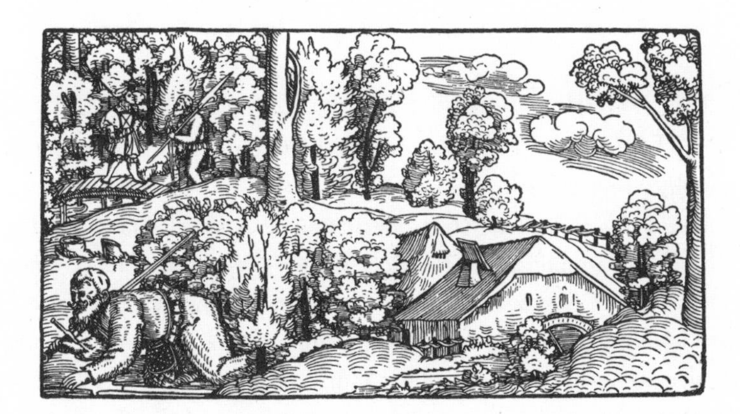

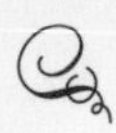

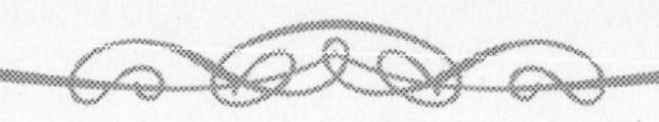

Ash

Fraxinus excelsior, Fraxinus americana

NION, TREE OF KNOWLEDGE, TREE OF LIFE, TREE OF SPEECH, WORLD TREE, YGGDRASIL

Parts Used: leaves, branches

Ash trees grow tall and slender, with oval leaves in clusters. Ash is one of the most important trees for Wiccans and witches. It represents healing and the element of water. Its main magickal power is protection, though it can also prompt prophetic dreams. A rich lore of magickal tradition surrounds the ash. It is used in many magickal applications, including the wand, medicine bundles, staffs, and amulets. It is said that if you would like to see a unicorn, you must take your ash wand out into the woods at dusk. Ash is one of the trees honored at winter solstice as well as Beltane. It is also one of the nine sacred woods burned in ritual fires in the Celtic tradition. Planetary and deity associations for ash include Neptune, Mars, the Sun, Thor, and Poseidon.

Magick Wand

An ash tree branch and a clear quartz crystal are the natural substances that will help you align your magick with universal energy; they have been used in rituals and spellwork for centuries. Clear quartz crystal is a well-known and popular energy conductor in modern and ancient times. Clear quartz directs energy and clears the body and physical space from all negativity. Any other items you add to your wand will act as mental cues, energy enhancers, and personal amulets that connect you to Spirit. They also serve your creative muse; after all, this is your wand, and it must speak to you artistically as well magickally. Your wand is your personal calling card to let the deep mind know that you are now entering sacred space.

Creating your own magickal tools is both a meditation and a magickal act. Choosing and handling natural materials like the ones suggested below, utilizing

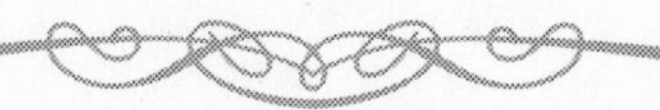

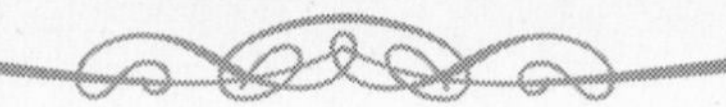

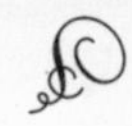

symbolism and color correspondences, brainstorming, and assembling the finished product all serve to infuse tools with your personal energy, so they can better serve as your intent. Making your own tools actually teaches a powerful magickal concept: all magick starts as a thought before it manifests on the physical plane.

Ash tree branch
Clear quartz crystal with a point
Copper or silver wire
Hemp cord
Gems, beads, bells
Charms and other symbols
Leather or sinew laces
Ribbons, feathers, and floss
Wood-burning tool (optional)

THESE SHADY TREES LIKE FULL SUN. MOST SPECIES CAN WITHSTAND A VARIETY OF TEMPERATURES AND SOIL. ASH IS NATIVE TO EUROPE AND NORTH AMERICA.

Trim the ash branch to a length that matches the distance from the tip of your index finger to the crook of your elbow. Whittle an indentation to fit your crystal into the wand. Secure it with a good energy-conducting wire, like copper or silver. You can also secure it with hemp cord and a little glue.

After the basic wand is cut to your desired length and the crystal is set in place, take some time to visualize how you want your wand to look. Be careful to choose colors, textures, and added objects that appeal to you. You might also want to use a wood-burning tool to add astrological signs, Theban script, runes, or other sigils that are meaningful to you. Spend at least an evening with this project. After all, this magickal tool is an extension of yourself and your power.

Once you have completed it, bless and consecrate your wand on the night of the next full moon. Say,

Blessings upon you tool of air
Bring to me magick good and fair
I infuse this wand with pure love
With the guidance of spirit from above
By my will so mote it be.

Your wand is ready for use!

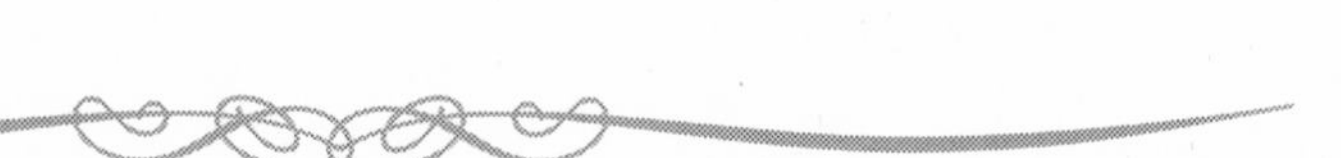

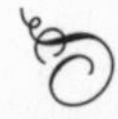

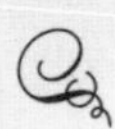

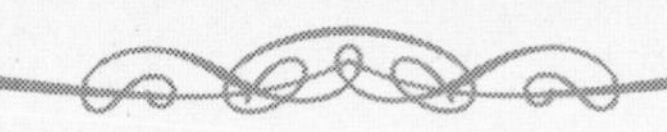

Avens

Geum urbanum, Geum chiloense, Geum triflorum

BLESSED HERB, GOLDEN STAR, HERB BENNET, CLOVEROOT, STAR OF THE EARTH, WILD RYE

Part Used: root

Avens is used in purification, protection, and cleansing rituals. Avens has wiry stems and fruit covered with hooks; sometimes it yields yellow, five-petaled flowers that grow atop a single long stalk with three leaves. In the Middle Ages, the graceful trefoiled leaf and the five golden petals of the blossoms were thought to symbolize the Holy Trinity and the five wounds of Christ. Avens has been associated with St. Benedict and is noted for its tremendous protective powers. By the fifteenth century in Europe, it was widely accepted that if avens root was in the house, evil would be rendered powerless; thus the herb was often worn as an amulet.

Avens is an astringent; is used as a gargle for sore throats; and treats diarrhea, dysentery, colitis, colds, chills, fevers, chronic and mild hemorrhages, gastric irritation, and headaches. The roots are traditionally gathered three to four days after Ostara. Avens is associated with Jupiter, the Romans' supreme god and the planet of the powers of expansion. Magickally the herb is associated with cleansing, love, purification, and spirituality.

Imbolc Soap

MAKES 4 BARS

The star shape of the avens flower is reminiscent of the snowflake, which is a symbol of the Imbolc sabbat. Each snowflake is pure and absolutely unique. Similarly, the concept of creating from a pure space is at the center of Imbolc, which honors the generation of new ideas. Imbolc is the time to nurture your inspiration, recognizing that first light has arrived. By your divine nature you are always pure and innocent. Purification rituals are performed as physical reminders of your true self.

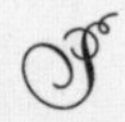

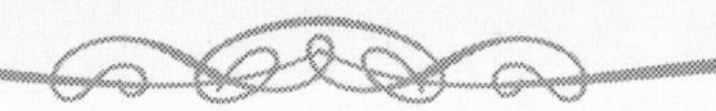

Purge yourself of negative thoughts. Holding them in your consciousness produces toxins and sends them through your body, and it removes you from your innate loving state. Make this soap during a waning moon, and wash with it to awaken you to a pure and innocent state of being. This is particularly important to do before any creation rituals of spring.

Sunflower oil
1 round soap mold with embossed snowflake design
4 ounces white glycerin melt-and-pour soap base
10 to 12 drops avens oil
10 to 12 drops peppermint oil
12 ounces clear glycerin melt-and-pour soap base
Teal or blue gel colorant
Glitter or powdered mica

Avens is a perennial herb, which grows best in sun or partial shade. In warm climates, avens needs regular watering. It is native to the British Isles and other parts of Europe.

Cover your work surface with waxed paper. Apply a thin, even coat of sunflower oil to the mold. Cut the white soap base into 1-inch squares and place in a microwave-safe container. Heat it in the microwave 40 seconds. Stir. Continue to heat and stir for 10-second intervals until the soap base is completely melted. (You can also choose to melt it on the stove top.) Allow it to cool. Stir in 3 to 5 drops each of the avens and peppermint oils, a drop at a time, until the desired scent strength is reached. Spoon the white soap base into the embossed area of the mold. (If you spoon in too much, just scrape away the excess with your fingernail.)

Melt the clear soap base according to the instructions above. Allow it to cool. Stir in 5 to 6 drops each of the avens and peppermint oils, a drop at a time, until the desired scent strength is reached. Add the desired amount of glitter and color gel, stirring constantly until the soap base is evenly coated. Pour the mixture into the mold to fill it. The glitter will sink to the bottom of the mold, giving a nice shimmer to the surface of the soap. Allow the soap to cool for 24 hours before removing it from the mold.

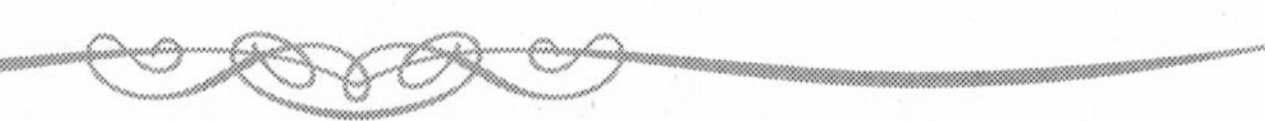

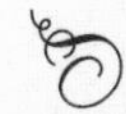

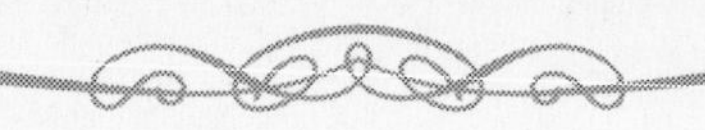

Balm of Gilead

Commiphora opobalsamum, Cedronella canariensis

Mecca balsam

Part Used: buds

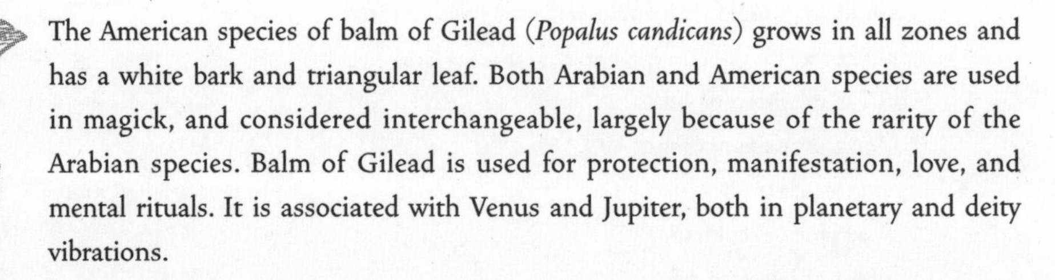

The American species of balm of Gilead (*Popalus candicans*) grows in all zones and has a white bark and triangular leaf. Both Arabian and American species are used in magick, and considered interchangeable, largely because of the rarity of the Arabian species. Balm of Gilead is used for protection, manifestation, love, and mental rituals. It is associated with Venus and Jupiter, both in planetary and deity vibrations.

Heart Renewed

The attributes of balm of Gilead make it effective for warding against a broken heart—be it a broken heart caused by a lover, a family member, a friend, or life itself. A broken heart is caused by a dream of a future that did not come to pass. With this spell you can use the restorative powers of the herb to rebuild your hope and trust in your passions. Sometimes we dream big and set ourselves up for disappointment, but without our dreams we cannot create. Your life is designed with you as cocreator.

This ritual can be performed during any phase of the moon, as it is a spell of need. If the moon is waxing, concentrate on your heart center and see it growing strong. If the moon is waning, focus on your heartache departing from you. In any case, ask for guidance to accept the situation as is and see the blessing within.

1 (3 by 4-inch) piece of pink fabric
1 (24- to 30-inch) piece black silken cord
2 tablespoons dried balm of Gilead buds
2 tablespoons dried rose petals
Small rose quartz

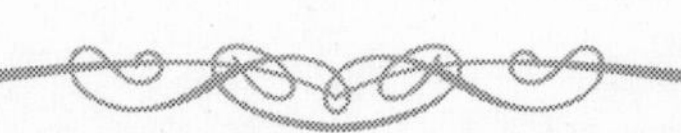

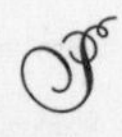

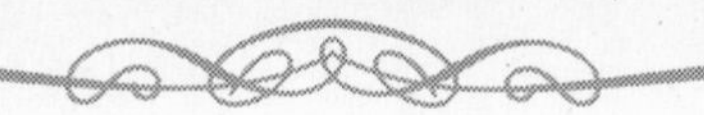

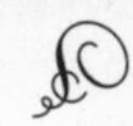

Fold over ½ inch of the top and bottom of the pink fabric. Sew a hem along the bottom edge, leaving enough room to pass a thin cord through. Fold the material up, with the sewn edge facing out. Beginning below the hem, sew the two sides together. Turn inside out. Take the cord and pass it through the top of your pouch (you can use a safety pin to guide the cord through). Make sure the cord is long enough that the pouch sits over your heart when hung around your neck. Mix together the balm of Gilead buds and rose petals. Place a small rose quartz in the middle of the herbs. Hold your hands over the herbs and crystal and say,

Love lost never more
Mend my heart ever more
By my will, so mote it be
Three times three times three.

Put the contents in the pouch and place the cord around your neck until you feel mended.

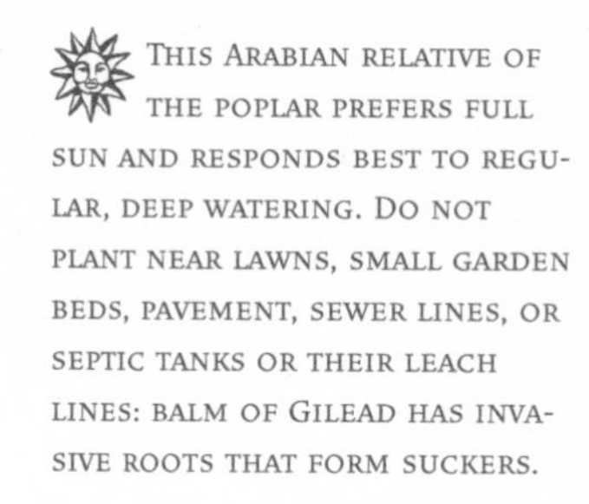

This Arabian relative of the poplar prefers full sun and responds best to regular, deep watering. Do not plant near lawns, small garden beds, pavement, sewer lines, or septic tanks or their leach lines: balm of Gilead has invasive roots that form suckers.

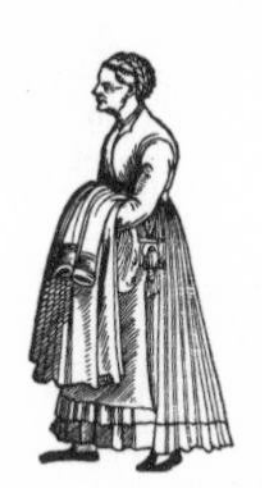

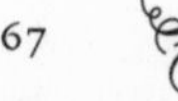

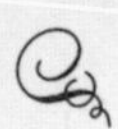

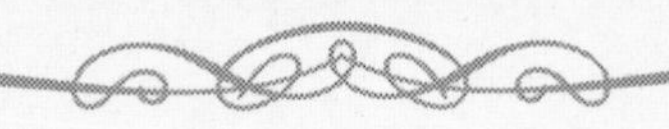

Basil

Ocimum basilicum

ALABAHACA, AMERICAN DITTANY, OUR HERB, ST. JOSEPH'S WORT, SWEET BASIL, WITCHES' HERB

Parts Used: leaves, flowers

Basil has whorls of small, white-hooded flowers and shiny oval leaves. It is found in woodlands and along riverbanks, as well as in many gardens. The herb was introduced to Europe in the sixteenth century and has since been used extensively. Basil is associated with Brigid's Day and carries the magickal powers of peace, protection, purification, cleansing, tranquillity, business success, love, and money.

Drinking basil tea can relieve nausea, vomiting, and indigestion and stimulate the immune system. The leaves can be rubbed on the skin to relieve the bites of snakes, scorpions, and spiders. In ayurvedic medicine, basil is used to relieve chills, coughs, snakebites, skin irritations and infections, and earaches. Basil is associated with the Hindu Sun god, Vishnu, the deity and planet Mars, and the astrological sign of Scorpio.

DO NOT USE BASIL OIL EXTENSIVELY FOR TODDLERS OR PREGNANT WOMEN.

Nirvana Tomato-Basil-Garlic Pasta

SERVES 6

As you prepare this dish, allow yourself to create a new world in which peace reigns. Slow down long enough to light a candle. Allow any frustrations, worries, or concerns to be transformed through the light. The candle's flame represents the spark that is you—containing individual nuances—while at the same time containing the intelligence of the Universal Source. Enjoy the peace of focusing on one task at a time. There is a richness and a timelessness that comes from observing your life in this way. You have the opportunity to create a world of joy within the very hearth of your home, where household tasks no longer appear as duties,

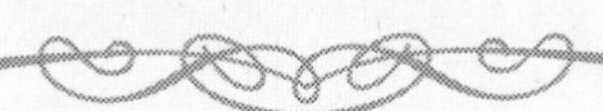

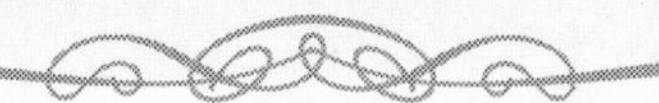

but rather as opportunities to rediscover the expansive creativity inherent in all things. (Sara Nelson, who has loved cooking since her childhood, offered this recipe.)

- ¼ cup extra virgin olive oil
- 12 to 14 garlic gloves, thinly sliced
- 1 cup fresh basil leaves, chopped
- 8 medium tomatoes or 10 plum tomatoes
- 16 ounces angel hair or vermicelli pasta

In a bowl, combine the oil, garlic, and basil. Cut a shallow X in the bottom of each tomato. Blanch tomatoes in a pot of boiling water for 1 minute. Place the tomatoes in cool water until they are cool enough to handle. Peel off the tomato skins. Chop the tomatoes and add to the basil mixture. Cover the bowl with plastic wrap or cheesecloth. Let stand in a warm place at least 3 hours and up to 1 day.

Bring 8 cups salted water to a boil in a large pot. Add the pasta and cook 7 to 10 minutes, until tender but still firm to the bite. Drain the pasta and return to the same pot. Add the tomato-basil mixture and toss with the pasta. Serve hot.

THIS ANNUAL HERB PREFERS FULL SUN AND REGULAR WATERING; OCCASIONAL OVERHEAD WATERING WILL PRODUCE BRIGHT, CLEAN FOLIAGE. SOW BASIL SEED IN EARLY SPRING, PLANTING SUCCESSIVELY TWO WEEKS APART. SPACE THE PLANTS TEN TO TWELVE INCHES APART. FERTILIZE ONCE DURING THE SUMMER MONTHS WITH A BALANCED FERTILIZER. MOST PEOPLE PREFER TO PINCH OUT THE FLOWER SPIKES TO KEEP FROM SETTING SEEDS. PLANT NEAR PEPPERS AND TOMATOES TO ENHANCE VEGETABLE GROWTH (THIS WORKS: IN DECEMBER I STILL HAVE TOMATOES!). BASIL IS BELIEVED TO BE INDIGENOUS TO INDIA.

Winter Blues Banishment

Basil's association with Brigid's Day makes it an ideal herb to use during the dark months of winter. This spell is intended to remind you of the peace and importance of relaxation during the dark times, especially if a wicked case of the winter blues hits. You can harvest and freeze basil leaves in the summer so that you have a ready supply for making basil oil in the winter. If you cannot find basil oil in a magickal shop, you can fill a jar with a tight-fitting lid with fresh, clean basil leaves. Pour olive oil over the leaves and allow the mixture to sit for at least six weeks before using.

For this meditation, you will need a yellow and a blue candle. Anoint both with basil oil. Carve the word *light* into the yellow candle and the word *peace* into the blue candle. Light the yellow candle and visualize the first rays of sunlight coming back to your corner of the world. Imagine the warm sun on your face. Know that this same light burns within you. Light the blue candle and breathe deeply of peace and tranquillity. Say the word *serenity* three times. What would peace look like in your life? Know that the calm of peace resides within you.

Note: Use any remaining basil oil within a year.

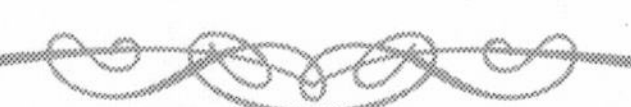

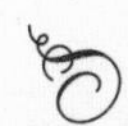

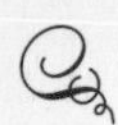

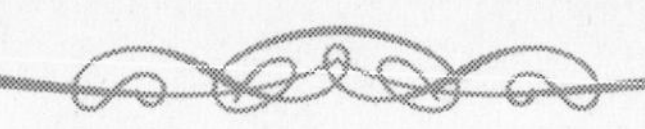

Bay Laurel

Laurus nobilis

BAY, BAY TREE, GRECIAN LAUREL, ROMAN LAUREL, SWEET BAY

Part Used: leaves

Bay leaves are oval, shiny, and gold-flecked. The flowers are round and green, and the berries are dark. Down through the ages, the majestic, aromatic bay tree has come to represent glory, respect, and admiration. In ancient Greece, bay branches were woven into wreaths to honor great athletes, artists, and heroes. To be presented with and wear the laurel wreath was a highly regarded attainment. Sacred groves of bay were cultivated near the healing temples because of the herb's particularly strong curative powers. Magickally, it is believed that your wishes and success can come to pass if you smell the invigorating scent of bay leaves or hang a bay laurel wreath on your door. A tree that is native to the West Coast, the California bay or Oregon myrtle (*Umbellularia californica*), can be substituted in some situations, though its leaves are more pungent than those of the bay laurel. California Native Americans hang its boughs about their homes to keep them free of insects, especially fleas.

Bay creates a therapeutic warming effect, both in the atmosphere and your own temperature. For traditional housewarming parties, bay oil is anointed on candles and bay leaves are thrown into the hearth fire to bathe the home and all who enter in an affectionate, welcoming aura. Bay leaves release a heady, vitalizing scent that physically warms the body as well, which can infuse love or lust into a room. The herb can be used in an oil, incense, or in a prepared dish to revive an intimate relationship. Bay is associated with Apollo, Ceres, Cerridwen, and the sun.

Itch Relief Bay Tea

Bay's healing properties are used to aid with the colic, stomachaches, headaches, and diarrhea, and as an insecticide. It is also known to extract the poison from poison oak rashes, bee stings, or irritation from stinging nettle. If you have come

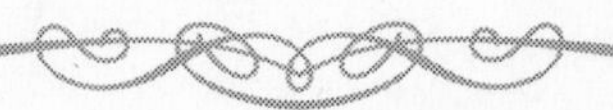

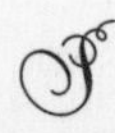

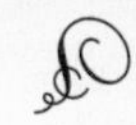

into contact with poison oak or nettle, apply the tea as soon as you can to the affected area (do not drink it). The heating element of the bay extracts and dries out the poison, eliminating the itching.

20 to 30 bay leaves
2 cups water

In a pot, combine the bay leaves with the water. As you mix the ingredients together, say,

I call upon bay's healing power
To aid me this very hour.

Bring the water and leaves to a boil. Turn off the heat and let the mixture sit until the water has turned brown, about 20 minutes. Use a cloth to apply the tea to infected areas. Leftover tea can be kept, covered, in the refrigerator for up to a year.

Bay seeds often grow moldy and cuttings are difficult to root, so you may prefer to buy a young tree from a reputable nursery. Bay trees, which are evergreen shrubby trees, prefer moderate temperature and soil, very good drainage, and ample sunlight. They can be clipped into topiary shapes or hedges. Bay is native to Mediterranean countries.

Money from a Tree

Bay's magickal powers include clairvoyance, promoting healing, love, prosperity, protection, purification, success, wishes, and victory. As an evergreen, this tree is associated with the concept of constant abundance within the universe. It is always available, pointing to the fact that prosperity and affluence are consistently accessible. Gaining entry to this prosperity is only a matter of opening the portals between our limited physical world and the spiritual world of infinite possibilities. This ritual is designed to make you feel rich and supported, while recognizing that there are many avenues to the perspective of abundance. (The prosperity oil used in this spell is an oil made by a magickal practitioner with the intent of prosperity.)

Parchment paper
9 dried or fresh bay leaves
Prosperity oil (see page 98)

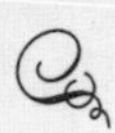
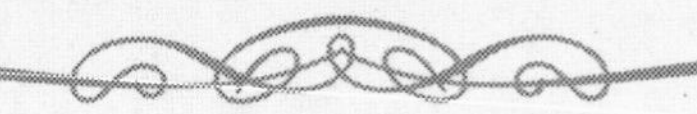

During the waxing of the moon, write down on a piece of parchment paper some words about what makes you feel prosperous or draw pictures of the same. It can be a type of environment, a particular balance in your savings account, or little luxuries such as a ready supply of bath oils, incense, or candles. Crush the bay leaves in a mortar with a pestle, moving the pestle in a clockwise direction. As you do this, chant,

Prosperity as my divine right
I call upon you tonight
Bless me with protected light
Security and abundance are in sight.

Sprinkle the leaves on your paper and drop 9 drops of prosperity oil on the paper. Set the paper on an east-facing altar or windowsill: the direction of east evokes creation and new beginnings. When you have achieved your desire, bury the paper.

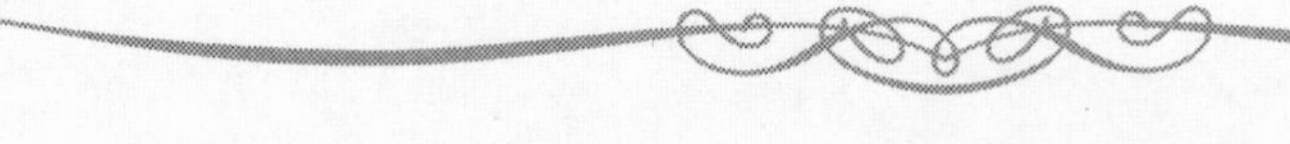

Bergamot

Citrus aurantium bergamia

BEE BALM, GOLDEN MELISSA, HORSEMINT, INDIAN NETTLE, OSWEGO TEA

Parts Used: fruit, rind

Bergamot, also commonly known as bee balm, has flowers that are known to attract hummingbirds. Bergamot is often used to flavor teas, especially Earl Grey tea. In aromatherapy practice, bergamot oil is considered cheerful, uplifting, and balancing. It relieves anxiety, reduces tension, stress, and mood swings, and works as an immune system booster. Bergamot is used in prosperity and protection rituals, especially in situations of sexual harassment. It can be added to baths, potpourris, and perfumes.

DO NOT USE BERGAMOT IF YOU HAVE LIVER PROBLEMS OR ARE PREGNANT.

BERGAMOT PREFERS RICH, MOIST, HUMUSY SOIL AND FULL TO PARTIAL SUN. AS A MEMBER OF THE CITRUS FAMILY, BERGAMOT CAN BE ANNUAL, BIENNIAL, OR PERENNIAL, DEPENDING ON LOCATION AND GROWING CONDITIONS. PLANT NEAR TOMATOES AND IT WILL ENHANCE THEIR GROWTH. THE BERGAMOT TREE IS NATIVE TO THE MEDITERRANEAN.

Chakra-Balancing Ritual

Bergamot is best known for its ability to create balance in your life, so it is an ideal magickal herb to use when balancing your chakras. Chakras are energy vortexes or centers that focus on states of being. There are seven main chakras, but many more have been discovered. To work with the seven chakras, you should begin with clearing and balancing these initial centers; they govern over basic elements that, once attuned, foster and help awaken the others.

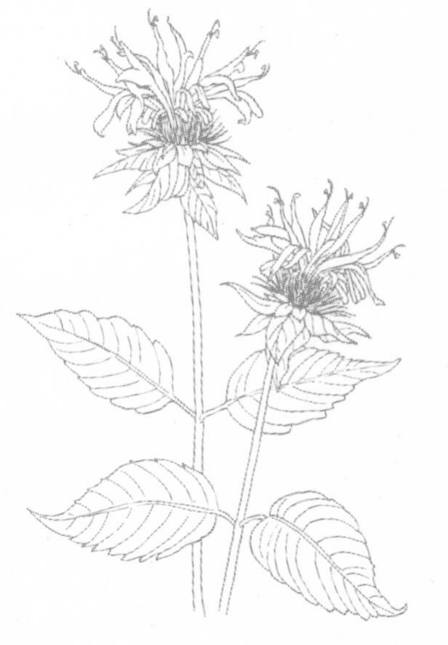

The root, or first, chakra rules over your trust in survival. It governs your physical locations and energy level, ensures that your basic physical needs are being met, and grounds you. It is located at the perineal floor.

The sacral, or second, chakra governs feelings, creativity, and duality. It rules desire, sexuality, birth, emotions, intimacy, and acceptance or awareness of polar opposites. It is located in the region of your sexual organs.

The solar plexus, or third, chakra governs acceptance and awareness of personal power. Within this sacred center, located at your navel, lies your instinct, will, and

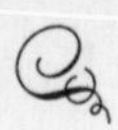

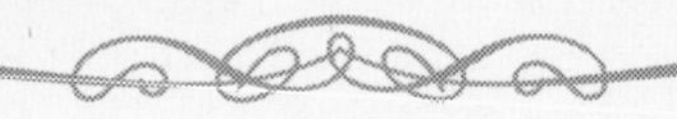

ability to exert and bring your gifts to the world.

The heart center, or fourth, chakra concentrates on emanating unconditional love. This energy vortex, located at your heart, seeks out love without an opposite attachment (or strings). Here you learn to trust yourself as Spirit incarnate.

The throat, or fifth, chakra rules communication. Located at the base of your throat, it is where you discover how to bring feelings into words, and allow your Divine essence to be expressed in action.

The third eye, or sixth, chakra allows for insight—knowledge of the truth that is the wisdom of the Divine manifested. Located just below the middle of your forehead, it is the portal for your intuition.

The crown, or seventh, chakra is the opening to the Divine. Here you receive guidance on how to bridge heaven and earth. This chakra is at the top of your head.

The seven chakras work together and are interconnected, passing energy through the heart center. The first and seventh chakras work together as do the second and sixth chakras, and the third and fifth chakras. These connections balance heaven and earth, because the first three, or lower chakras, concentrate on base needs and desires of the earthly nature while the last three, or higher chakras, focus on the etheric realms. Harmony between the two realms is essential. Without the higher chakras one will never know oneself as God/Goddess; without the lower chakras, one may become too spiritual to be of any earthly good.

Bergamot oil

Rainbow-colored advent candle

7 scarves, each a different color of the rainbow—
red, orange, yellow, green, blue, indigo, violet, and white

Use the bergamot oil to anoint the candle, your third eye, your heart center, and both palms. Light the candle. Close your eyes and concentrate on your breathing. Take 10 deep breaths. Focus on your perineum floor. Imagine a cord leaving this area and growing down into the ground. Once the grounding cord has reached the center of Mother Earth, allow white light energy to come back to you. When that energy reaches the perineum, focus on your root chakra. Visualize the

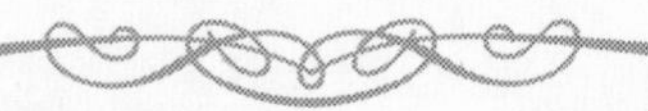

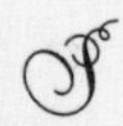

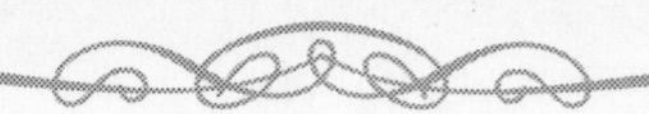

color red and concentrate on a word or energy field that you can associate with this energy vortex; for example, I think of action or force. Watch the light move to the second chakra—the lower abdomen—below your belly button. Visualize the color orange and concentrate on a word or energy field that you can associate with this energy vortex, possibly balance, trust, or faith. When you have a clear picture of the qualities this chakra can impart to you, watch the white light move up your core center to the third chakra—the seat of life—located underneath the diaphragm. Imagine the color yellow. Focus on a word or energy field that symbolizes this area, such as power or will. The light now travels to the heart center, which resonates with a green light. Feel the love emanating from this vortex. Notice the courage it takes to open this chakra. The energy continues upward until it settles in the throat, in front of the thyroid. Blue is the color of this area, and freedom of expression is associated with this energy field. Now the light moves to your forehead, between and just above your eyebrows. This area is often referred to as the third eye. The color of this sixth chakra region is indigo or purple. Intuition is a name given to this energy. Now imagine the top of your head opening up to light descending from above. This is the crown chakra, and it is white. Here you receive divine inspiration, which makes it clear whether the ideas in your head are Spirit or ego talking. Visualize a white light connecting all the chakras in a line.

Now it is time to move, which will reinforce this ritual, which is balance. Play varied music with slow and fast beats, deep and high resonances. Dance with all the scarves, 1 at a time and all together. Dance skyclad (naked) if possible: the natural state of nakedness is believed to enhance the spiritual connection.

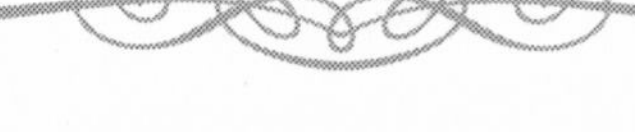

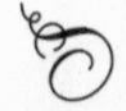

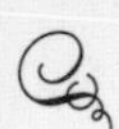

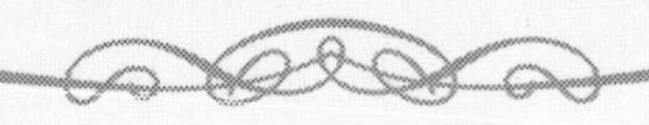

Birch

Betula (various species)

MOUNTAIN MAHOGANY, LADY OF THE WOODS

Parts Used: leaves, buds, catkins, bark, branches

Birch is a deciduous tree with small, fine-toothed (serrated) leaves. Its botanical name is derived from the Sanskrit word *bhurga,* which means "that which is written upon." In past centuries, birch bark was often made into paper.

During the old days, druid priests and priestesses of the Goddess wove their knowledge of the plants into their holy day ceremonies. Plants were so central to their lives that the letters of the British Isles' early alphabet, ogham, were named for them. Birch was known as *beth* and symbolized the letter *b*.

Birch can be applied to open wounds and skin irritations. It is an effective diuretic, antiseptic, tonic, and detergent. The oil, which dissipates quickly when exposed to heat, can be used as aftershave lotion or massage oil. Beer can be made from the inner bark of the sweet birch (*Betula lenta*). Native Americans made syrup from the sap of the tree.

Birch represents new beginnings and often is used to construct maypoles. Its protective powers are highly regarded, to the point that baby's cradles are often made from its wood. Birch is used in protection and blessing ceremonies and is associated with Thor, the Goddess, and the planet Venus.

Monthly Deep Meditation for Women

During our menses, women need to be still. It is best to not take on any new projects for the three heaviest days, and to avoid taking in new information. Try not to cook, clean, or do heavy excercise. You are in ceremony of the most sacred kind and need to honor it as such. The following ceremony allows for cleansing and purification of all ways that no longer serve your highest good.

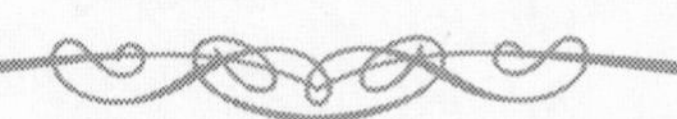

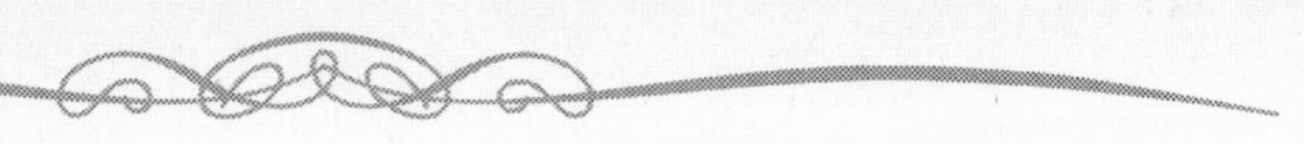

Red candle
Fire-retardant pentacle
Birch oil
Birch branches

During your menses, on your heaviest day, set aside at least one hour when you can just be still. If you do not have a menses, then designate one Saturday a month for this process. Light a red candle on an altar and place it atop a fire-retardant pentacle. Anoint the candle with birch oil.

Birch prefers full sun and rainy climates or ample watering. Birch trees are common in Europe and temperate regions of Asia and North America.

Take a moment to bring your awareness into your body. Imagine your feet growing roots. Visualize these roots growing deep into Mother Earth. Place birch branches around your candle. As you sit, meditate on releasing all that no longer serves you. Know that your blood holds all your energy, and focus on cleansing your mind and your body. This is the time to release and give birth to new directions. Imagine this blood being released through you into Mother Earth. She will transform its impurities to be reused for a positive purpose. Visualize where you would like to see this regenerating energy sent, such as to a poverty- or war-stricken environment or a threatened part of nature. If you do not have any place you want to send it, ask the Great Mother to send it where it most needs to go. Write in a journal about your thoughts, dreams, or your surroundings. Rest for a while. Only by slowing down can you truly experience the gifts of Spirit.

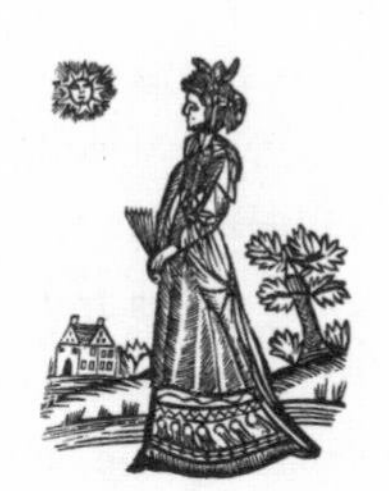

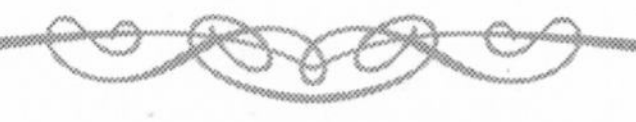

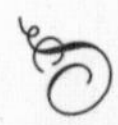

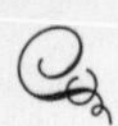

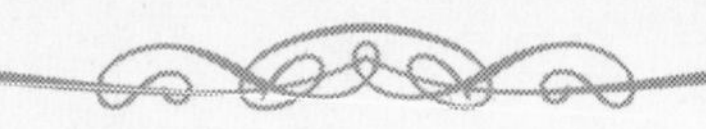

Black Haw

Viburnum prunifolium

AMERICAN SLOE, STAG BUSH, SWEET VIBURNUM, SHEEP BERRY, NANNY BERRY

Parts Used: root bark, fruit

Black haw is a shrub with black and red edible berries; serrated, oval leaves; and clusters of white flowers. For centuries, black haw has been used all across North America for its ability to prevent miscarriage. This herb contains four powerful active ingredients: salicin, a compound responsible for aspirin's anti-inflammatory and pain-relieving benefit; valerianic acid, a sedative; saponin, a hormone producer; and scopoletin, a uterine relaxant. The combined active components in black haw make it quite effective for relieving menstrual and post-partum cramps and for easing bleeding after childbirth.

BLACK HAW CONTAINS OXALATES. IF YOU HAVE A HISTORY OF KIDNEY STONES, YOU SHOULD CONSULT YOUR PHYSICIAN BEFORE USING IT.

New Mama's Tonic Tea

MAKES 1 CUP

When using herbal tonic teas, keep in mind that it takes time for the effects to manifest. Using herbal remedies as a means to improve general health or to aid a particular system will work as long as you are an active participant in your health. Herbs cannot override the negative effects of daily misuse of your mind, body, and spirit. Herbs such as black haw will help you become more in tune with your body.

One of the best ways to maximize effects from teas is to monitor your timing. Teas can take from ten to twenty minutes to take effect after you drink them. When taking this herbal tonic to relax muscle tension or to relieve cramps, take it fifteen minutes before nursing. Alternatively, drink the tea before you put the baby to rest, when the time has come for you to slow down and relax.

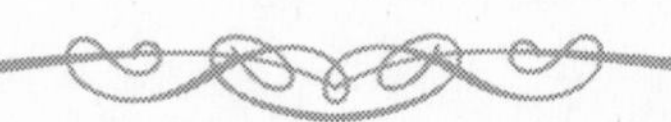

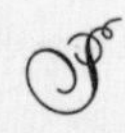

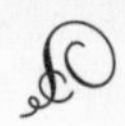
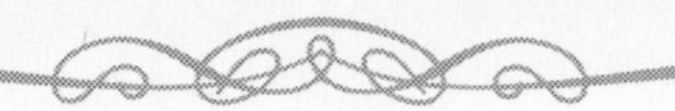

You can make this tea as strong as you need it to be. Begin with the following weaker version, and if needed, you can gradually add more until you reach one heaping tablespoon of bark to one cup of water.

1 teaspoon fresh black haw root bark
1 cup purified water

In a small pot, simmer the bark in the water for 20 minutes. Remove from the heat and steep 15 minutes. Strain the bark out of the tea and discard. Begin with ½ cup to test how your body responds to it.

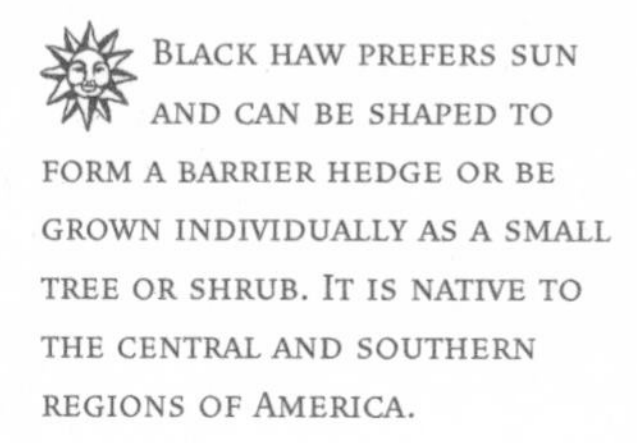

Black haw prefers sun and can be shaped to form a barrier hedge or be grown individually as a small tree or shrub. It is native to the central and southern regions of America.

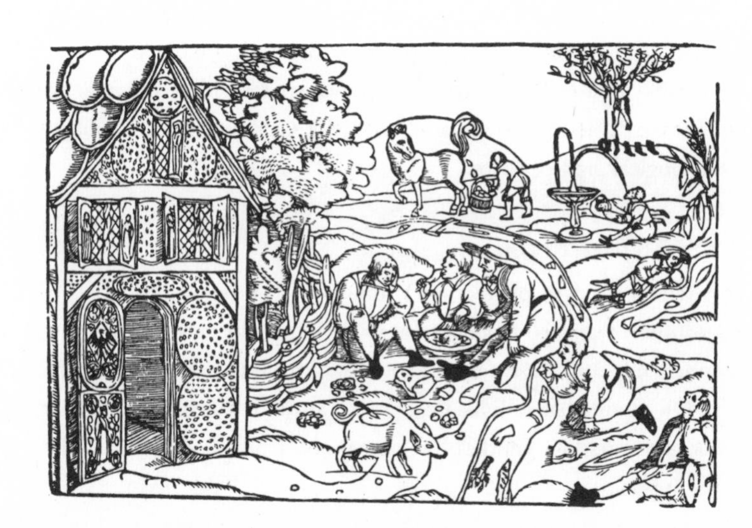

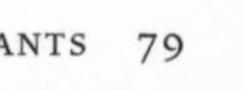

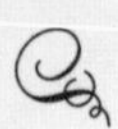

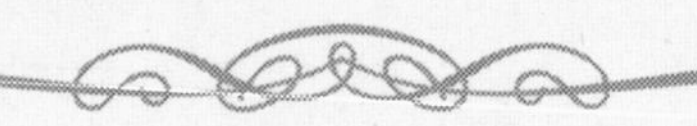

Blessed Thistle

Cnicus benedictus

HOLY THISTLE, SPOTTED THISTLE

Parts Used: leaves, flowers

Blessed thistle is found in wastelands and waysides. The plant's flowers are yellow or purple and its leaves are spiky. There are many varieties of thistle, and not all have the same properties; it is best not to harvest wild-growing plants unless you are absolutely certain which species they are. The entire plant is edible; trimmed of their prickles and coarse outer layer, the leaves make a delicious salad. The roots are eaten as a vegetable, and the heads are consumed like artichokes, before flowering. Blessed thistle treats depression, memory loss, and ailments of the stomach, liver, and kidneys, and it is an excellent blood purifier. Blessed thistle is also known to increase milk production in lactating women and regulate irregular menstruation. Blessed thistle is associated with the God and Pan, the planet Mars, and the astrological sign of Aries.

Mabon Potpourri

Blessed thistle is used in protection rituals and corresponds to the Mabon or autumnal equinox festivals. *Equinox* means "equal night." The two equinoxes are the time when day and night are equal in length—the scales are perfectly balanced. The full moon that falls nearest to the autumnal equinox is known as the harvest moon because its gentle blue cast enables people to harvest their crops late into the night.

Mabon is a thanksgiving celebration that revolves around gathering crops, blessing the abundance of the harvest, and taking part in rituals to ensure the success of the next year's harvest. It is the second in a trilogy of Wiccan harvest festivals, and it marks the completion of the grain harvest begun at Lughnasadh.

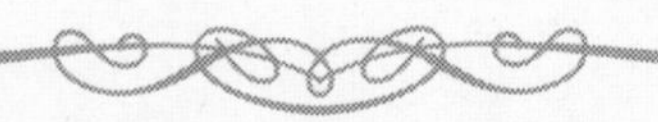

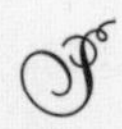

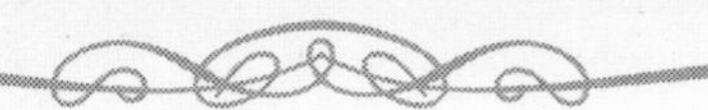

We celebrate the story of Mabon ap Modron, "the son of the mother"—the Divine Youth, the Son of Light, a figure who appears in many traditions.

Mabon festivities honor the need for death so that new life may eventually thrive. It is a time of great joy and great sorrow, the two necessary halves to the whole of our lives, and the energy that dances between life and death. We embrace the darkness that will soon enfold us, knowing that the Mother will hold the seed of light in her womb until it is time for rebirth. We are physically reminded that our time is a spiral, not linear; there is no end without beginnings.

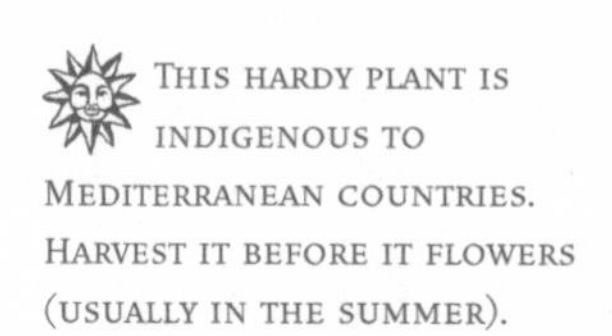

This hardy plant is indigenous to Mediterranean countries. Harvest it before it flowers (usually in the summer).

Make this potpourri to remind you to savor the last hours of the bright light of the year. Allow it to be a remembrance of your many blessings and abundance.

- ¼ cup dried blessed thistle leaves
- ¼ cup dried orrisroot (see page 201)
- ¼ cup dried calendula flowers
- ¼ cup dried rose petals

Mix all the ingredients together. Place in a muslin pouch or a glass container with ventilated lid. Sit and write a list of all the things for which you are grateful.

Variation: You can substitute any of the traditional Mabon plants such as apple, balm of Gilead, cypress, mugwort, myrrh, oak, passionflower, pine, or sage.

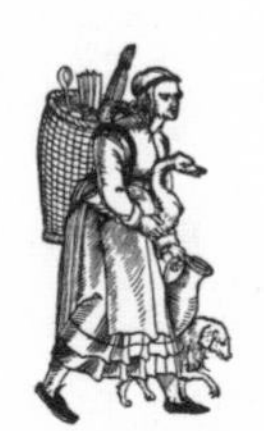

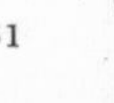

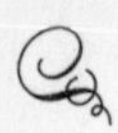

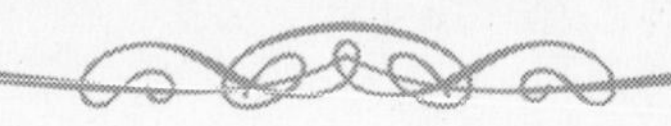

Broom

Cytisus scoparius

BANAL, GENISTA, IRISH BROOM, LINK, SCOTCH BROOM

Parts Used: flowers, twigs

Broom is a shrub with tiny, oval-shaped leaves on green stems and strongly scented yellow flowers. It grows on sandy commons, heaths, and rocky hillsides. Broom has been used to treat jaundice, dropsy, kidney and bladder disease, and to expel venom from poisonous bites. The Spanish gypsies make cologne from the aromatic flowers. Magickally, broom is used for wind and rain spells, protection, and purification. Broom is associated with the deity and planet of Mars.

BROOM IS POISONOUS IF TAKEN INTERNALLY;
NO PART OF THE PLANT SHOULD BE INGESTED.

Return to Sender

There are times when we can feel negative energy being sent directly toward us and we assume we know who the sender is. This feeling can be deceptive; sometimes we set people up to attack us by giving off victim attitudes or by being aggressive. We rarely have all the pieces to the puzzle. The ritual here will use the winds of change to send negative vibrations away from you. During this spell, do not picture anyone specific; you are not a judge or punisher. Let the universe take care of it. (I have never suggested casting a spell against another person, and I never will.)

What I do offer is a spell that helps. With it, you proclaim that you cast off the victim role; you no longer welcome adverse situations or people in your life. This spell will send any harmful vibrations to Spirit, where they can be transformed. Remember, falling into a role of being a victim makes you feel power, but true power comes from love, not fear.

Get a black and red candle, preferably with black on the top and red on the

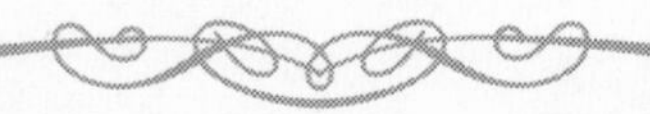

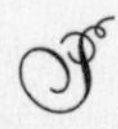

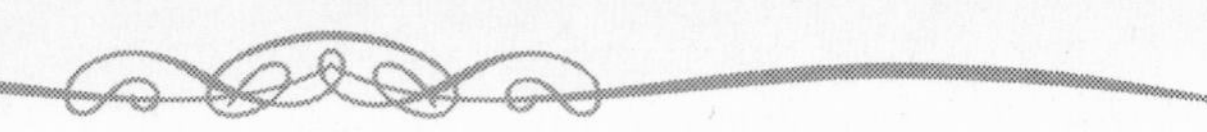
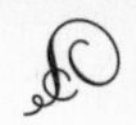

bottom, in a glass container. (This is like a seven-day advent candle.) If you need to use two candles (one red and one black), tie them together with a black cord. If you can find reversing oil, anoint your candle with three drops of it. Sprinkle broom flowers around the candle. Alternatively, you can gently heat broom sprigs and olive oil for 5 to 10 minutes, allow to cool, and use this as your oil. On a piece of parchment paper with a red pen or dragon's blood ink, write "Return to Sender." Roll the paper away from you and place under the glass candle. Light the candle. Visualize the negative energy hitting a protective shield around you and shooting up into space, where it dissipates. Douse the flame and repeat the ritual for the following two days.

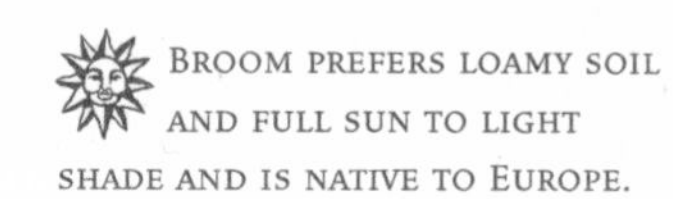

Broom prefers loamy soil and full sun to light shade and is native to Europe.

On the third day after performing the ritual, allow the candle to burn down. Throw a handful of broom flowers in the air and yell,

By my will, *be gone!*

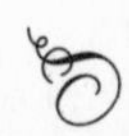

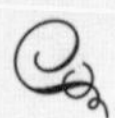

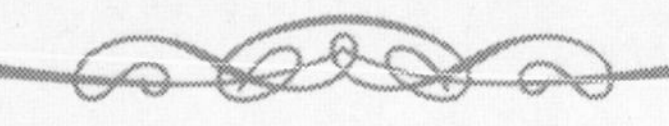

Burdock

Arctium Lappa

BEGGAR'S BUTTONS, CLOTBUR, CUCKOLD, FOX'S CLOTE, HAPPY MAJOR, HARLOCK, PERSONATA

Parts Used: leaves, roots, burrs, seeds

Burdock grows on wasteland and by roadsides. It has large leaves and thistlelike lavender-colored flowers. The flowers are shaped like burrs and attach to clothing and animal fur. Seventeenth-century herbalist Nicholas Culpeper believed that burdock worked wonders against bites from serpents or mad dogs. Burdock has a long-standing reputation for boosting the immune system, aiding kidney or bladder disorders, and purifying blood. Today, its diuretic and mild laxative qualities gently remove toxins from the system, which may be responsible for its effectiveness in healing skin problems such as psoriasis, eczema, and acne. Lay crushed leaves over burns, skin irritations, or ringworm. For an anti-inflammatory and nerve-fortifying drink, steep equal parts of burdock root and hawthorn berries. Burdock is used in protection and purification spells and is associated with Venus in both her planetary and goddess vibrations.

Meatless Meatball Soup

SERVES 4

I like to use Gardenburger brand meatballs for this recipe, but any meatless meatballs will work equally well. (Melinda Listening Deer Rodriguez, a Reiki master teacher, drum-circle facilitator, and certified spiritual counselor donated the recipe for this delicious dish.)

2½ quarts thyme vegetable stock (see page 239)
Salt
Pepper
1½ pounds meatless meatballs
1 burdock root, chopped

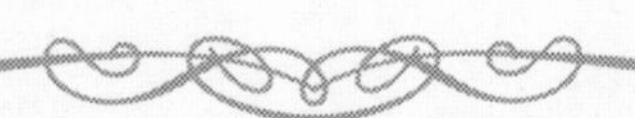

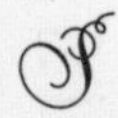

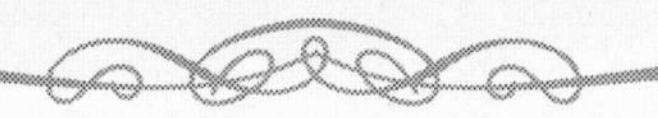

10 green onions, green parts chopped
1 cup thinly sliced celery
1 cup thinly sliced carrots
½ small head cabbage, shredded
2 tomatoes, peeled and cut in ⅛-inch pieces
½ cup rice
1 bay leaf
2 tablespoons chopped fresh parsley
1 tablespoon chopped fresh basil
2 or 3 tablespoons soy sauce

In a large pot, bring the broth to a simmer. Drop in the meatballs. Season with salt and pepper to taste. Add the burdock root, green onions, celery, carrots, cabbage, tomatoes, rice, bay leaf, parsley, and basil. Cover and simmer for 35 minutes, stirring occasionally. Remove the bay leaf. Stir in soy sauce to taste and serve.

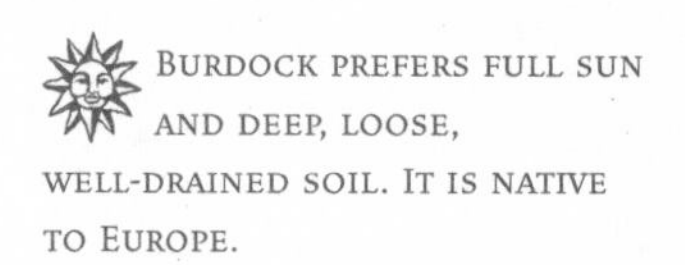

Burdock prefers full sun and deep, loose, well-drained soil. It is native to Europe.

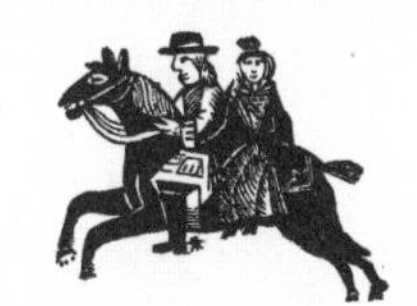

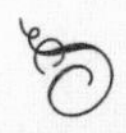

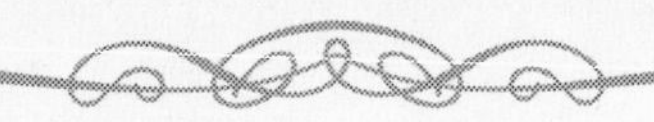

Calendula

Calendula officinalis

BRIDE OF THE SUN, GOLD BLOOM, POT MARIGOLD, SUMMER'S BRIDE

Parts Used: flowers, leaves

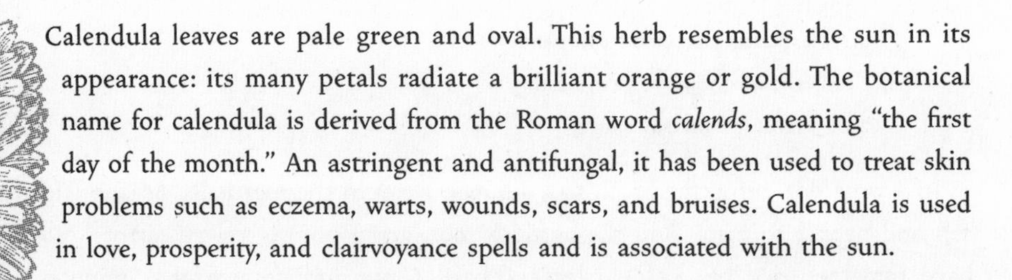

Calendula leaves are pale green and oval. This herb resembles the sun in its appearance: its many petals radiate a brilliant orange or gold. The botanical name for calendula is derived from the Roman word *calends*, meaning "the first day of the month." An astringent and antifungal, it has been used to treat skin problems such as eczema, warts, wounds, scars, and bruises. Calendula is used in love, prosperity, and clairvoyance spells and is associated with the sun.

A NOTE OF CAUTION: CALENDULA (*Calendula officinalis*) IS THE EDIBLE PLANT USED IN FOOD, BEAUTY PRODUCTS, AND MAGICK. THE PLANT MORE COMMONLY CALLED MARIGOLD IN PLANT STORES IS ONE OF VARIOUS SPECIES OF *Tagetes*, THE MEXICAN MARIGOLD (SOMETIMES CALLED FRENCH OR AFRICAN), AND THESE PLANTS ARE FOR THE MOST PART TOXIC.

Calendula Facial Steam

Pliny and Dioscorides referred to calendula as an excellent skin healer, while medieval healers called it plainly magickal. It was believed that if you rubbed a concoction of calendula and honey over your body before going to sleep, your future mate would appear in a dream. Alternatively, sprinkling one's bed with pot marigold petals was believed to induce prophetic dreams. Calendula is best known today for its skin-soothing properties. The following steam will leave your skin glowing and refreshed. Those who suffer from acne, acne rosacea, or spider veins should take care: steams can aggravate these conditions.

- ½ cup fresh calendula flowers
- 2 tablespoons fresh chamomile flowers
- 2 tablespoons fresh lavender flowers
- 2 tablespoons fresh rose petals
- 2 tablespoons fennel seeds
- 3 cups water

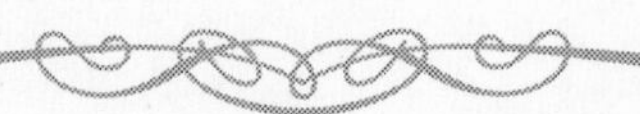

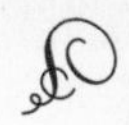

Bring water to a boil in a pot. Carefully pour the boiling water into a wide heat-proof bowl and add the herbs. Drape a large towel over your head and lean over the bowl, keeping your face about a foot above it. Allow sweat to build, and steam your face for 10 minutes. Splash cold water on your face and follow the treatment with a mask or the comfrey toner on page 103.

Eczema Salve

The high mucilage content in calendula makes the plant an excellent resource for aiding the complexion. You can add one part bruised calendula leaves to two parts of your favorite face cream or moisturizer for added benefit. The following salve will provide soothing relief to those who suffer from eczema.

CALENDULA PREFERS FULL SUN AND MODERATE WATERING. IT CAN THRIVE IN ALL ZONES AND LASTS DAYS AS A CUT FLOWER. PLANT NEAR POTATOES, ROSES, AND TOMATOES TO ENHANCE THEIR GROWTH. CALENDULA IS NATIVE TO SOUTHERN EUROPE.

⅓ cup fresh calendula flowers
⅓ cup fresh chickweed (*Stellaria media*)
⅓ cup fresh St. John's wort flowers
¾ cup extra virgin olive oil
¼ cup beeswax
6 to 8 drops tea tree oil
6 to 8 drops essential oil for fragrance, such as lavender or rosemary

In the top half of a double boiler set over simmering water, heat the calendula, chickweed, St. John's wort, and olive oil for 1 hour. Do not allow the mixture to boil. Strain the mixture through muslin or cheesecloth into a stainless steel pot. When the cloth is just cool enough to handle, wring out as much oil as possible, with the herbs still wrapped in the cloth. Add the beeswax to the oil and heat until melted. Check for the desired consistency by placing a tablespoon of the mixture in your freezer for 1 minute. (If it's too soft, add more beeswax; if it's too hard, add more oil.) When the desired consistency is reached, immediately remove from the heat and add the tea tree oil and whatever fragrant essential oil you desire. Pour the mixture into small glass jars and store in a cool, dark place. When properly stored, this salve will last for a year.

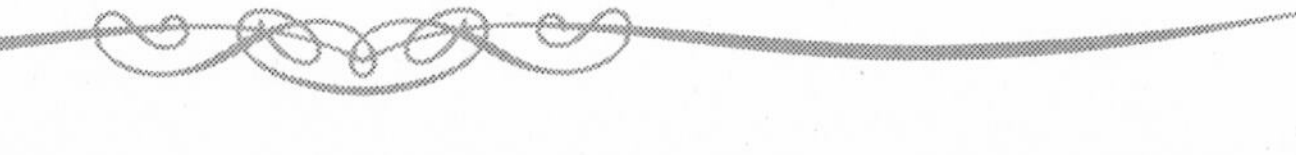

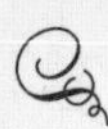

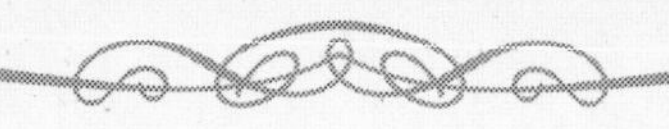

Catnip

Nepeta cataria

CAT'S WORT, FIELD BALM

Parts Used: Leaves, flowers

Catnip is often found growing along hedges. The flowers are hooded, white or lavender, and the leaves are downy and grayish. It is an ancient medicinal herb used to aid the minor ailments of babies and young children, digestion, and menstruation. Catnip treats spasms associated with colic and whooping cough. It is used in love spells and in rituals to contact animals and familiars (a familiar is a guardian creature who has vowed to protect and accompany you). Catnip is associated with the goddesses Bast, Sekhmet, and Venus—including Venus's planetary vibrations.

Joyous Creation

As all cat lovers know, cats love this herb and adore rolling around in it. The following ritual for cat lovers is one for security, and calls on your familiar. Bast, an Egyptian goddess, represents the beneficial power of the sun and is associated with laughter, joy, music, dancing, and protection; you will be calling on her during this ritual.

- Cat hair
- ¼ cup dried catnip
- 3 drops Bast oil (see page 260)
- 1 black cat candle
- 3 cups salt water
- 1 piece charcoal
- Catnip incense (see page 260)
- 1 white candle
- 1 sage bundle
- 1 pink candle
- Dragon's blood incense (see page 260)

For best results, cast a full circle before beginning this ritual. Pet your cat, and ask him or her to help you bless your home with joy. Listen quietly for an answer. If permission is granted, you may begin; otherwise, try again at a later date.

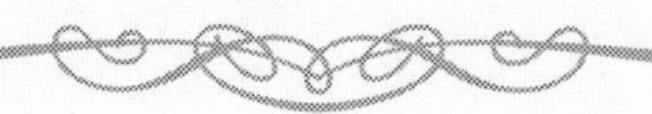

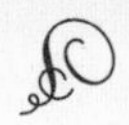

Stroke your cat from head to tail in 1 long, sweeping motion. Place cat hair collected from petting in a cauldron with the catnip and Bast oil. Dip the black cat candle in salt water and then dry it off.

Beginning in the middle of the candle, rub on some of the catnip mixture, working outward from the center. Infuse your thoughts of banishing stale or negative vibrations from your home into the candle. Light the candle. Place charcoal in a fire-retardant container; sprinkle catnip incense over it. Carry the candle, salt water, and incense 3 times in a counterclockwise direction (often called widdershins) around the house, either inside or outside depending on your preference. Sprinkle the salt water on the ground. Say,

Stale or negative vibrations hear me now
You have no right in this realm; be gone!

Imagine that you are gathering up a black ball of unwanted energy. Roll the ball out the door. Tell it to go beyond where you can see, then twice that distance to a space you cannot sense, then thrice beyond that until it is no more.

Play some light-hearted music. Light a white candle and burn a sage bundle. Walk 3 times clockwise (called sunwise or deosil) around the house. Say,

I infuse light, music, and joy here
By my will, so mote it be.

Light a pink candle and burn dragon's blood incense. Walk 3 times clockwise around the house. Say,

I infuse peace, laughter, and harmony in this dwelling
By my will, so mote it be.

Say farewell to the guardians, quarters, God, and Goddess and take down the circle.

This herb prefers full sun, light to moderate water, and a lot of space. It is a vigorous plant that does well in light soil. Catnip is native to Europe and has naturalized in North America.

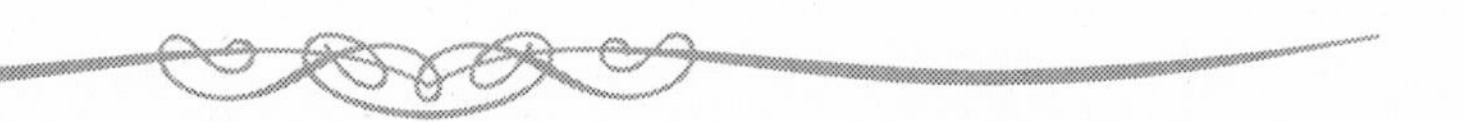

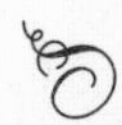

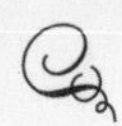

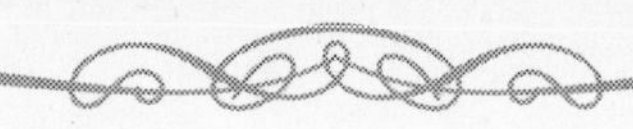

Cayenne

Capsicum annuum

CHILE PEPPER, HOT PEPPER, TABASCO PEPPER

Part Used: pod

Cayenne is found wild in Africa, Central America, Mexico, and South America, and is cultivated in hot climates elsewhere. It has oval, shiny green leaves and small drooping white flowers that develop into green pods, which turn bright red when ripe. *Cayenne* derives from the Greek word *kapto* meaning "I bite." Cayenne has been added to unpasteurized milk to fight bacteria, sprinkled inside socks to keep toes toasty during the winter, and scattered in vegetable beds to ward off animals and crawling pests. It has been used to relieve heart attacks, chills, and sore muscles, as an antispasmodic, and to treat rheumatism, jaundice, and arthritis. Powdered cayenne can be sprinkled over infected or old wounds. It will sting for a brief time, but is harmless and highly curative. Cayenne is known as a tonic for all organs of the body.

Cajun Shrimp

SERVES 4

Cayenne is associated with Mars, the Roman god of war and war's ruling planet. Mars is an activating force, giving a boost to any incantation or dish that uses cayenne.

Prepare this dish when you are in need of motivation or courage. The energy of Mars activates boldness and has been associated historically with agriculture and uniting people. In early Roman times, Mars was called Marspiter, Father Mars, or Mars Gradivus (from *grandiri,* meaning "to grow"). Concentrate on the concept of victory for all. When going to battle, be clear about your intent. Make sure you are a spiritual warrior, moving toward the higher good of our global community, not merely an aggressor seeking your own way.

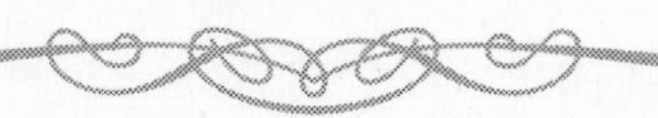

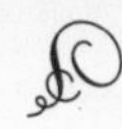
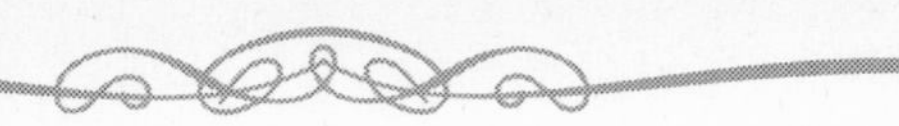

¼ cup extra virgin olive oil
5 cloves garlic, minced
2 pounds large shrimp, peeled, deveined, rinsed
¼ cup minced fresh parsley
2 tablespoons freshly squeezed lemon juice
¼ teaspoon cayenne pepper
¼ teaspoon salt

In a skillet, heat the oil and garlic for 2 minutes over medium heat. Increase the heat and add the shrimp. Cook, stirring occasionally, until the shrimp turn pink, about 7 minutes. Remove from the heat. Stir in the parsley, lemon juice, cayenne pepper, and salt. Serve immediately.

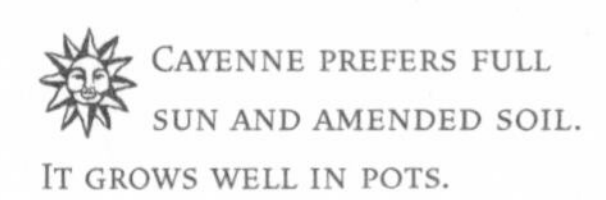

CAYENNE PREFERS FULL SUN AND AMENDED SOIL. IT GROWS WELL IN POTS.

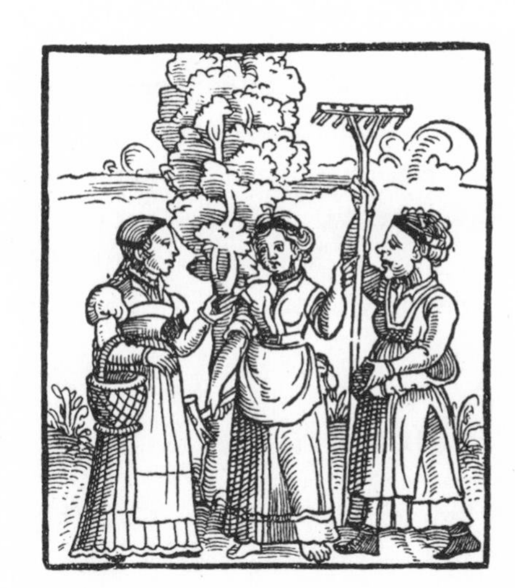

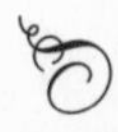

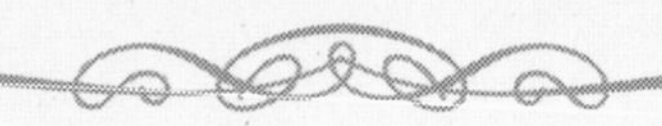

Chamomile

Chamaemelum nobile, Matricaria recutita

CAMAMYLE, CHAMAIMELON, GERMAN CHAMOMILE, GROUND APPLE, MANZANILLA, GOLDEN BALL, ROMAN CHAMOMILE, WHITE STAR

Part Used: flowers

Chamomile leaves are feathery, and its fragrant flowers are white, small, and daisy-like with yellow centers. It has been used for two thousand years to counteract irritation, soothe stomachaches, protect against ulcers, fight bacterial and fungal infections, and calm the nervous system. Chamomile works best for those who are restless, impulsive, highly sensitive, and suffer from pain but are unable to accept help. According to folk medicine, chamomile is known as "childbed flower" for its many useful pediatric remedies.

A variety of different plants are sold under the name *chamomile* at nurseries, and you should be careful to obtain the one appropriate to your purpose. The flowers of German chamomile (*Matricaria recutita*) are the best for making tea. Some plants sold under the name *Matricaria* are actually varieties of *Chrysanthemum parthenium* (see Feverfew, page 122) and should not be used. Roman chamomile (*Chamaemelum nobile*) is used in shampoos, cosmetics, and as hair highlighter. Chamomile is used in prosperity rituals and to aid meditation and is associated with the sun.

Calming Chamomile Tea

MAKES 1 CUP

Chamomile tea is excellent for calming and soothing. This is a strong medicinal tea and should be diluted for children. It can be given to colicky babies or to babies with gas; place a few drops of diluted tea on their tongues. Damp chamomile tea bags can be placed on the eyes to relieve sties and soreness.

1 cup fresh chamomile flowers
1 cup boiling water

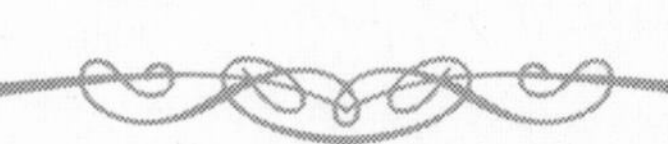

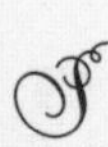

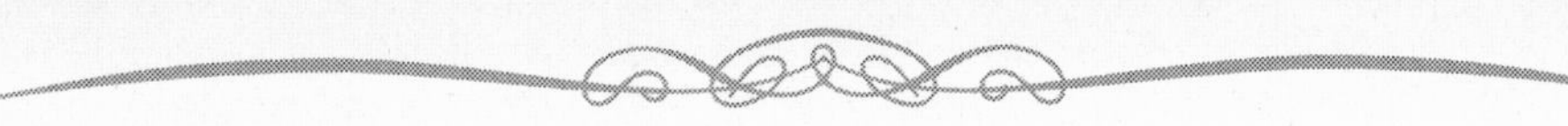

Add the flowers to the boiling water and let steep for 5 minutes. Strain and drink.

Relaxing Eye Pillow

Chamomile's well-known calming abilities are very effective as an aid to meditation. When you shut out the busy schedule of your life, you can better hear the words of wisdom from your soul. When you learn to take care of yourself, you come to understand the importance and value of being gentle and slowing down. With a little tenderness toward yourself, you show others how to appreciate you.

1 cup flaxseed
10 to 12 drops chamomile essential oil
1 (10 by 3-inch) piece satin or silk fabric

Pour the flaxseed into a small bowl. Add the essential oil and mix with the seeds.

Iron the fabric. Fold it lengthwise, with the outer surface of the fabric on the inside. Using a small stitch, sew a seam along the bottom and side, ¾ inch from the edge, leaving the top open. Sew a second time over the original stitching. Turn the pillow right side out. Fill the pillow half full with the seed mixture. Turn down the top so that the outer surface of the material is once again facing inward. Hand-sew or machine-finish the top. You now have a beautiful eye pillow!

Lie down on your back in the most comfortable way. You can put a pillow under your knees, or try putting the soles of your feet together, allowing the knees to drop down. Both of these positions help the lower back sink into the bed or ground. Place the eye pillow over your eyes. Turn your palms up and bring your forefinger and thumb together in what is known in yoga practice as the Om position. Allow your body to melt into its support. Let all your worries go. You can relax this way until you feel worry-free, or at least less stressed.

Note: Test the fabric's softness by placing it over your eyes. If it is thin, strengthen the pillow before you sew it shut with an additional layer of stronger material, such as muslin, on the inside. If you add too many flaxseeds, the pillow will be too heavy and will not conform to the contours of your beautiful face.

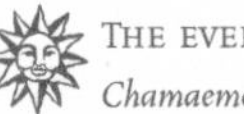

THE EVERGREEN PERENNIAL *Chamaemelum nobile* (FORMERLY KNOWN AS *Anthemis nobilis*) PREFERS FULL SUN TO PARTIAL SHADE AND DRY, SANDY, WELL-DRAINED SOIL. IT CAN BE PLANTED BETWEEN STEPPING STONES. THE SUMMER ANNUAL SPECIES KNOWN AS *Matricaria recutita* NEEDS LITTLE WATER ONCE IT IS ESTABLISHED AND LIKES FULL SUN. SOW SEEDS IN LATE WINTER OR SPRING. WHEN GROWN IN PROXIMITY TO THEM, THE HERB BENEFITS CUCUMBERS AND ONIONS AS WELL AS MOST HERBS. CHAMOMILE IS NATIVE TO EUROPE.

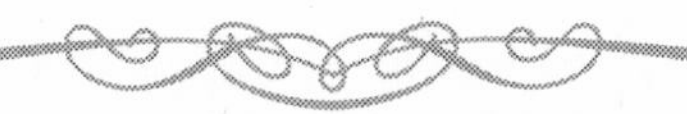

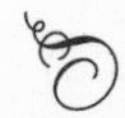

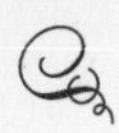

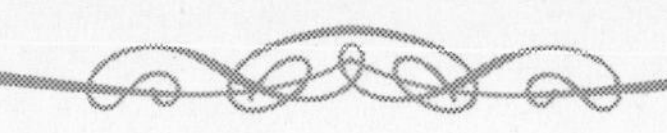

Cinnamon

Cinnamomum zeylanicum

CASSIA, CEYLON CINNAMON, SWEET WOOD

Part Used: inner bark

For centuries, cinnamon has been highly sought after and the reason for world exploration and conquest. Native to East Asia, it was once valued beyond gold and was as rare and precious as frankincense. The Egyptians used the spice in their embalming. Medieval physicians used cinnamon to treat coughs, hoarseness, and sore throats. It was also valued for its preservative effect on meat; this is due to the phenols it contains, which inhibit the bacteria responsible for spoilage. The aroma also masked the stench of aged meats. It has been used to reduce fevers, regulate menstrual cycles, reduce stress and anxiety, and combat infections, killing various bacteria, including staphylococcus, *E. coli,* and salmonella, for nearly five thousand years. For a simple, but beautiful potpourri, combine cinnamon sticks with rose petals. Cinnamon is also an aphrodisiac and is associated with Uranus.

DO NOT USE CINNAMON IN MEDICINAL AMOUNTS WHILE PREGNANT.
AVOID PLACING CINNAMON DIRECTLY ON YOUR SKIN.

Lughnasadh Corn Dolly

The corn dolly was made in ancient times to preserve a part of a year's successful harvest. It was made in the form of a female figure or "grain mother" to ensure abundance for the next year's crop. *Corn,* in this case, is a generic term for any grain. The dolly itself could be made of wheat stalks, corn husks, or other materials. Corn dollies are traditionally fashioned during the sabbat of Lughnasadh (Lammas) from the last sheaf of corn to be harvested. They are kept until the spring, when they are plowed back into the field to breathe the life force of the corn back into the soil. The corn dolly is dedicated as a symbol of abundance and is used as a house decoration to usher in the fall.

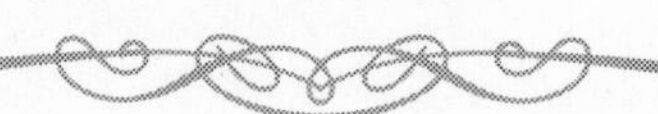

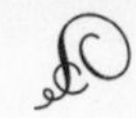

No matter where you live, make one of these festive dolls to remind you of the year's abundant harvest—whatever it may be. Whether your personal harvest was completing an education, finishing a project, growing a garden, or just getting through a difficult year, let this symbol remind you of the abundance in your life. As you sprinkle the doll with cinnamon, call on the herb's ability to bring protection, healing, prosperity, love, intuition, and purification.

1 corn broom (natural household broom)
12 stalks wheat
9 strands (or more) uncolored raffia
4 strands colored raffia (perhaps rust or burgundy)
1 small candle
Some sprigs of dried flowers
Feather
Small dish water
Clay bead
Cinnamon oil

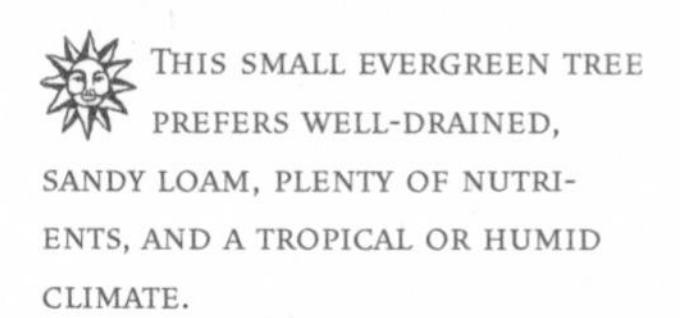

This small evergreen tree prefers well-drained, sandy loam, plenty of nutrients, and a tropical or humid climate.

Take the broom apart carefully and set the pieces aside. Boil a kettle full of water. Place the broom straw and the wheat in a large flat-bottomed pan. Pour enough boiling water over the material until it covers. (Do this in the bathtub or outdoors.) Set something heavy on the materials, such as a brick, so they don't float. Let the materials stand for 20 minutes. While they soak, put the 9 strands of uncolored raffia together and tie a knot at the end. Separate into 3 sections, make a braid, and set aside. Gather some of the damp broom straw into a bundle 1 inch thick (you will have extra). Trim the bundle to 1 foot long and tie off each end to hold the bundle together. This bundle will form the doll's arms. Set aside. Gather another bundle of broom about 2 inches thick. Trim to 18 inches long and add the wheat around the bottom to make a skirt. Tie with a strand of colored raffia about 3 inches down from the top. Pull the larger bundle apart near the top and slide in the arms. Secure under the arms with more uncolored raffia. You might need to tie the dolly here and there with bits of uncolored raffia to secure it; these will blend in with the straw and wheat. This is the basic doll.

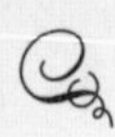

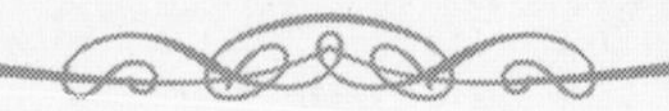

Now it is time to give her some personality. Take some time and a few deep breaths. Put on your favorite autumnal music (I like *Shakin' down the Acorns* by Tony Elman). Light the candle, representing the element of fire, and get a sense of the Harvest Lady. Meditate on the goddess Demeter, Grain Mother. Think about the abundance of the earth and how earth relates to your life. How did abundance manifest in your life over the past year? Feel the gratitude in your body. Now hold the doll and let some of that gratitude infuse into her. Wrap another strand of colored raffia around her neck (like a shawl), and be grateful for your own warm coat. Tie the braid on the top as her hair and poke in the dried flower sprigs around the head area, pausing to be grateful for your best physical attributes.

The corn dolly is now ready to be blessed. Take the feather, which represents the element of air, and fasten it into her shawl. Wave the candle over the dolly. Sprinkle her with a little water. Now tie the bead, which stands for the earth element, to her shawl, where you started. You've come full circle. Dab cinnamon oil onto a cotton ball to anoint her head, hands, and womb and say,

Mother Earth
  I bless your head
For fruit and grain
  Our daily bread

Terra Mater
  I bless your hands
As you hold the children
  Of your land

Mother Demeter
  Your womb I bless

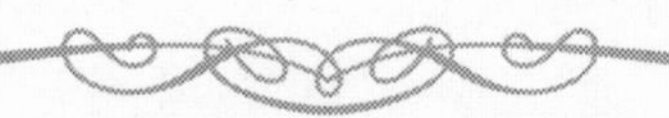

All life begins
In your great abyss

Let us remember
An abundant year
And the Harvest Lady
We hold so dear.

Enjoy your corn dolly and all the blessings of Lughnasadh.

Romance Incense

This incense will have such kick that you must focus on your desires very carefully. Cinnamon is a powerful catalyst in incense mixtures. You may be familiar with incense sticks rather than the powder form. To burn powder incense, you must first place a charcoal in a fire-retardant container, then light the charcoal until it sparks. Add the incense once the charcoal is lit (some people wait until the charcoal turns white; test to see what works best for you).

1 teaspoon ground cinnamon
½ teaspoon ground cloves
½ teaspoon sandalwood chips
½ teaspoon dried patchouli leaves
½ teaspoon dried rose petals

In a small bowl, stir together the cinnamon and cloves. Grind the sandalwood chips individually in a mortar with a pestle; add to the spices. Repeat with the patchouli and rose. Use 2 pinches on your incense burner. Add more as needed.

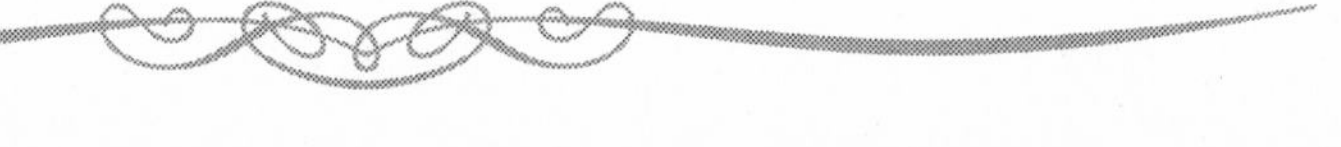

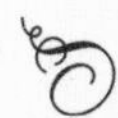

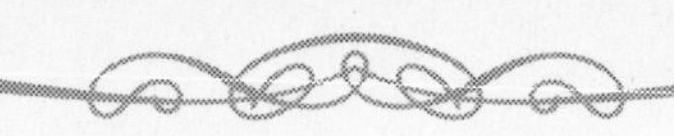

Cinquefoil

Potentilla tabernaemontani (often called Potentilla verna)

CENTURY PLANT, FIVE-FINGER GRASS, SUNFIELD

Part Used: flower

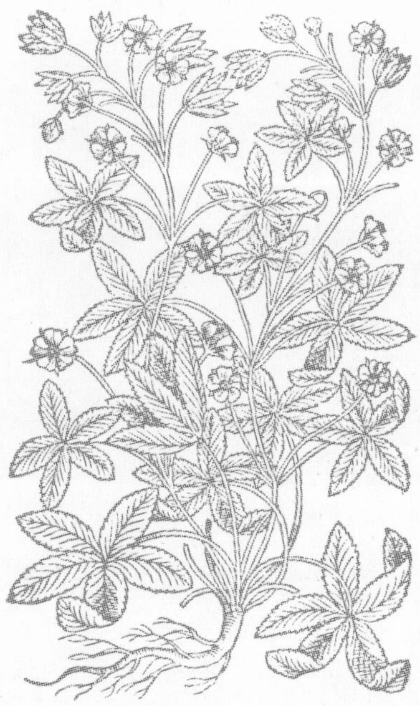

Cinquefoil is found along roadsides and in wastelands. Its silver, five-fingered leaves shaped like palm fronds, and the flat, yellow flowers composed of five petals characterize the plant. Its botanical name is derived from the Latin word *potens,* meaning "powerful," which alludes to its medicinal efficacy. Cinquefoil makes a wash for all wounds, including sore gums and mouth, a nerve sedative, and a general astringent. Cinquefoil is used magickally for protection, love, luck, prosperity, health, power, and wisdom. It is associated with Jupiter and Mercury's deity and planetary vibrations.

Prosperity Burr

There are times when you need an exact amount of money, offering you an opportunity to be very specific about your intent. As you emphasize the exact amount needed, also allow yourself the freedom to receive it. Do not obstruct future abundance by focusing on limiting thoughts of unworthiness. Instead, focus and create the life you want. (Witches' burr can be found in magickal stores; it is made from the resin of sweet gum trees [*Liquidambar styraciflua*], which are also commonly known as liquid amber trees. I collect mine from trees in local parks.)

1 tablespoon dried cinquefoil flowers
1 tablespoon dried calendula flowers
1 patchouli leaf
2 tablespoons extra virgin olive oil
1 witches' burr
Gold sand
1 green candle

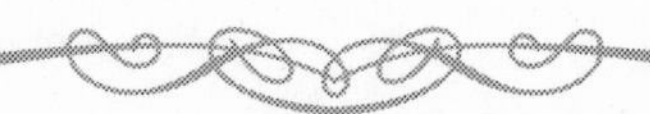

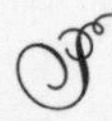

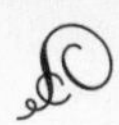

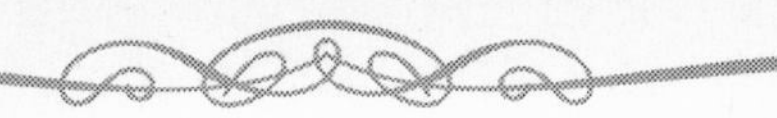

Cinquefoil prosperity oil
Red mojo bag, or pouch
Green cloth

Fill a small jar with the cinquefoil and calendula flowers and the patchouli leaf. Pour the olive oil over the herbs and cover with a tight-fitting lid. Let sit for 6 weeks. Strain the oil and reserve: this is cinquefoil prosperity oil. On a Thursday, sprinkle a witches' burr with gold sand. Carefully melt green candle wax over the burr. After the burr has cooled, anoint it with the cinquefoil prosperity oil. Place in a red mojo bag or any pouch. Tie the pouch's cord in five knots, symbolic of good luck. As you do this, say,

> Witches' burr, sand of gold
> Candle green, to seal the three
> Money to come, in needed sum
> Blessed be

Place the bag on a green cloth on your altar until the spell has worked, or as long as you like.

CINQUEFOIL NEEDS SUN, PARTIAL SHADE IN HOT SUMMER AREAS, AND LIGHT TO MODERATE WATERING. IT IS PLANTED FOR GROUND COVER AND IN GARDEN BORDERS.

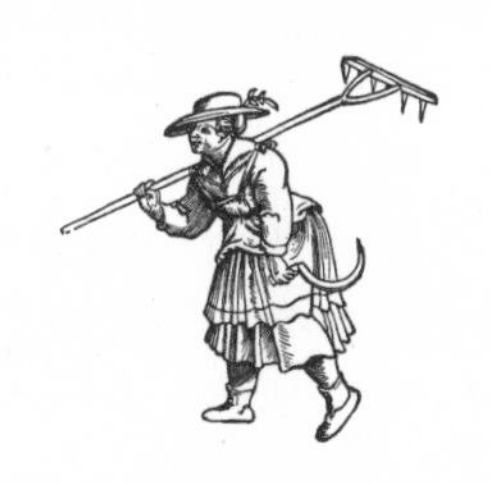

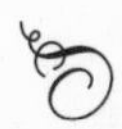

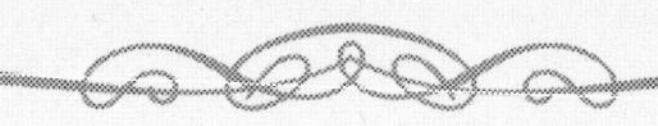

Clove

Syzygium aromaticum

Part Used: bud

Clove's magickal properties include purifying an area and removing negative energy, memory strengthening, protection for young ones, and relief from malicious gossip. Clove resonates with the fire elements: it draws on the heat and healing aspect of the sun, making it an excellent herb to represent the Father aspect of God. Today, cloves are used medicinally to ease toothaches. Clove is associated with the planet and deity of Uranus.

Father's Spice Pillow

Fathers play a major role in the balance of nurturing and raising children. They symbolize the faith in the seed of our desire that will find its home, root, grow, and thrive.

With the awareness of the father's great strength and willingness to be the backbone of our physical needs, a warm glow—like sunlight—shines over our hearts and heals the petty wounds of the day. Sunlight heals with its promise to nurture our seeds and desires.

It comes as no surprise that Father's Day falls near the summer solstice, when the sun at its peak. The sun is representative of male energy. Father's Day and summer solstice are times to honor the gifts the male facet brings to our life. This is a season of outward abundance, a time for a declaration of faith and ripeness.

Make this pillow when you need to feel the foundation, strength, and security the male energy provides. Understand that you possess this protective energy for yourself and all your loved ones. Alternatively, give this present to a new father or father figure in your life as a representation of that person's guiding light.

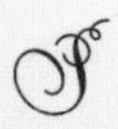

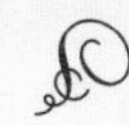

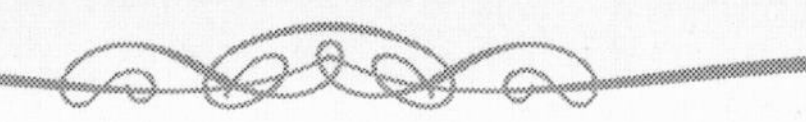

2 tablespoons whole cloves
2 tablespoons whole allspice berries
2 cinnamon sticks
2 cups uncooked long-grain rice
1 (20 by 10-inch) piece of fabric

Grind the cloves, allspice, and cinnamon in a mortar with a pestle in a clockwise (often called sunwise) direction. As you grind, direct the healing warmth of the sun into your spices. In a small bowl, combine the spice mixture and the rice. Take the fabric cloth and fold it in half. Sew up the two long sides. Pour the rice and herb mixture inside. Sew up the opening. You can microwave the pillow for 2 minutes for a comforting, warm pillow, or place it in the freezer overnight to make a cold pack.

THE CLOVE TREE IS NATIVE TO VERY WARM CLIMATES, AND IN AREAS THAT DON'T HAVE FROST IT DOES WELL IN ORDINARY SOIL AND FULL TO PARTIAL SHADE. IT IS NATIVE TO INDONESIA.

Orange Pomanders

Pomanders were extremely popular (and necessary!) in the Middle Ages. The wealthy class often used elaborate metal holders of silver or gold that they filled with strong, sweet-smelling spices, herbs, or perfumes. Most people, however, would have used a more modest container or poked spices in a piece of fruit. The pomander would be strung on a ribbon or chain and worn around the waist or neck. The sweet scents delighted the senses and drove off the sometimes strong odors of waste, animals, or sickness. Most people used pomanders as medicine or charms to ward off sicknesses. Cloves were believed to be particularly effective protection from the plague.

You can make your own pomander to provide a beautiful air freshener for your home. The recipe here makes enough spice mixture for three pomanders. Pomanders make beautiful Yule presents and decorations. The orrisroot called for in the recipe is available at most health food stores. (This recipe was donated by Tara S. Seefeldt, who cowrote *The Wicca Cookbook* with me. Tara teaches university courses in English History, European Witchcraft, and Medieval History.)

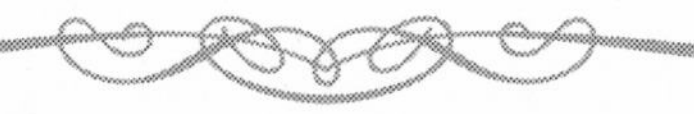

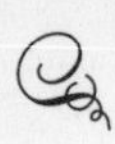

1 cup ground cinnamon

½ cup ground cloves

¼ cup ground allspice

¼ cup ground nutmeg

¼ cup ground orrisroot

2 cups large whole cloves

3 small, unblemished, thin-skinned oranges

1 thin knitting needle

1 brown paper lunch bag

In a bowl, mix together the cinnamon, cloves, allspice, nutmeg, and orrisroot. Set the mixture aside. Insert the whole cloves into the fruit in an orderly pattern by piercing the skin of the orange with the knitting needle and then inserting a clove. Cloves should be placed close together (approximately 5 mm) but not crowded; if too close, the fruit will split. Repeat the process on the remaining 2 oranges.

Finish your pomanders on the day you start them. Unfinished areas of the fruit may begin to rot if left overnight. When you have finished, the fruit should be completely covered with nearly touching cloves. Roll the fruit in the bowl of ground spices, then place them in the brown paper bag. Hang the bag in a well-ventilated area until the pomanders have dried and hardened, about 2 to 5 weeks. You can clip the paper bag to a wire hanger with a clothespin and hang it on a towel rack near a heating duct to speed up the drying process. Once cured, your pomander can be decorated with velvet or satin ribbon to suit particular festive occasions.

Pomanders can also be made with apples, pears, limes, or grapefruit.

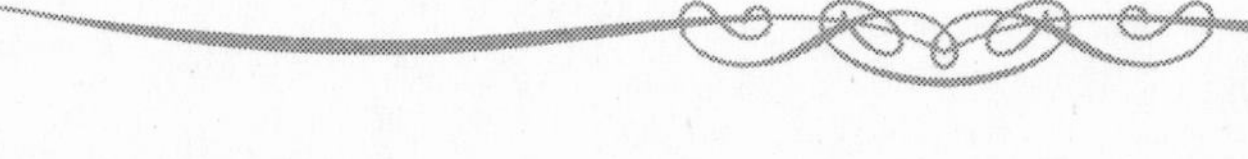

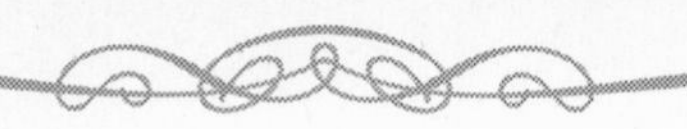

Comfrey

Symphytum officinale

BONESET, BRUISEWORT, HEALING BLADE, KNITBONE, SLIPPERY ROOT

Parts Used: leaves, stems, root

Comfrey is found wild in damp places throughout its native habitat in Europe, and is cultivated in other parts of the world. It has pale blue, or sometimes yellow, bell-shaped flowers that droop in clusters. This herb's curative powers, when it is used in compresses, poultices, and ointments, have been healing wounds for millennia. In both Latin and Greek the word for comfrey means "to grow together," referring to its amazing ability to knit fractured and broken bones and strengthen weak or strained ligaments and muscles. Magickally, it is best known for its protective powers, especially in relation to travel. Comfrey is associated with the astrological sign of Capricorn and the planetary and deity associations of Saturn.

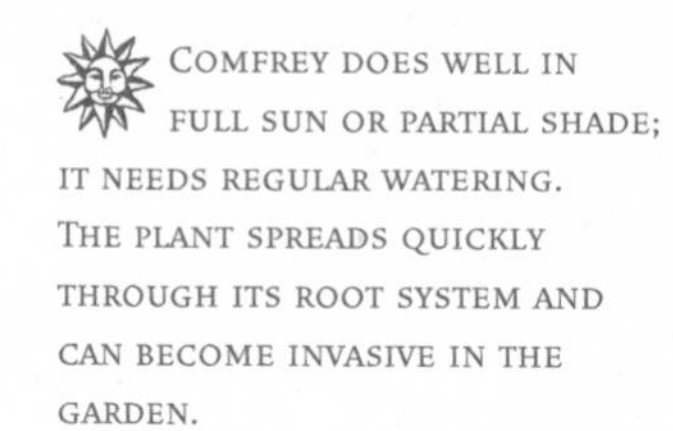

COMFREY DOES WELL IN FULL SUN OR PARTIAL SHADE; IT NEEDS REGULAR WATERING. THE PLANT SPREADS QUICKLY THROUGH ITS ROOT SYSTEM AND CAN BECOME INVASIVE IN THE GARDEN.

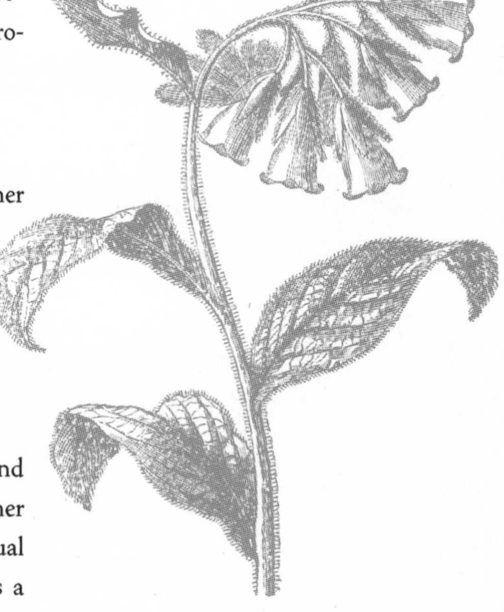

Revitalizing Toner

Comfrey's skin-calming protective elements are perfect for use in a refreshing toner that awakens you to the beauty of life in a safe, secure way.

2 cups fresh comfrey leaves, slightly bruised
2 cups apple cider vinegar
2 tablespoons witch hazel astringent lotion
16 cups distilled water

Pack the comfrey leaves into a 1-pint-capacity glass jar. Pour the vinegar in and close the lid tightly. Let stand for 3 to 6 weeks. Pour the liquid through a strainer into a bowl. Add witch hazel. Pour ¼ cup of the mixture into each of 8 individual glass bottles. (You can also pour the mixture into a misting bottle and use as a spritzer.) Add 2 cups distilled water per bottle. Shake well. This toner can be used for up to a year. Mother vinegar, a slimy coating, may appear on the surface; just spoon it off and use the toner—it doesn't affect the quality.

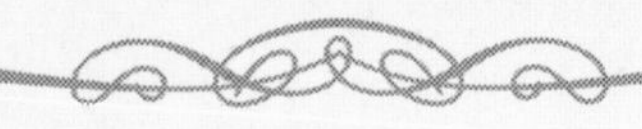

Coriander

Coriandrum sativum

CHINESE PARSLEY, CILANTRO, CULANTRO

Part Used: seeds

Coriander grows in fields and around gardens. It has fanlike, dark green leaves with pink-white flowers in umbrella-shaped clusters. It has a fetid scent when the leaves are bruised—hence the name of the herb, which relates to the Greek word for bug. As a tonic, coriander aids chronic indigestion and stomach or bowel pains, including those associated with childbirth. Fresh coriander leaves (commonly called cilantro) can be eaten raw in salads or dips and are used as a flavoring in many cuisines worldwide. Coriander is associated with the moon and the planetary and deity vibrations of Mars. Coriander resonates with the element of fire.

Spicy Nuts

MAKES 2 CUPS

These nuts are a delicious treat to keep on hand to share when visitors arrive at your home. I especially like to eat this mixture by the fire during the long, cold nights of winter.

- 2 cups raw cashews
- 1 tablespoon sugar
- 1 teaspoon salt
- ¼ teaspoon ground coriander
- ¼ teaspoon ground cumin
- 1 teaspoon curry powder
- 2 tablespoons raisins
- 2 tablespoons water
- 1 teaspoon brown sugar
- 1 tablespoon unsalted butter

Position 1 rack in the center of the oven and preheat to 350°F. Line a jelly-roll pan with parchment paper and spread cashews in the pan in an even layer. Bake 5 minutes; rotate the pan, and then bake 5 minutes longer. Meanwhile, stir the sugar, salt, and spices in a medium bowl; add the raisins. Remove the nuts from the oven and cool in the pan on a wire rack.

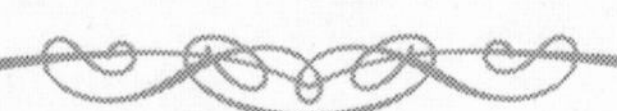

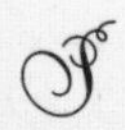

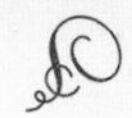

In a saucepan, bring the water, brown sugar, and butter to a boil over medium heat, whisking constantly. Add the nuts, stirring to coat completely until all the liquid has evaporated. Stir the glazed nuts into the spice mixture. Cool on a parchment-lined baking sheet.

Courageous Love Dish

Serves 4 as an appetizer or 2 as a main course

Mars, the planet associated with coriander, encourages the development of the will and courage. The influence of Mars helps you to be assertive and express your needs. Its energy represents freedom, independence, enthusiasm, and determination. Use this force to expand your horizons, take risks, and test your limits in trusting intimacy.

Besides containing Martial resonances, coriander also carries the power of love. If your instinct is telling you that you have found that special someone but you fear emotional closeness, use this recipe to follow your heart. Tuesday is the day of Mars and new beginnings. Try serving this dish to that special someone in your life on a Tuesday. Go for it!

Coriander prefers moderately rich, light, well-drained soil and full sun to partial shade. Do not plant near common parsley or fennel, as these strong herbs will crowd out coriander's delicate stalks. Coriander enhances anise growth. It is native to southern Europe and western Asia.

- 2 cups French green beans (haricots verts), stems removed
- 3 tablespoons olive oil
- 1 teaspoon mustard seeds
- ½ cup chopped onion
- ¾ cup sliced miniature carrots
- ½ teaspoon fresh minced ginger
- 1 teaspoon ground coriander
- ½ teaspoon salt
- 2 teaspoons freshly squeezed lemon juice

Bring 6 cups water to a boil in a saucepan. Add the haricots verts and cook for 3 minutes. Drain and rinse the haricots verts under cold water; set aside. Heat the olive oil in a skillet over medium-high heat. Add the mustard seeds and sauté until they begin to pop, about 2 minutes. Add the onions, carrots, and ginger. Cook, stirring frequently, until the onions are translucent and carrots are tender-crisp, about 5 minutes. Add the coriander and salt. Reduce heat to medium-low and add the haricots verts. Cook until the haricots verts are thoroughly heated, about 3 minutes. Remove from heat, sprinkle with lemon juice, and toss before serving.

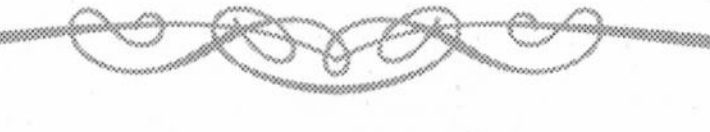

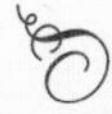

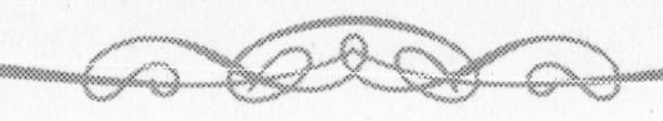

Cypress

gopher wood, cupressus

TREE OF DEATH

Part Used: branches, leaves, cones

Cypress is an evergreen conifer with tiny scalelike leaves set closely together on cordlike branches. Its cones are round with shield-shaped scales. Cypress is an anti-spasmodic and general tonic. It is used to treat colds, flus, sore throats, and muscle aches. Planetary and deity associations for cypress include Aphrodite, Hercules, Persephone, Pluto, and Saturn. Cypress vibrates with the earth element and is often used to remember and honor those who have crossed over to the other side. It is known for its powers of protection and consecration.

DO NOT TAKE CYPRESS INTERNALLY WITHOUT THE SUPERVISION OF A HEALING PRACTITIONER.

Cypress Sea Salt Scrub

Cypress is used in this exfoliating sea scrub as a reminder of the fact that you have the opportunity to create yourself anew. Everyone is dying and living at every moment. Allow yourself to shed old ideas and perceptions so that you can embrace a paradigm shift in awareness. Freeing yourself of old ideas can help you let go of judgments. Only when you have forgiveness and peace of mind can you see the Divine in every person, thing, and situation.

When you use this scrub, imagine yourself shedding all your grudges, preconceived ideas, judgments, and fears. Sea scrubs exfoliate dead skin, making you feel soft and silky. Some experts believe that scrubs assist the lymphatic system to eliminate toxins by breaking down fatty pockets in the skin. (This also helps to get rid of cellulite.) For an effective releasing ritual, use this scrub during a waning moon.

2 cups coarse sea salt
15 drops cypress essential oil
1 cup avocado, almond, grape seed, or olive oil

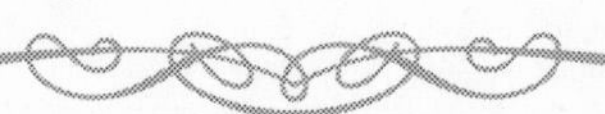

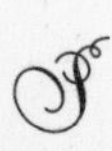

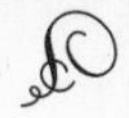

Pour the salt into an airtight jar with a hinged, sealable lid. In a small bowl, combine the two oils, adding the cypress oil drop by drop. Pour the mixture into the jar. Mix well and then seal the lid and shake vigorously.

To use, apply the scrub to a long-handled back brush or a loofah mitt. Start at your feet, brushing with long sweeping movements. Work up your legs, across your hips and tummy. Stroke upward toward your heart, avoiding your breasts. Move to your hands and arms and stroke upward to your shoulders. Continue the process, stroking back toward your heart, and other areas in need of exfoliation. Store the scrub in a cool, dry place and use within 1 year.

CYPRESS TREES PREFER FULL SUN AND REQUIRE LITTLE WATER ONCE ESTABLISHED. THESE EVERGREEN TREES ARE FAST GROWERS AND NEED ALMOST NO PRUNING. CYPRESS TREES ARE NATIVE TO TURKEY AND ARE WIDELY CULTIVATED IN THE MEDITERRANEAN.

Spicy Cypress-Oatmeal Soap

MAKES 3 BARS

Cypress carries a woodsy scent. As an essential oil it can be worn or breathed at funerals or on Samhain to raise our awareness that death is but a portal to another experience of growth. Death represents a crucial stage that allows regeneration and rebirth to occur. This soap is easy and quick to make. It's the perfect homemade present to give a friend.

Sunflower oil
1 (5-ounce) rectangular soap mold
1 pound clear glycerin melt-and-pour soap base
4 to 6 drops cypress essential oil
4 to 6 drops apple essential oil
4 to 6 drops sandalwood essential oil
2 cups old-fashioned oats, ground in the blender

Cover a work surface with waxed paper. Apply a thin, even coat of sunflower oil to the mold. Cut the soap base into 1-inch squares and place in a microwave-safe container. Heat the soap base in the microwave 40 seconds. Stir. Continue to heat and stir for 10-second intervals until the soap base is completely melted. (You can also melt it on the stove top.) Add the oils 1 drop at a time until the desired scent is attained. Stir in the ground oats. Pour the soap base into the mold. The oatmeal will sink to the bottom. Allow soap to cool 24 hours before removing from mold.

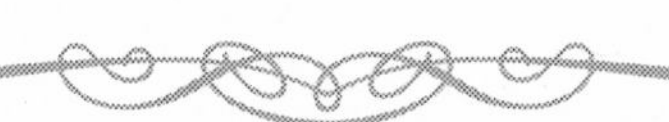

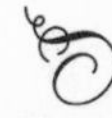

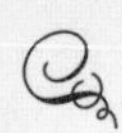

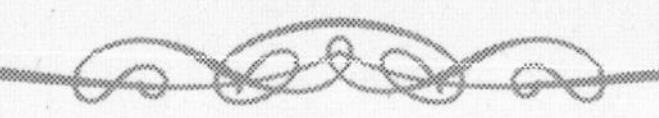

Dandelion

Taraxacum officinale

BLOW BALLS, DENT DE LION, GOAT'S BEARD, LION'S TOOTH, PEASANT'S CLOAK, PEE-A-BED, WILD CHICORY

Parts Used: leaves, roots, stems

Dandelions are found in waysides and meadows. Their flowers are long and yellow and heavily honey-scented. *Dandelion* comes from a French root meaning "tooth of the lion." Its botanical name may originate from the Greek words for *disorder* and *remedy.* It is known to remineralize the body and can be helpful to menopausal women. It is a blood tonic, blood cleanser, and lymph cleanser. The herb is also a strong diuretic, hence the folk name pee-a-bed—do not drink dandelion tea right before bedtime!

Dandelion is quite effective in treating disorders of the liver and bile, especially jaundice. The white juice, extracted from the leaves and stems, can relieve bee stings, warts, old sores, blisters, and hard pimples. Dandelion contains eudesmanolides—compounds not found in any other herb—along with flavonoids, mucilage, and sterols. The combination of these compounds stimulates bile, a fluid that graciously aids fat digestion. The leaves must be chewed, passing over the back of the tongue. Receptors there signal the presence of a bitter that will begin the digestion process. Eating dandelion greens also treats diabetes, excessive sleepiness, and obesity. The dried roots and leaves make an excellent tea, and are also available in a tincture. Dandelion is associated with the planet and deity Jupiter and the astrological sign of Sagittarius.

BE CAREFUL NOT TO USE DANDELIONS HARVESTED FROM LAWNS THAT HAVE BEEN TREATED WITH INORGANIC FERTILIZER OR HERBICIDES.

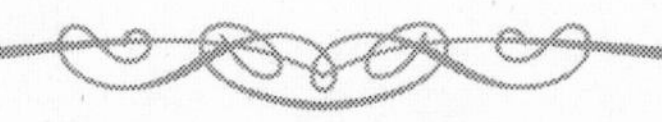

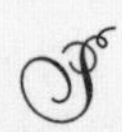

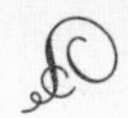

Shadow Dancing

Dandelions are often referred to as weeds. We pluck them, often without regard to their gifts. They can teach us a lesson that applies to our shadow selves: if we engage in the act of constantly denying an aspect of ourselves, it will only grow. That which we resist persists.

Any of the sabbats during the darker months of the year present a great opportunity to make friends with our shadow selves. When we ride the seasons, we find that as the weather cools we are ready to hunker down and be still. But sometimes when life gets quiet, our minds cannot stop and they begin to tell us falsehoods about ourselves. When the chatter begins, we yearn to push it away. This only serves to divide us, pushing us away from the dark self. This aspect of you only wants to dance in the light. It doesn't really want to be trapped in the darkness any more than you want to hear the negative self-talk. The guided meditation that follows helps you begin to reconcile with your shadow self.

Dandelions prefer full sun and regular watering. Invite them into your garden; don't just treat them as weeds lest they react like their shadow selves and proliferate where you least desire. Dandelions enhance fruit trees' growth.

Light a white candle. Cleanse yourself by directing the smoke from a smoldering bundle of dried sage over your body. Take several deep breaths to bring your awareness to the present moment. Visualize a cord leaving your root chakra (located in the perineum) and descending to the depths of Mother Earth, where her energy is. Draw that energy back to you. Be still for a moment.

Imagine that a black cloak shrouds you, blocking all light, except for the tiniest pinhole of light in the far distance. You may be in a cave or a dark closet. Hold the space to allow the smallest part of you to speak its truth. Do not pass judgment or try to "fix" this small part of you; just allow it to talk. Imagine the color, smell, or taste of this part of yourself. Feel yourself surrounded by the pain and sadness of feeling small, alone, unheard, or sad. Visualize this imagery in its worst possible scenario. It appears there is no way out.

Visualize a small child of your gender holding a candelabrum containing three lit candles. He or she beckons you to follow, but you resist. You remain passive, blaming someone else for not responding to your pain and rescuing you. Now imagine a symbol of the person you want to blame standing before you. Allow the small self to react to the blamed one—anything is acceptable because the blamed

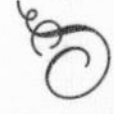

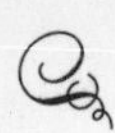

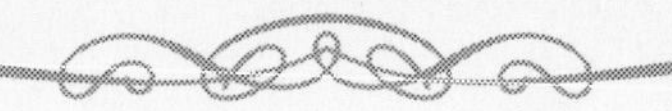

one represents an archetype or relationship pattern, not a particular person who can be harmed. Release all of your anger or sadness.

The child with the candelabrum appears before you again. Again you are asked to follow. Now you find that you can. The child hands you three flowers. By the candlelight you can tell they are dandelions; they represent the past, present, and future. The child leads you up a hill toward a light.

As you reach the light, you find you are in a beautiful garden. You can hear the wind speak, saying, "I carry your dreams." At your feet, a beetle says, "Come, visit my home. We shall have tea." A robin asks, "Have you seen how well my children fly?" Sunlight plays on a spider's web; pumpkins grin fat-cheeked smiles. The garden of spirits is alive with voices and colors, all teeming with life.

The child turns to you and smiles. Take note of the child's face. Do you recognize yourself? See his or her wonderment and pure belief in all things possible. The child represents knowledge of the power of creation and the interconnectedness of all living creatures. The child carries faith and self-love, recognizing love as all things; this wisdom is accessible only when you accept all parts of yourself as beautiful and holy. The joy and light you desire already exists; you only need open yourself to it.

Look down at your dandelions. They are now white puffs of seeds. Blow the intent of living your joy into the fluffy seed heads. Watch the small seeds float to the four corners of the world. By your will, so mote it be!

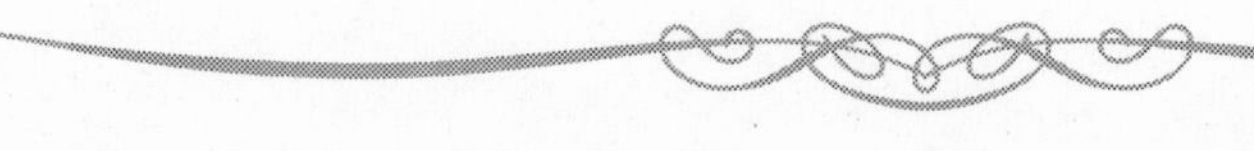

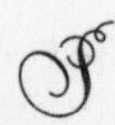

Dragon's Blood

Dracaena draco

DRAGON TREE

Part Used: gum

Dragon's blood is a small, evergreen, palmlike tree with broad, curved ribbonlike leaves, a stout trunk, and greenish white flowers. Dragon's blood increases the power of most spells. Its basic powers include purification, protection, and energy manifestation. It can be used in love or lust rituals. Dragon's blood is associated with the gods and planets Pluto and Mars.

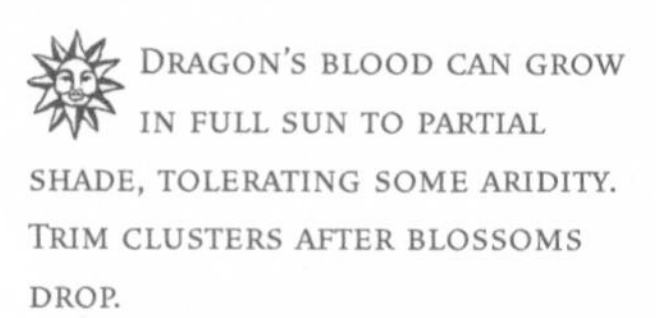
DRAGON'S BLOOD CAN GROW IN FULL SUN TO PARTIAL SHADE, TOLERATING SOME ARIDITY. TRIM CLUSTERS AFTER BLOSSOMS DROP.

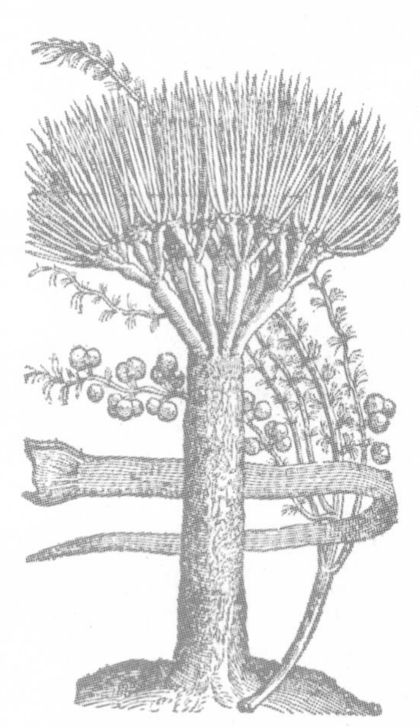

Slay the Stress

Design a two-column list of payoffs or rewards and consequences or penalties for stress. The benefits of stress revolve around how you think you are supposed to feel. Stress is an ugly, dirty garment placed over a pristine being. Cast this spell on a Saturday during a waning moon. If you need this spell immediately, it will work regardless of the day or time of the month. Building a spell around a specific time increases the spell's potency, but the most important element will always be your intent.

Combine equal parts of dragon's blood incense (for potency and energy), sage incense (for purification), and frankincense incense (for exorcism) in a cauldron placed on the floor. Take off your clothes, one garment at a time. (Leave on undergarments if doing so makes you feel more comfortable.) As you remove them, drag the clothes over your skin. Concentrate on the area of your body where you have locked your stress. Imagine the anxiety peeling away from you. When you are done, stand over the smoldering cauldron, face upward, and inhale the Divine. Breathe out through your mouth, expelling negativity. Step over the cauldron three times. Say,

I let go of the stress I feel
Releasing it as no part of me
I am free and light of mind
By my will, so mote it be!

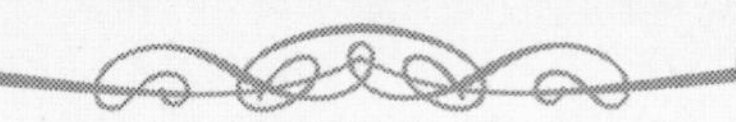

Echinacea

Echinacea angustifolia, Echinacea purpurea

BLACK SAMPSON, KANSAS SNAKEROOT, MISSOURI SNAKEROOT, PURPLE CONEFLOWER

Parts Used: flowers, roots

Echinacea grows wild along pathways and hedges. The herb has rough, hairy leaves and purple flowers. Native Americans use the roots of this plant against snakebites, rabies, and toothaches, and to remedy women's ailments. Today, it is a popular herb for combating the flu, colds, slow-healing wounds, infections, and inflamed skin conditions.

This herb treats laryngitis, bronchitis, pneumonia, tonsillitis, chronic sore throats, indigestion ailments, skin irritations and infections, rosacea, and psoriasis. It boosts the immune system by activating white blood cell production and is often taken at the onset of a viral or bacterial infection. It is believed that echinacea stimulates the lymphatic system through the mouth; if you are taking it as a tincture, hold it in the mouth for a bit before swallowing. Echinacea is effective for those who tire easily, avoid conflict, procrastinate, and find difficulty relaxing unless absolutely silent. Avoid it if you have an autoimmune disorder such as multiple sclerosis or lupus.

Maiden Tea Ritual

The three herbs used in this ritual are all top blood purifiers. Our jewel-red blood contains the power of life, a representative of creativity, abundance, and energy. During her menstrual cycle, a woman is extra-powerful. She is engaged in a natural cleansing process that has long been regarded as a sacred ceremony in many indigenous cultures.

Celebrating the first menses welcomes maidens to womanhood, creating a strong, tender, and supportive foundation. This support encourages them to embrace their womanhood; they can feel safe to search for their individual powers

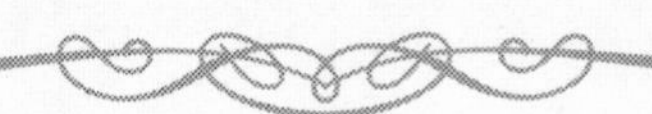

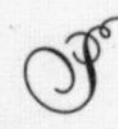

within their feminine identity and be encouraged to outgrow their elders.

Host a circle for a young maiden right after her first moon cycle (menstrual period). Explain that this ceremony is intended to honor the maiden within each one, and especially for the initiate who has just entered the first stage of her womanhood. Present a red garment to the maiden. (If you are in a ritual circle, this blessing would be offered at the time of cakes and ale.) Have maiden tea (see the recipe below) in a pitcher. Hold it up to the sky and say,

> Dear God and Goddess, we offer you this drink that we may honor thee
>
> In love we ask that you cast your blessings upon our Maiden ceremony
>
> And by your guidance we may learn the mysteries of love and light
>
> And the magic of earth and all young and innocent delights.

Pour the tea into individual chalices. After everyone has a drink, say,

> We honor the maiden present tonight
>
> We honor our blood as our birthright
>
> We honor our power, strong and true
>
> We honor [the maiden's name here], blessings to you!

1 quart water
¼ cup dried echinacea flowers
¼ cup dried dandelion leaves
¼ cup burdock root, ground to a powder
Honey

Bring the water to a boil. Place the echinacea, dandelion, and burdock in a bowl. Pour the boiling water over the herbs and let steep 15 to 20 minutes. Strain the herbs out of the tea. Add the desired amount of honey.

This perennial is easy to grow in full sun to light shade in fertile, well-drained soil. It is native to the central United States.

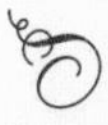

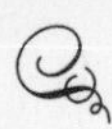

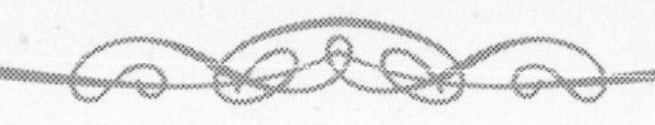

Elder

Sambucus nigra, Sambucus canadensis

BATTREE, BOUR TREE, ELDERBERRY, OLD GAL, PIPE TREE, TREE OF DOOM

Parts Used: root, berries, bark, flowers

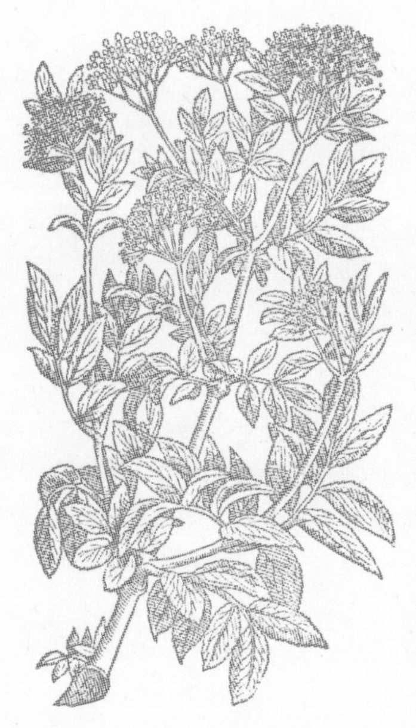

Elder is the common name for a variety of species of trees and bushes; not all species bear edible berries. Only the blue or black berries are medicinal. The European species name is *Sambucus nigra,* which has a long history of use as both a food and a medicine, going back to Hippocrates. In Denmark, the tree is believed to house Hylde-Moer, the Elder Tree Mother, who haunts anyone found harming it. The American elderberry, *Sambucus canadensis,* produces the best-tasting berries, used in pies and (with the flowers) to make wine.

Medicinally, the flowers are used to treat eyes, the root helps lymphatic and kidney problems, the leaves are brewed as a tea for an itch remedy, and the berries are used in wine as a healing remedy for sore throats, as a laxative, and to relieve the pain of burns. The most common medicinal uses for elder are for relief from colds, flus, sore throats, herpes breakouts, and swollen glands. The berries contain vitamins A, B, and C plus various flavonoids, including quercetin; but these substances alone cannot account for its remarkable effect in reducing the symptoms of a cold or flu. Teas made from elder flowers can be taken as a diuretic and a purgative, or used externally as a wash for acne.

For magickal purposes, use elder in protection, love, and purification rituals. The branches can be made into wands. In olden days, the branches were sometimes hung on doorways for general protection. You can scatter the leaves and berries in the four directions as a quick and easy way to protect and purify an area. The elder is sacred to the Crone aspect of the Goddess and is associated with Samhain. Elder is associated with the planet and deity Venus.

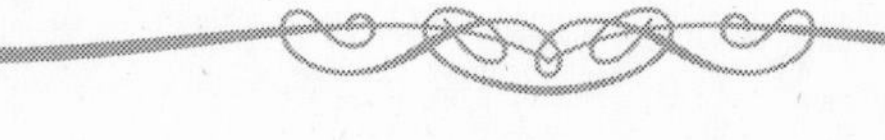

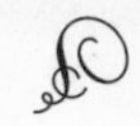

Elder Purification Meditation

Elder is a sacred tree that has long been used as a connection to dryads and faeries, as a tool for blessings, and in purification ceremonies. It is associated with the goddess Venus, who represents love, harmony, equilibrium, and appreciation for aesthetics and relationships. She is also the goddess of spring and rebirth. As you take this sweat bath, ask Venus to help you gently rid yourself of toxic thoughts and energy. Release all that no longer serves you. Come to recognize the love that the Divine Source holds for you in the cadence and impermanence of life. Relax into this rhythm and know that the universe supports you in awakening to the greatness within.

Elder grows well in full sun or light shade with moderate watering. It is fast growing and benefits from a good pruning every year during its dormant season. Elder is native to Europe.

2 tablespoons elder flowers
2 tablespoons peppermint flowers and leaves
2 teaspoons ground ginger

Combine equal parts elder flowers and peppermint flowers and leaves. Cover with boiling water and let steep 10 minutes, then strain. Run a hot bath while the tea is steeping, adding about 2 teaspoons of ground ginger to the water. Soak in the hot bath while drinking the tea. This will induce a good sweat, helping the toxins release from the body.

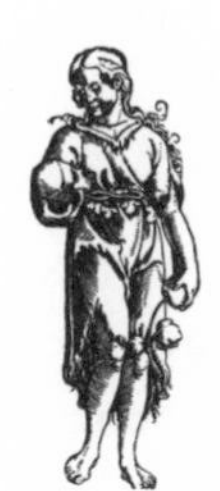

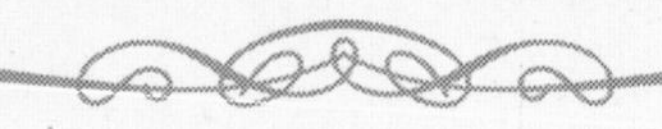

Eucalyptus

Eucalyptus (various species)

BLUE GUM, FEVER TREE

Part Used: leaves

Indigenous to Australia, this aromatic tree was transported en masse to America to protect groves of orange and lemon trees from wind. *Eucalyptus globus* contains a chemical called eucalyptol, or cineole, that is responsible for relieving bronchial and nasal congestion and fighting infection. The fragrant oils made from eucalyptol act as an antiseptic and expectorant, while the tannins relieve inflammation. Eucalyptus essential oil can be rubbed over fingernails to strengthen them. In aromatherapy practice, eucalyptus is used to cool the body in the summer and protect it in the winter. Eucalyptus is found in disinfectant, insect repellent, and products that provide relief from sore muscles and sinus problems.

You can make a flea collar for your pet with this aromatic oil. Take an extra-wide shoelace and drip onto it a few drops each of eucalyptus and pennyroyal oil; place around your pet's neck after it has dried. Watch for skin irritation, however, as some animals are hypersensitive.

The tree's medicinal powers are so potent that its healing powers carry over to the magickal realm as well. Include fresh eucalyptus leaves with the color blue in any healing ritual you do. Eucalyptus is associated with the moon and the deity and planet Pluto.

Depression-Lifting Candle

Even Witches get the blues sometimes. We are healers, and sometimes we come across a situation in which we absorb too much negative energy. When you need a quick pick-me-up, create this candle. The combination of the herbs in this recipe is used for the following reasons: eucalyptus for healing, cloves for driving away negative energies, thyme for health and energy, rosemary for purification, marjoram for happiness, mint for protection, and lavender for peace. Wax crystals and wicks

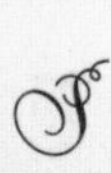

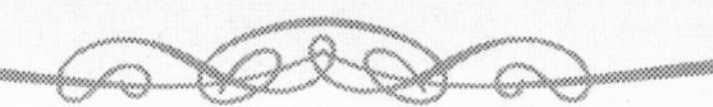

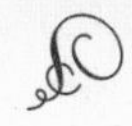

can be found at candle supply and arts and crafts shops. (This recipe comes from Jeannine Marie, an eclectic Witch who began her Wiccan path at the age of nine.)

- ¼ teaspoon eucalyptus oil
- ¼ teaspoon ground cloves
- ¼ teaspoon dried thyme
- ¼ teaspoon dried rosemary
- ¼ teaspoon dried marjoram
- ¼ teaspoon dried mint
- ¼ teaspoon dried lavender
- ½ cup (112 grams) colored wax crystals (choose a color that brings you happiness)
- 1 prewaxed wick

The root system of this tree is very shallow, so don't plant too close to your house or sidewalks. This tree likes full sun and can tolerate aridity extremely well.

Combine the eucalyptus oil and all of the herbs and grind them in a mortar with a pestle to create a fairly fine powder. Set the mixture aside. Place the wax crystals in a small bowl, add the herb powder, and mix together with your fingers. Say,

> By the blessed moon
> O root, o soil,
> No longer will my soul toil
> I am happiness, I am love
> I am charged by the stars above!
> So mote it be!

Take the mixture and pour it carefully into a wide-mouthed glass jar (baby food jars works great). Insert the wick straight into your candle and gently pat the wax down around the wick. Trim the wick short enough so the flame will be in balance with your wax creation (about ¼ inch). Light and enjoy. (Remember never to leave a candle burning unattended.)

Magick Hearth Broom

In ancient Rome, the broom was associated with female magick, mysteries, and wise woman traditions. Midwives would sweep the threshold of a home after childbirth to drive away evil spirits. Women also "rode" their brooms, jumping up and down between the rows of crops to insure fertility for the year's harvest. This might be one of the reasons people thought witches flew on broomsticks!

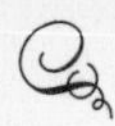

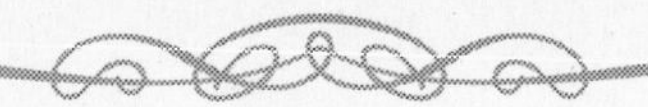

Traditionally the broom was made of ash wood for the handle, birch twigs for the brush, and willow for the binding. These materials and their associations all contain fertility symbolism, which they bestow on the broom.

The symbolism for a hearth broom is quite different. This broom—with its eucalyptus—emphasizes sacred women's work. Protecting the spiritual sanctity of the home and its inhabitants, as well as their physical well-being, was and continues to be an honored role for the priestess and wise woman of the home. The broom can also be used in place of a wand when casting a circle. When working with a ritual, don't let the broom touch the actual floor: you are sweeping out negative energies, not dust bunnies! (These broom instructions come from Cindy Cox, who has been exploring the spiritual and metaphysical through art and craft for over twenty years.)

1 (4- to 6-foot) eucalyptus branch, 2 to 3 inches in diameter
Oak or birch twigs, 5 to 6 inches long
Bunch of eucalyptus leaves
Glue
Heavy wire
Dried flowers and herbs
Ribbons, gemstones, and other decorative material
Paint or wood-burning tool (optional)

When you gather the branch for the broom, try to find one that has already fallen. If you must cut a branch, make sure the tree is offering it to you. You might want to sit by the tree for a few minutes and bond with it. You will know in your meditations and visualizations if the tree is offering you a branch. In any case, always leave an offering of thanks for the tree; a fertilizer stick, a small gemstone, or a libation (wine or other liquid poured on the ground around the tree) is appropriate.

Gather some oak or birch twigs, trim to the desired length, and set aside. Now you're ready to ponder your broom decoration and think about its home. Will it be sitting alongside the fireplace, by the front door, in the kitchen? Knowing the broom's permanent place in your home will help you decide how it should be

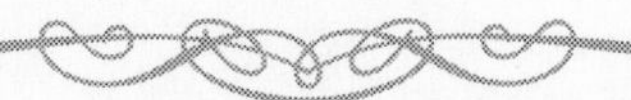

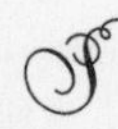

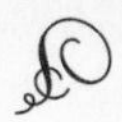

decorated. My broom, which stands by the front door, is carved with protective rune symbols and some tumbled, unpolished amethyst, and it has a small bag filled with dried lavender flowers attached. It has burgundy- and lavender-colored ribbons and raffia tied to it as well. These colors can be changed seasonally: red and green for Yule, tied with a small bag of fresh mistletoe; spring colors with a bag of rose petals; or bay leaves for Imbolc are some seasonal options.

Arrange the eucalyptus leaves and oak or birch twigs around the branch. Secure them with glue and wrap tightly with the wire. Set the broom aside and let the glue dry for 20 minutes. Next, decorate it with the items you have chosen. Use colors, gemstones, herbs, and other items that will correspond to the purpose you have in mind for your broom. These items are the things that make the broom powerful and personal to you.

Your broom is now ready to bless and consecrate as one of your most versatile magick tools. Say,

> *I bless this instrument of wind and change*
> *To expand my magick in breadth and range*
> *Bring to me light and love*
> *And the highest blessings from above*
> *By my will, so mote it be!*

It is important to let your broom change and grow with you. Use it in ritual often, especially in ritual and gatherings involving family and friends. This seems to keep a positive flow of energy going into the broom. Set it outside on a sunny day or under the full moon to cleanse it and charge it anew with energy. My favorite use for the broom is to sweep negative energy right out the back door or into the fireplace; the broom really seems to enjoy this important job! Be gentle with this important magick tool, and it will serve you well for years to come.

Note: For convenience, you can disassemble a natural corn broom from the grocery store and use its twigs instead of using oak or birch twigs.

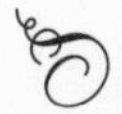

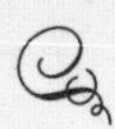

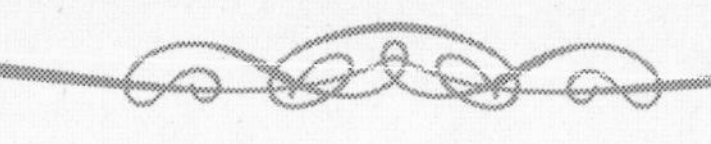

Evening Primrose

Oenothera biennis

CURE-ALL, GERMAN RAMPION, SCABISH, SUN DROP, TREE PRIMROSE

Parts Used: oil from the seeds, roots

EVENING PRIMROSE PREFERS FULL SUN AND LIGHT WATERING. IT IS NATIVE TO NORTH AMERICA.

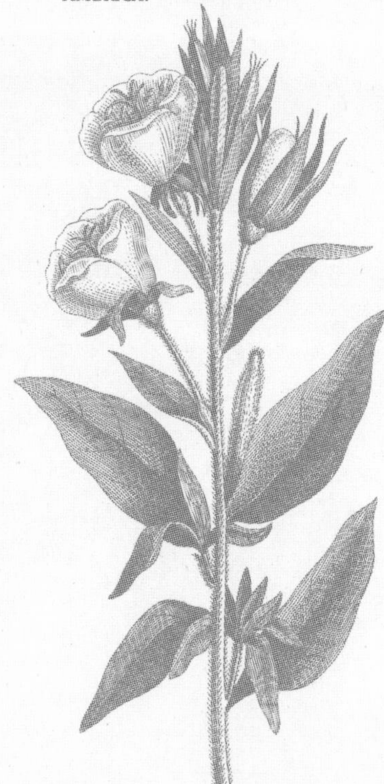

Evening primrose grows in rough places. The herb has showy, four-petaled silky yellow flowers; other species of *Oenothera* have rose pink or white flowers. The plant's mucilage is used to aid eczema, dry skin, hay fever, asthma, and arthritis. It is also used to combat free radicals. Evening primrose is known to oxygenate the blood, speed fat digestion, improve skin conditions, lower blood pressure, alleviate arthritis, calm nervousness in active children, reduce cholesterol, stimulate metabolism, strengthen the immune system, regulate body temperature and stomach acids, and relieve premenstrual and menopausal conditions. Native Americans from the Cherokee to the Iroquois used this edible plant to soothe hemorrhoids. Evening primrose is associated with Freya and both the planetary and deity associations of Venus.

Vertigo-Relief Smoothie

MAKES 1 SMOOTHIE

Used in a morning smoothie, evening primrose oil (sometimes found combined with flaxseed and borage oil) relieves vertigo, which can be caused by a vegetarian diet. Not getting enough essential fatty acids, which aid in prostaglandin production can bring on a case of vertigo. You can drink this smoothie in the morning as a pick-me-up alternative to coffee.

- 1 tablespoon evening primrose oil
- 6 to 8 strawberries, hulled
- 1 banana
- ½ peach, peeled, pitted
- ½ cup (125 ml) coconut-pineapple juice
- ¼ cup (60 ml) apple juice
- 1 cup (250 ml) ice

Process all the ingredients in a blender until smooth, then pour into a glass and enjoy!

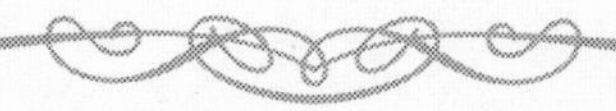

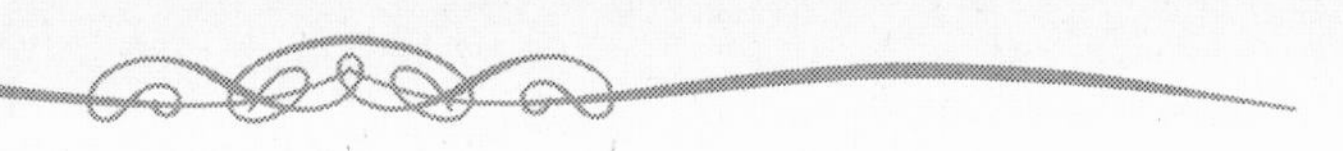

Fennel

Foeniculum vulgare

SWEET FENNEL

Parts Used: fresh stems, seeds, leaves, roots

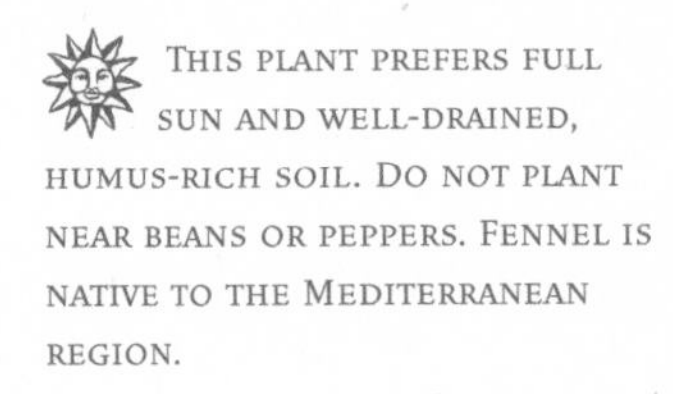

THIS PLANT PREFERS FULL SUN AND WELL-DRAINED, HUMUS-RICH SOIL. DO NOT PLANT NEAR BEANS OR PEPPERS. FENNEL IS NATIVE TO THE MEDITERRANEAN REGION.

Fennel is found on dry banks and hillsides, especially in coastal regions. It has feathery dark green leaves and a pungent scent. The herb's yellow-green flowers form umbels. This herb, which tastes a bit like licorice, has been used all over the globe from China to Jamaica to Africa to relieve ailments ranging from diarrhea to lethargy. Fennel leaves are used to treat gastric ailments, obesity, cramps, and rheumatism, and to help sore eyes and diabetes. They also improve the memory. The root is a fine laxative, and the seeds expel poison from the body. The plant's volatile oils soothe and stimulate the digestive system, increase breast milk production, and fight infection. The lure of catnip is well known, but in actuality, 20 percent of dogs and cats don't like it because of its minty scent; they prefer fennel, which is just as useful. Fennel is associated with Mercury.

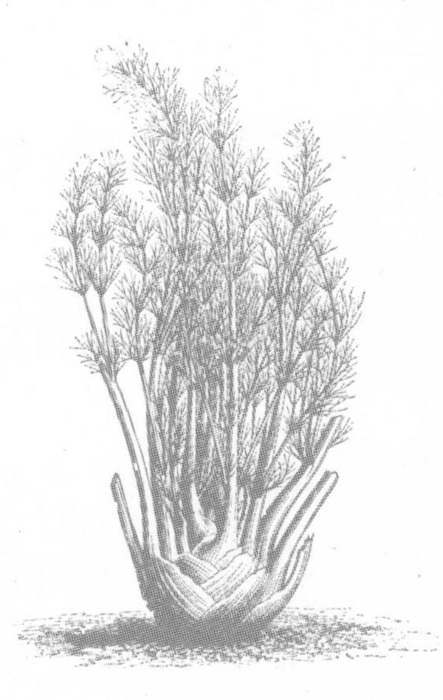

Fennel Salad

SERVES 4 TO 6 AS A FIRST COURSE

Fennel links to the planet and god Mercury, opens up communication with the spirit realms, and increases intuition and trust in healing. Create this salad for additional help with speaking your truth clearly and honestly.

- 1 medium fennel bulb (about 1 pound), peeled, leaves discarded, cut into thin strips
- 1 red bell pepper, julienned
- 1 yellow bell pepper, julienned
- ¼ cup extra virgin olive oil
- ½ cup balsamic vinegar
- 2 teaspoons cracked black pepper

Toss the fennel and all bell peppers in a bowl. In a small bowl, whisk the oil, vinegar, and pepper. Pour over the salad and mix well to coat. Cover and refrigerate the salad for 1 hour before serving.

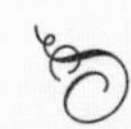

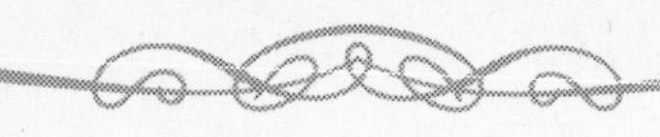

Feverfew

Chrysanthemum parthenium

FEATHERFEW, FLIRTWORT, VETTER-VOO

Part Used: leaves

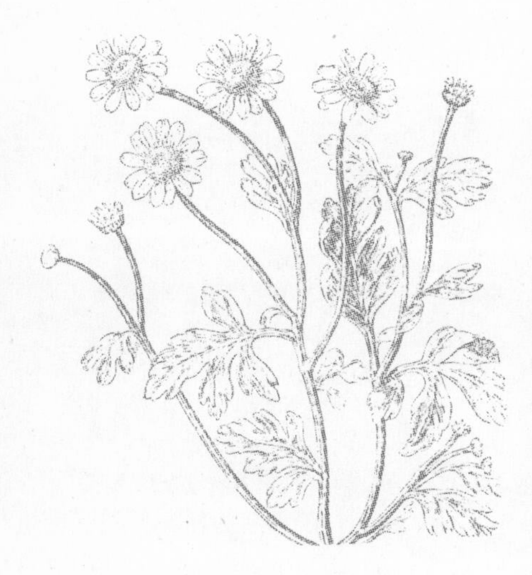

Feverfew is found in wastelands. Its leaves are feathery and its white and yellow, daisylike flowers have a pointed center and bear a resemblance to chamomile flowers. As a member of the daisy family, feverfew grows easily as a hardy, vigorous biennial. It stands straight up with finely furrowed stems. The herb is quite aromatic. Feverfew has been used medicinally to treat headaches and migraines for at least four hundred years. It contains the active ingredient parthenolide, which restricts the release of serotonin, a natural antidepression neurotransmitter that constricts blood vessels. The fresh leaves can be taken daily in a tea or added to a salad as a preventive for chronic headaches. Feverfew resonates with the sixth chakra (the area on your forehead where the third eye resides), and it's often recommended that you chew one or two leaves a day to ward off migraines. Dioscorides, an ancient Greek doctor, praised feverfew's effectiveness on problems relating to the uterus. It is a good herb for women, as it aids female infertility, helps prevent miscarriages, and relieves difficult labors. Feverfew is associated with Venus, in her planetary and deity vibrations.

Women's Moontime Ritual

Pick a handful of feverfew leaves early in the morning. Sprinkle the leaves around a chalice of your moon blood (menstrual blood). You can collect moon blood either by putting a used pad or tampon into a cauldron of water, or simply by squatting over a container and later pouring the blood into the chalice. (I know how this sounds, but trust me, this is a very empowering ritual for increasing intuition.)

Take several deep breaths. Imagine roots growing from the bottoms of your feet into the deep soil of Mother Earth. Pull on her energy and visualize her white

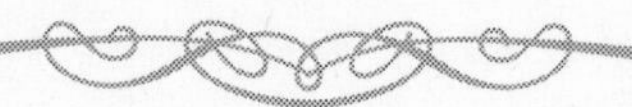

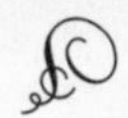

light coursing through your body. Raise your hands to the sky, and ask that the energy from the Father descend into your awareness. Light a red candle. Ask that God, Goddess, and your guardians be with you. Take as much time as you need. Begin in the east. Anoint your third eye (in the center of your forehead) by dipping a finger in the chalice and touching it to your forehead. Say,

> By my blood, I bless my sight
> So that I may see Spirit's divine light.

FEVERFEW DOES WELL IN FULL SUN OR LIGHT SHADE WITH REGULAR WATERING.

Turn to the south. Anoint your heart chakra by dipping your finger in the chalice and touching your chest with a drop of your blood. Say,

> By my blood, I bless my love and heart
> So I will know from Spirit I never part.

Turn to the west. Anoint your solar plexus by dipping your finger in the chalice and touching your abdomen just above your navel with a drop of your blood. Say,

> By my blood, I bless my power
> With love and temperance this very hour.

Turn to the north. Anoint your root chakra by dipping your finger in the chalice and touching your perineum with a drop of your blood. Say,

> By my blood, I bless my human journey
> And trust the Spirit's channel as me.

When you reach the east again, sit or stand still. Take three deep breaths. Say,

> My thanks to God, Goddess and my guardians
> for being with me
> Return to your home, or stay if you wish.
> Hail and farewell. Blessed Be.

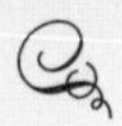

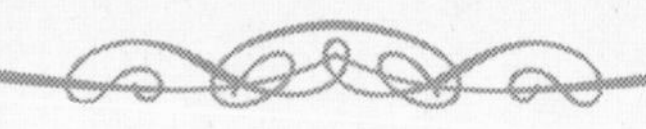

Flax

Linum usitatissimum

LINSEED, LINTBELLS

Part Used: seed

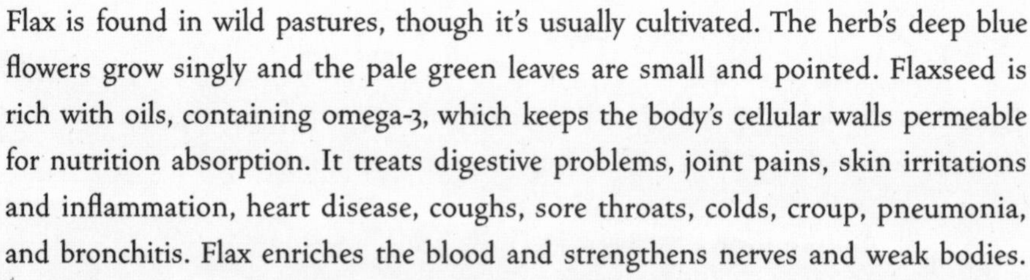

Flax is found in wild pastures, though it's usually cultivated. The herb's deep blue flowers grow singly and the pale green leaves are small and pointed. Flaxseed is rich with oils, containing omega-3, which keeps the body's cellular walls permeable for nutrition absorption. It treats digestive problems, joint pains, skin irritations and inflammation, heart disease, coughs, sore throats, colds, croup, pneumonia, and bronchitis. Flax enriches the blood and strengthens nerves and weak bodies.

Flaxseed oil is an effective laxative for babies and can relieve constipation. Flaxseed is very perishable and should be sealed and stored in a cool, dark place. Do not heat the oil, as this will cause it to lose its nutrient properties.

For relief from coughing or respiratory ailments, soak flaxseed overnight. Drain off the water, retaining the seeds. Infuse 1 cup of seeds in 2 cups of fresh water and let stand in a warm place for several hours. Strain and discard the seeds; add a teaspoon of honey to the liquid and drink. You can also pour warm flaxseed oil over steamed vegetables or grind seeds in a spice grinder to sprinkle over salads.

Flax is associated with Mercury in both his planetary and deity vibrations. In magick, flax is used in protection, banishing, and cleansing rituals. Flax is a good plant for the home and house blessings as it brings blessings and good health. Perform house blessings when moving into a new house, for cleansing after an argument, or for releasing negative energy.

IMMATURE FLAX SEEDPODS ARE VERY POISONOUS, SO THE SEEDS MUST BE HARVESTED WITH GREAT CARE.

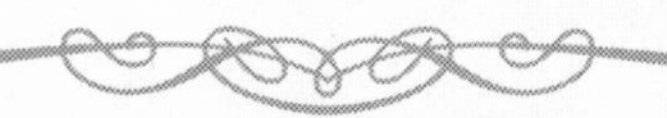

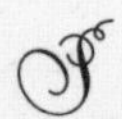

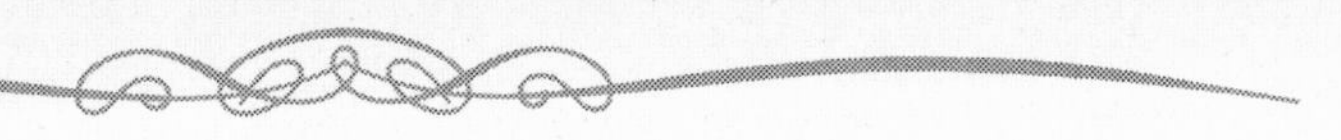
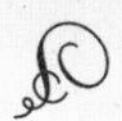

Go Nutty

Makes 12 to 16 balls

The following recipe makes a great high-protein snack. To grind the flaxseeds, I like to use a mortar with a pestle, which releases the seeds' oil.

½ cup almond butter
½ cup ground flaxseed
½ cup tahini
¼ cup protein powder
¼ cup ground sunflower seeds
¼ cup dried apricots, chopped
¼ cup maple syrup
½ cup dried shredded coconut

Flax does well in full sun with some aridity. It is native to temperate regions of Europe and Asia.

Combine the almond butter, flaxseed, tahini, protein powder, sunflower seeds, apricots, and syrup in a bowl. Roll the mixture into balls about the size of small walnuts. Roll the balls in the coconut. Keep refrigerated until ready to eat, but consume these treats within a week.

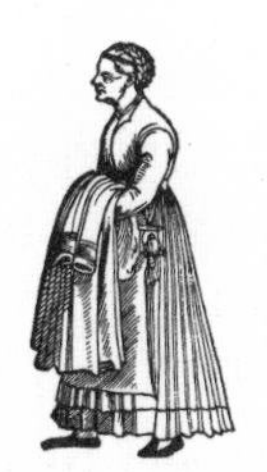

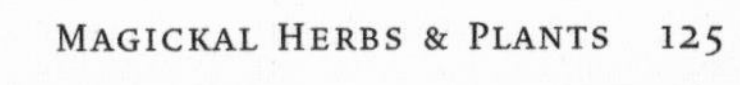

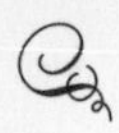

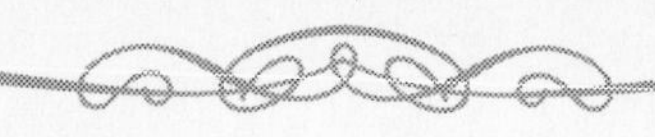

Foxglove

Digitalis purpurea

FAERY CAPS, FAERY GLOVE, FAERY THIMBLES, WITCHES' GLOVES

Part Used: leaves

Foxglove is found in hedgerows and deep ditches but most often grows in woodlands and shady gardens. Multiple tubular, thimble-shaped flowers bloom in purple, lavender, pink, and white on tall spikes. The hairy, grayish, oval leaves grow in clusters at the base of the plants. Foxgloves often attract hummingbirds.

Foxglove is a potent plant. It has poisonous qualities, as well as medicinal ones. A widely used heart medicine is produced from the powdered leaves. Externally the leaves can be applied to reduce inflammation and headaches. Foxglove can also increase blood pressure and a powerful diuretic. Foxglove is associated with Pluto and Venus, both the planets and deities.

EATING A SINGLE LEAF OF FOXGLOVE CAN CAUSE PARALYSIS AND SUDDEN DEATH, AND ALL PARTS OF THE PLANT ARE POISONOUS. IT SHOULD NEVER BE USED MEDICINALLY UNLESS PRESCRIBED AND THE DOSAGE CONTROLLED BY A HEALING PROFESSIONAL.

Root Survival

I include this herb purely in honor of the faeries, who call the pastel-colored flower home. Faeries, elves, and other little people have long been associated with the foxglove, as the folk names indicate. Faeries are earth angels who protect the plant world. They remind us of the beauty found in this earth plane. They point the way to the space between the mundane and the Divine, and are the holy spirit between creator and created. Trusting the guidance of the faeries will lead you to have faith in your ability to manifest heaven on earth. You will align with Spirit, and will be filled with abundance beyond measure.

If you are insecure about your basic needs being met, try the following ritual. For instance, are you afraid to explore living an artistic life outside the main-

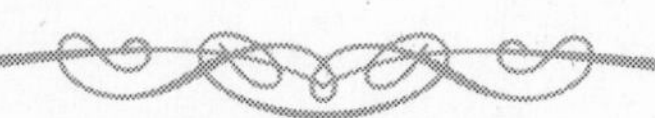

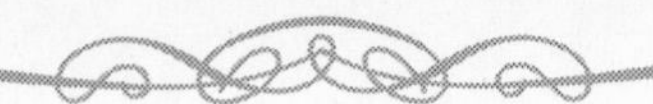

stream, because you assume you will not be able to pay your bills? Or maybe the rent or mortgage is due in five days and it's two weeks from payday, or you have a perpetual feeling that the rug (in the form of home, food, clothes, or a job) will be pulled out from under you. You may be tempted to manipulate your environment, including the people in it, to make sure your needs are met. You lack trust that the Universe will provide for your safety.

Divine Love always has met, and always will meet, every human need (Mary Baker Eddy). This is true for everyone. We may have made a sacred contract before incarnating that we would live life at a "primarily basic need" level, yet still we can never really be harmed. The most harm or unsafety that can come to us is caused by unkind or vicious words we believe to be true about ourselves.

FOXGLOVE IS A BIENNIAL PLANT THAT DOES WELL IN ALL ZONES. IT PREFERS LIGHT SHADE AND REGULAR WATERING. AFTER THE FIRST FLOWERING, DURING THE WANING MOON, CUT THE FIRST SPIKE FOR A FULLER LOOK. FOXGLOVE IS NATIVE TO EUROPE.

You can test for the feeling of distrust by checking out your root chakra. Imagine a red ball at your perennial floor (the area of the perineum). This energy vortex connects you with your survival and ability to ground and feel safe on the earthly plane. If the ball feels small or dense, go out and buy a foxglove. Let the faeries heal you.

Before you plant it, ask the faeries or nature devas (the spirits of the flower's essence) where they want the flower to be planted. Everyone has the power to communicate with the invisible realms. Trust your instincts. As soon as you hear the small voice, perceive the knowing guidance, or see the sparkle of light, you will know where to plant the flower. Don't argue with your instincts or messages from the faeries—this will only serve to confuse you.

Take three deep breaths. As you dig a hole for the plant, imagine a spark of pure, white light glowing from your heart center. Allow the light to grow. Watch it spread down your arms, up to your head, and through your legs, until it fills your entire being. See the light extend out to your aura (anywhere from one to four feet away from the physical boundaries of your body). This is your true self—pure light and love. Imagine what it would be like to be weightless light, able to move backward and forward through time and space. This was your only state of existence before you committed to a body, personality, and life situation.

Now massage the roots of the foxglove gently. As you do this, visualize sending a tendril of light from your aura to examine your parents, the home you will live

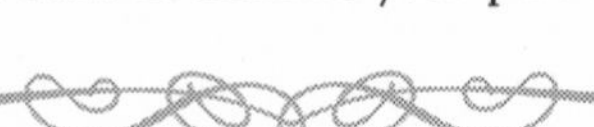

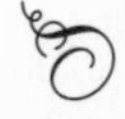

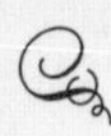

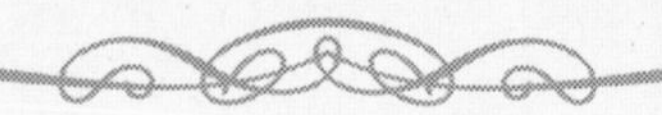

in, and any other surroundings as they were prior to your birth. What do you see, smell, hear, taste, or feel? Hold your finger up toward the sun until it glows red. Close your eyes and imagine what it was like before you were born, visiting your new body in utero. With your mind's eye, imagine the sun shining through your momma's belly, just as it did through your finger. Feel the sun's glow warming you. This is one of your first pleasurable encounters with the outside world. Hear your mother's heartbeat and tender voice. Play with your buoyancy.

Now retreat into your light self. Make a conscious decision to be part of the human tribe. Place the plant in the earth. Visualize your light swirling into the body of you as a baby. Watch as you are born. See the host of guardians and angels surrounding the birth. Imagine the plant's roots as your root chakra going into the earth. Send the energy about one foot below the soil and out horizontally to meet and merge with the energy flowing through all Mother Earth. You can now receive and give energy to all plants, deserts, mountains, oceans, people, animals—all of creation. You are part of a connected system that always supports you and your needs.

As you fill in the dirt around the plant, see your light shine from within the babe that is you. Know that no matter what physical being you occupy, your essence is always light and fully supported. You are one who chose to grow and thrive on this earthly plane for an incarnation. To get upset about the limitations of your body or state of awareness would be as fruitless as dreaming about being a fox who wishes to be an eagle. Either enjoy the gifts of fox, or change the dream.

Now feel your heart center. Feel the love and light grow in this area. Visualize the energy growing huge until a bright green ball fills your chest. When it is complete, imagine a white spiral door spinning open at the crown of your head. All knowledge and ability to manifest dreams and thrive in the human world passes through this energy vortex. You need only keep this door open to have access to divine wisdom from the true self of light and love. Imagine the energy moving from your crown chakra, through your heart, and down to your root chakra in a diagonal line. See the energy loop around and move back up to your crown chakra in a figure eight, the symbol of infinity and you, All That Is.

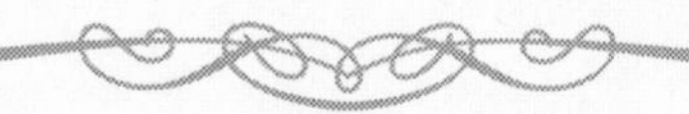

Frankincense

Boswellia sacra

INCENSE, OLIBANUM, OLIBANS

Part Used: gum

Frankincense has oblong, serrated leaves and white or pale pink flowers. Incense made from this tree's resin is often used in Hebrew, Catholic, and pagan religious practices. It invokes the deities Bel, Adonis, Apollo, and Demeter, who bring favor and success to the magickal practitioner. Frankincense incense is often wafted over magickal tools to consecrate or bless them with pure intent. This powerful protective herb is used in protection, purification, prosperity, banishing, manifestation, and consecration rituals or spells. It increases clairvoyance and concentration and is particularly successful when used in conjunction with the sun.

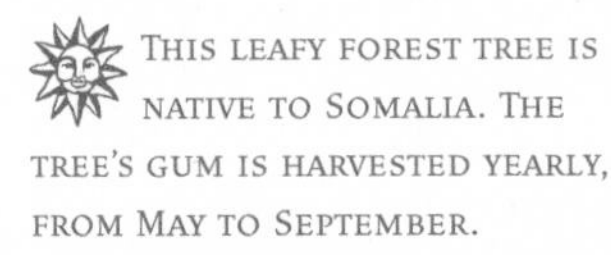
This leafy forest tree is native to Somalia. The tree's gum is harvested yearly, from May to September.

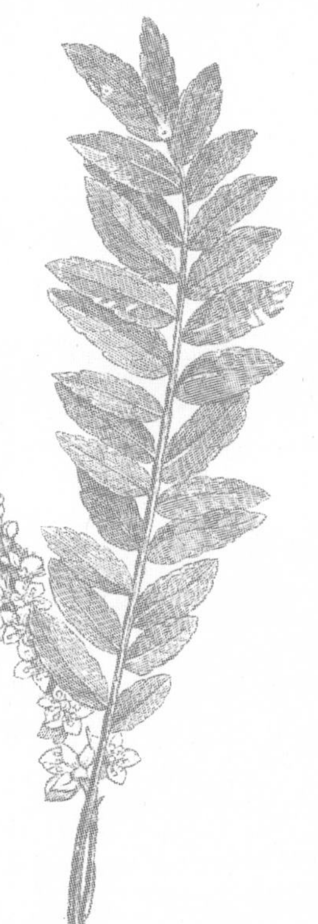

Jingle Bell Candle

Frankincense is associated with Yule and thus fits perfectly with the Yule-time craft described here. *Yule* is a Norse word meaning "wheel." The wheel of life represents a cyclical pattern of living. Moving deeper into the Wiccan craft and changing from the cerebral to the intuitive way of behaving and being can be scary. We have grown accustomed to following rules and the familiar way of things keeps us feeling grounded. The modern world is fast-paced, and we are learning life lessons faster; but not all of it makes sense to our logical minds. We must learn to be comfortable with not knowing all the answers immediately.

1 (12-inch) red or green pillar candle
4 drops myrrh oil
4 drops frankincense oil
20-gauge and 24-gauge gold craft wire
3 small gold jingle bells
1 silver jewelry headpin
Gold decorative paper

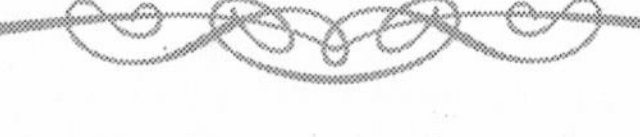

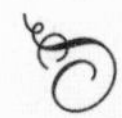

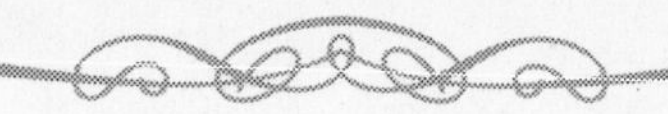

Anoint the candle with the oils. Cut four 4-inch lengths of the 20-gauge wire and bend into a spiral shape with handheld pliers. Cut one 12-inch length of 34-gauge wire and thread the jingle bells onto it, positioning them in the middle. Twist the wire a few times to secure, leaving a tail at both ends. Wrap the jingle bells around the headpin and curl the wire ends. Tighten the wire if necessary. Trim the headpin with wire cutters to about 2 inches long and insert spiral wire shapes and bells into the candle. Measure the circumference of the candle base and add ¼ inch to this measurement. Cut a strip of the gold paper 1½ inches wide and the measured length. Trim 1 edge of the strip with decorative-edged scissors. Wrap the paper around the base of the candle and glue at the back.

As you burn the candle, let your intuition develop and trust it. Living your life on the rhythmic mandala of Nature will provide an example of how to relax into the ebb and flow of energy. Let the power of frankincense catapult you into a world where you are one with the seasons, living as another spoke on the wheel.

Cleopatra Perfume

Frankincense can be used to alleviate jet lag and give you a jump-start when you're feeling the afternoon slumps. This perfume below is a bit costly, but when you are in the mood, it's worth it! Frankincense is a strong manifester. Before you wear the perfume, perform the following ritual to charge your essence with the ability to actualize or become all that you were meant to be. As you make this perfume, ask yourself what it is that you want. Record the following ritual and allow it to play in the background as you work. (Sharon Rettich, the creator of this ritual, is an artist-designer and founder of the website Legacy of the Cauldron. Michael Riley created the perfume.)

Become intimate with that part of you that desires; the part of you that knows you can manifest your dreams; it is your destiny to have joy. Become aware of that part of you that does not want fulfillment: the martyr, the victim, the long-suffering struggler. Know that if that part of you did not exist, you would probably already have your heart's desire. Know the possible "payoffs" that result in not having your heart's desire: the "opportunity" to blame, the "opportunity" to hold onto that anger.

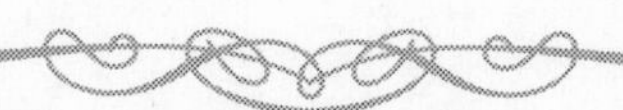

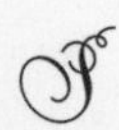

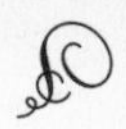

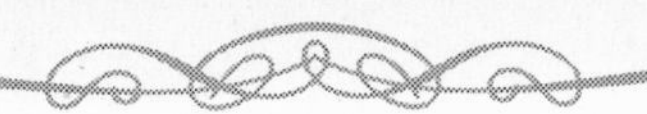

Success does not happen to those who deserve it, but to those who choose it. What choices have you been making? The power to choose lies at the very core of your being. From this place of power, know and understand that the choices really are yours to make. Make the choice to have your heart's desire! Go deep. Know thyself. To thine own self be true.

With the confidence and the dignity of knowing every desire comes the means to make it happen—in the presence of God, Goddess, and All That Is, your higher self and all your unseen friends—declare your desire with clear and precise intent. Release your desire to the creative womb of the Mother, represented by the cauldron. Know that as your desire blends with the energy of the cauldron and the energy of creation, it is given form. With harm to none. So mote it be!

Dab this perfume on your skin as a body scent, or add a little to the bath salts recipe on page 141. A drop on your handkerchief is a great magickal aromatherapy to remind yourself how powerful you are.

- 20 drops frankincense oil
- 7 drops myrrh oil
- 5 drops jasmine oil
- 3 drops musk oil
- 2 drops gardenia oil
- 1 drop sandalwood oil
- 1 drop honeysuckle oil
- ½ drop clove oil (optional)

In a glass bowl, gently mix all ingredients together. Pour into a glass bottle or vial with a tight-fitting lid and let stand for 2 to 3 weeks to blend. Stored in a cool, dark place or refrigerated, the perfume will keep for 2 to 3 years.

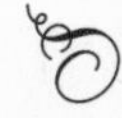

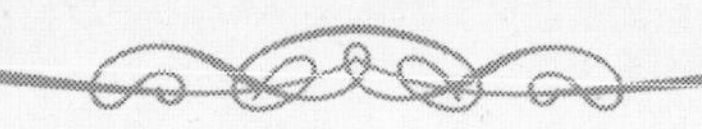

Gardenia

Gardenia jasminoides (also called Gardenia augusta)

Part Used: flower

Gardenia is an evergreen shrub; its white flowers contrast sharply with dark green, shiny leaves. Gardenia attracts love and passion. It has added potency when used in conjunction with the moon. If the moon is waxing, concentrate on beginnings, new love, increasing finances, and building friendships or partnerships. While the moon is full, focus on manifestation, the power of the present moment, and wishes. During a waning moon, banish negativity, initiate peaceful separations, and end undesirable habits. At the dark of the moon, rest, reflect, and rejuvenate. Gardenia is associated with the planet and goddess Venus.

Ostara Candle

Flowers abound during spring, celebrated at the sabbat of Ostara, also known as Earrach or Vernal Equinox. It is the midpoint of the waxing year when the spark of light—the sun—born at the winter solstice reaches maturity. This is the time of dawn, the festivals of the Grecian goddess Eos and the Old English Ostara (both goddesses of dawn), Persephone's return from the Underworld, and the rebirth of Adonis the beautiful.

Spring celebrations honor planting, abundance, and the greening of Mother Nature. The revitalization of the bright sunshine warms the earth and her children. Flowers bloom with rainbow colors, signifying that life has once again returned to the land of women and men.

Eggs have always been symbols of fertility, life, and spring. In the Ukraine, eggs were given as gifts, and each color represented a particular wish. Only women decorated these eggs during a spring ritual known as Pysansky. The women gathered eggs from hens who lived near a rooster; an infertile egg could bring barrenness to the home. The women worked unobserved, to keep evil away, transferring the goodness of the household into the designs on the eggs. Secret family recipes were

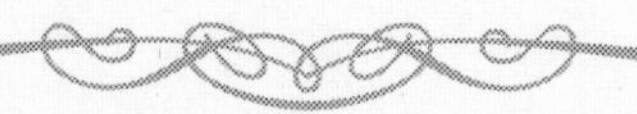

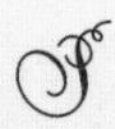

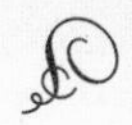

used for mixing the dyes and the women placed special blessings on each egg. The meanings of the colors varied from village to village; some examples are pink for success; purple for faith, trust, or spirituality; red for passion, love, courage, or hope; orange for tenacity, power, or drive; yellow for wisdom or the harvest; green for spring, rebirth, youth, or happiness; blue for health or calm; white for purity; and black for remembrance. Allow the color of the candle you choose to bring a special wish to you.

Decide in advance how you want to arrange the flowers on the candle, because you need to work quickly while the wax is soft.

1 bright jewel-colored pillar candle, any size
4 to 6 pressed gardenia flowers
Colorless granulated wax (without stearic acid)

Place an aluminum can that is larger than the candle in a warm place and fill it ¾ full with water. Heat the back of a spoon over a lighter or a lit match, and wipe away any soot that transfers to it. Using the warmed spoon, melt the sides of the candle slightly in the desired area and press the flowers into the wax.

Put the candle inside the aluminum can of water; be sure that it reaches to the bottom. Remove the candle from the water, and then scratch a mark inside the can to mark the water level. Pour out the water. Fill the can with granulated wax up to the mark, and place it in a pot of gently simmering water. Melt the wax until it reaches 180°F; you can use a candy thermometer to measure the temperature. (Do not allow the wax to get too hot, or the next step will not work.)

Using protective gloves, remove the can from the pot and place on a heatproof work surface. Using pliers, grasp the candle by the wick, and in one smooth motion, submerge the candle evenly into the melted wax, then lift it out. Repeat the dipping process to thicken the wax layer. (Dipping quickly creates a thinner layer, and dipping slowly creates a thicker layer.) After the candle cools a little, press the edges of the flowers into place under the coats of wax. Using the pliers, grip the wick and dip the candle into a bowl of ice water for a shiny finish.

Note: You can purchase granulated wax from an arts and crafts store.

This fragrant flower prefers sun on the coast, filtered shade in hot valleys, and moist soil. It can tolerate temperatures as low as 20°F, but in areas where the winters get colder, it should be grown indoors. Gardenia is native to the southeastern provinces of China.

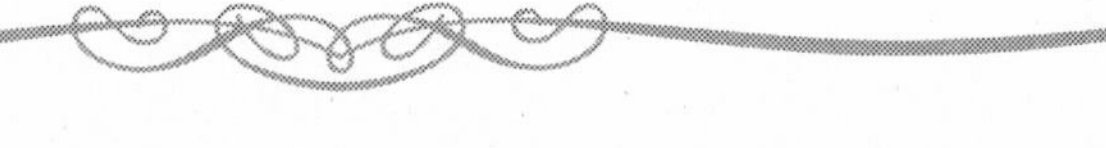

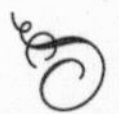

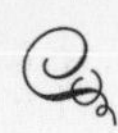

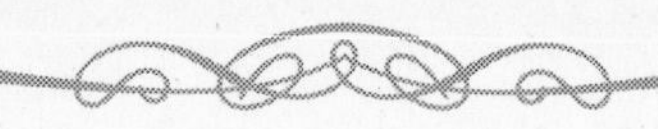

Garlic

Allium sativum

CLOVE GARLIC, POOR MAN'S TREACLE, STINKING ROSE

Parts Used: cloves, leaves, flowers

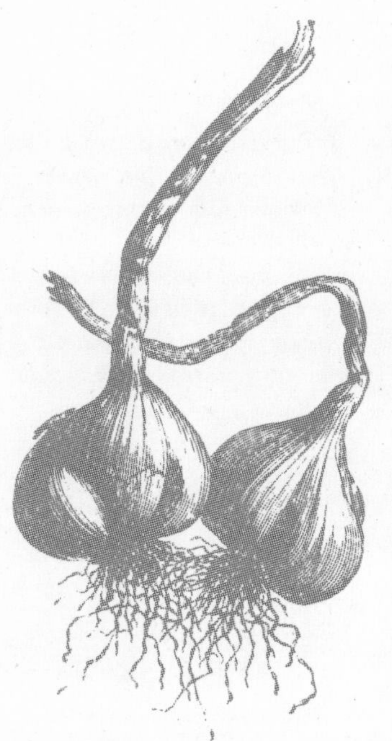

Garlic is widely cultivated, though wild relatives can be found in damp pastures and woodlands. It has a strong scent and oval leaves. Since the first century B.C., garlic has been known as an aid that "clears arteries and opens the mouths of veins," as stated by Dioscorides. Garlic's healing properties are revered by three classic healing systems: European medicine, Ayurvedic tradition, and traditional Chinese medicine. Some research has shown that garlic may help prevent cancer. Its main curative powers fight bacterial and fungal infections, lower high blood pressure and cholesterol levels, and aid the digestive system. Garlic is a strong antiseptic and works wonders on the mucous membranes. It is used to treat disorders of the blood and lungs, including tuberculosis. It protects the body and hair from parasites, wards off infections, and helps with asthma, high blood pressure, whooping cough, goiter, arthritis, sciatica, and rheumatism.

Garlic's powers are so pervasive that if you place a garlic clove in your shoe, within fifteen minutes the smell of garlic will be on your breath. Garlic powder or juice can be added directly to a dog's or cat's food to help them expel most types of parasites; but this must be done in moderation, especially for cats. Magickally, garlic is a powerful herb used for protection and banishing. Garlic is associated with the planetary and deity associations of Mars, Hecate, the moon, and the Triple Goddess.

Marvelous Marinara Sauce

MAKES 8 CUPS

There are so many recipes that can be made with garlic. From ice cream to main dishes to eggs, the choices appear endless. This stinking rose with its aromatic cloves is most memorable to me in Italian dishes, so I use it in this simple recipe for marinara sauce.

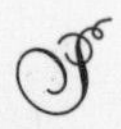

When possible, grow your own garlic, and make sure that the plants have plenty of sun. When I planted my bulbs last winter, I found out that spacing isn't a terribly important issue for garlic. I made pretty, neat rows of garlic and red onion, and then went inside for a glass of water. When I returned, my sons had dug holes throughout the patch of earth and dropped the garlic wherever they pleased. They covered them so quickly that the only evidence of their work was the empty bag. I let the garlic grow, allowing for the creativity of children, rather than digging up and replanting them. While the red onion suffered (I hardly got two), there was plenty of garlic. They grew on top of each other, smashed together, and underneath one another. I braided the stems and hung them in my kitchen. They turn out incredibly juicy—well worth the effort.

2 tablespoons olive oil
4 garlic cloves, chopped
6 cups diced and seeded plum tomatoes
1 (4-ounce) can tomato paste
2 tablespoons chopped fresh basil
2 tablespoons chopped fresh oregano
½ teaspoon nutmeg
½ teaspoon sugar

In a large heavy skillet, heat the oil over medium heat. Add the garlic and cook until soft, about 2 minutes. Do not brown. Stir in tomatoes, tomato paste, basil, oregano, nutmeg, and sugar. Simmer until the sauce thickens, about 30 minutes. Season with salt and pepper to taste.

Garlic Mashed Potatoes

SERVES 4

When you first come out of the broom closet, you may feel protective about your newly regained connection with nature. Some people will not understand; they may ask about ridiculous rumors such as witches flying on broomsticks. (Tell them that using brooms to fly is outdated: these days, we use vacuum cleaners for long distances and dust busters for short trips.)

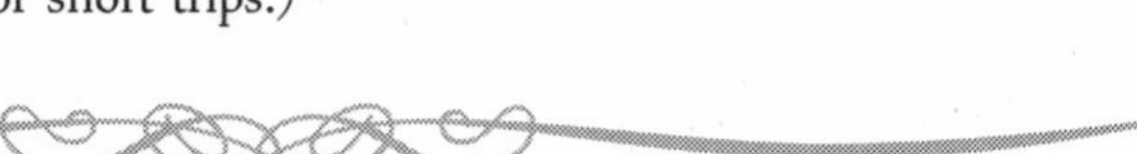

PLANT WHOLE BULBS OR INDIVIDUAL CLOVES IN THE WINTER AFTER THE GROUND HAS THAWED. HARVEST IN MID SEPTEMBER OR WHEN THE LEAVES HAVE TURNED YELLOW. GARLIC PREFERS WARM CLIMATES; FULL SUN; HUMUSY, COMPOSTED SOIL; AND REGULAR WATERING. TO KEEP APHIDS AWAY FROM ROSES, PLANT GARLIC NEARBY; PLANTED AROUND CARROTS, TOMATOES, CUCUMBERS, POTATOES, SPINACH, AND LETTUCE, IT WILL ENHANCE THEIR GROWTH. DO NOT PLANT NEAR CABBAGE, BEANS, OR PEAS. GARLIC IS NATIVE TO CENTRAL ASIA.

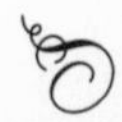

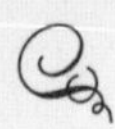

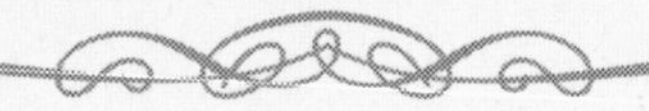

When you are faced with family, friends, or even a community who do not understand your religion, do not despair. It matters not if they understand, or think its funny and hip to put Quan Yin on the back of a motorcycle in an MTV music video. You must persist. The wise and healthy use laughter as their best medicine. Ultimately, you must discern your own worth. Repeat the affirmation "What you think is none of my business."

As you make this dish, allow Hecate's humor to help you lighten up and continue to breathe the gentle luminescent path. The seeds will fall where they may, and some will take root. Stay on your path; it will light you up.

2 medium heads garlic, cloves separated, skin left on
2 pounds russet potatoes, unpeeled, scrubbed
½ cup (1 stick) unsalted butter
1 cup half-and-half

In a small skillet over the lowest possible heat, toast the garlic cloves, covered, until they are brown-spotted and slightly softened; shaking frequently for about 20 to 22 minutes. Meanwhile, place the potatoes in a large pot and add enough cold water to cover. Bring to a boil over high heat. Decrease the heat to medium-low and cook, covered, for 20 to 30 minutes. Take the garlic off the heat and let cool 15 to 20 minutes until fully softened. When cooled, peel off the skins and cut off the woody root ends. Set aside. Drain the potatoes. Cut into large chunks. Mash the potatoes and garlic together. Whisk in the butter and half-and-half. Season to taste with salt and pepper.

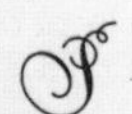

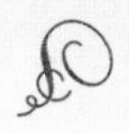

Geranium

Pelargonium (various species)

STORKSBILL

Parts Used: leaves, flowers

Traditionally, geranium is best known for its astringent properties and ability to clean and heal wounds. The flowers range in color from white to vibrant pinks and reds. Red geranium carries magickal protection powers, while white geranium promotes fertility.

Today geranium is used in a variety of home decorations. The flowers dry beautifully and are used in wreaths, potpourris, and soaps. There are many different kinds of scented geranium that will add a unique magickal and practical element to your spells and rituals. Geranium's highest magickal powers are fertility, healing, love, and protection. Its associated deities are Aphrodite, Isis, Gaia, Eros, Hecate, Venus, Mars, and the god known as the Horned One. Geranium resonates with the astrological sign of Libra.

Rose-Geranium Pound Cake

MAKES 2 CAKES

Rose geranium (the common name for various species and cultivars, including *Pelargonium capitatum* and *Pelargonium graveolons*) has citrus and rose scents that are quite pleasant. An essential oil made from it can be rubbed on women's wrists to ease menstrual cramps, depression, menopausal symptoms, hormonal imbalances, and fluid retention. When added to skin lotions and creams, it has been known to aid acne, eczema, and inflamed and infected wounds, and even to delay wrinkles. The rose component of this type of geranium imbues the plant with love's power.

A classic pound cake is made with a pound each of butter, sugar, flour, and eggs. Traditionally, the ingredients for a pound cake are listed in weight measurements,

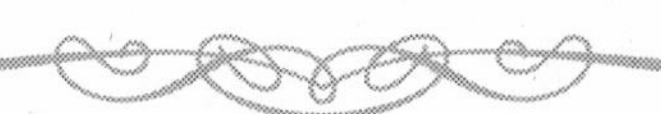

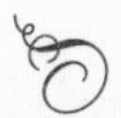

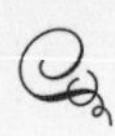
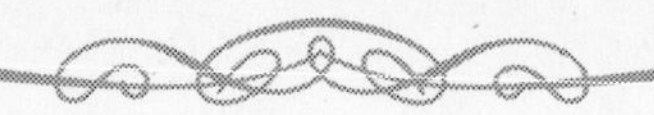

however, I have also listed the ingredients below in standard measurements for those who do not have kitchen scales. (This recipe comes from the archives of Joyce and Barbara Seidner at the Village Kitchen Shoppe in Glendora, California.)

Nonstick vegetable oil spray

12 to 16 organically grown rose geranium leaves, wiped clean, stemmed

1 pound (4 sticks) unsalted butter, room temperature

1 pound (2 cups) sugar

1 pound (2 cups) flour

2 teaspoons baking powder

9 large eggs, separated

2 teaspoons vanilla extract or almond extract

1 cup heavy whipping cream

Preheat oven to 325°F. Place a rack in the center of the oven. Spray two 9 by 4-inch loaf pans with nonstick spray and line with parchment. Arrange geranium leaves, with outside of leaves facing pan, along bottom and up sides of pan. Set aside.

Using an electric mixer, beat butter and sugar until light and fluffy, 2 to 3 minutes. In a separate bowl, mix together the flour and baking powder. With the mixer on low speed, add the yolks 1 at a time to the butter mixture, alternating with the flour mixture. With the mixer on medium speed, beat in the vanilla and cream (the batter will be thick). Transfer the batter to a large mixing bowl. Set aside. Using clean dry beaters, whip the whites until stiff peaks form. Using a rubber spatula, stir about ¼ of the whites into the batter to lighten. Fold in the remaining whites. Carefully spoon the batter into the prepared pans. Place additional leaves on top of the batter. Bake 80 to 90 minutes, or until a cake tester inserted into the loaves comes out clean. Let cool in pans on a wire rack for 1½ hours, and then remove from pans. Peel off the leaves. Wrap the cakes tightly in plastic wrap and keep at room temperature overnight; pound cakes always taste better served the day after they are baked.

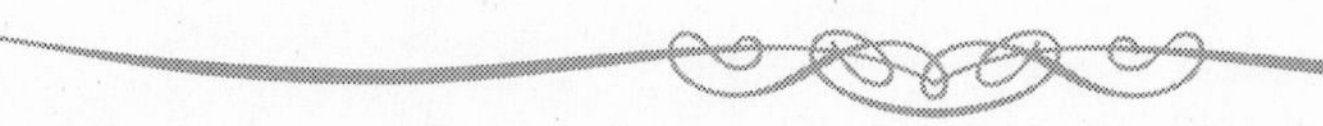

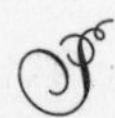

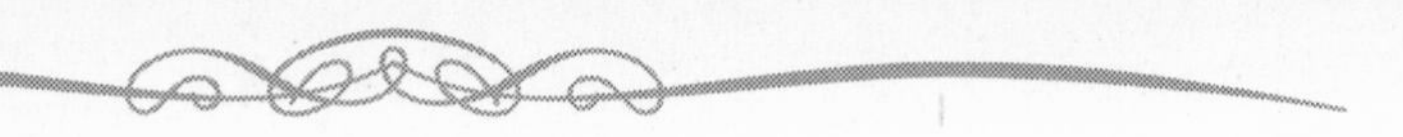

Love Powder

Creating homemade body treatments can be incredibly satisfying. Not only will you be sure the ingredients are safe and pure, but by imbuing the products with focused intent, your creations will be full of your personal energy. Once you have mastered this, you can substitute different oils and scents to match your moods. This silky homemade powder feels good on the skin and can be used to dry your body quickly or to slow down perspiration. Alternatively, it can be used for light tissue massages—usually quite erotic.

- ½ cup cornstarch
- ½ cup arrowroot powder
- 10 scented geranium leaves, washed, patted dry
- 2 or 3 drops geranium essential oil

Mix the cornstarch, arrowroot powder, geranium leaves, and oil in a wide-mouthed glass jar with a lid. Seal the lid and shake. Shake the container once every day for 4 days. On the fourth day, remove the leaves; your powder is ready to use. You can apply the powder with a puff or shake it from a flour shaker.

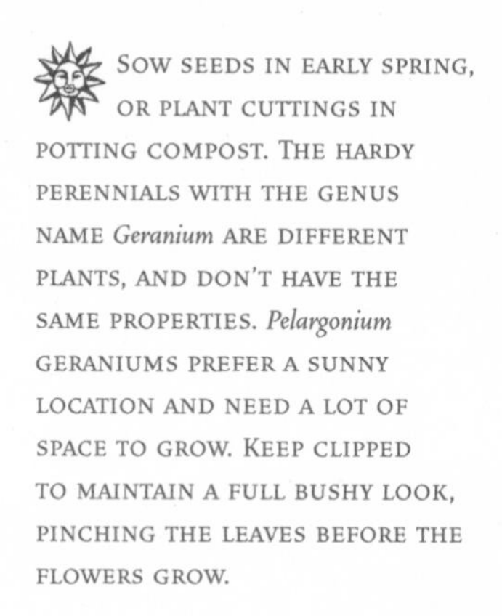

SOW SEEDS IN EARLY SPRING, OR PLANT CUTTINGS IN POTTING COMPOST. THE HARDY PERENNIALS WITH THE GENUS NAME *Geranium* ARE DIFFERENT PLANTS, AND DON'T HAVE THE SAME PROPERTIES. *Pelargonium* GERANIUMS PREFER A SUNNY LOCATION AND NEED A LOT OF SPACE TO GROW. KEEP CLIPPED TO MAINTAIN A FULL BUSHY LOOK, PINCHING THE LEAVES BEFORE THE FLOWERS GROW.

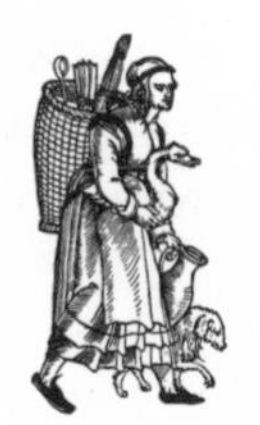

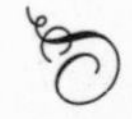

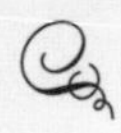

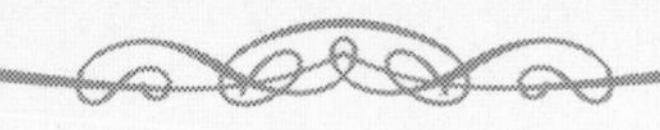

Ginger

Zingiber officinale

CANTON GINGER, TRUE GINGER

Parts Used: root, leaves

Ginger is widely cultivated but can be found in wild shady places, woodlands, and hedgerows. Its leaves are lance-shaped and it has plumelike golden flowers that are pleasantly fragrant. Ginger is highly praised in Chinese medicine, in which it has been used for its curative powers since 3000 B.C. Ginger's properties are warming, aromatic, stimulating, and digestive. Ginger is a general tonic for nerves and the digestive organs; its primary healing abilities are to quell motion sickness and prevent indigestion. To experience this relief, you can either drink an infusion as a tea or suck on candied ginger. Ginger eases pain from gas and diarrhea, ovulation, morning sickness, and menstrual cramps. It also relieves vomiting and stimulates saliva flow and digestive activity. The fresh leaves can be used in poultices. Ginger is associated with the moon.

Asparagus Seduction

SERVES 2 AS AN APPETIZER

Ginger has a hot element and when combined with passion-inducing incantations brings about a wonderfully seductive outcome. This recipe draws on the fiery male energy of the divine nature, and is used for enticing your lover. Balanced with the allure of the moon, ginger awakens necessary attributes for a rousing lovemaking session. Asparagus is a phallic symbol.

12 to 16 asparagus stalks
1 tablespoon butter
1 tablespoon grated peeled fresh ginger

Blanch the asparagus in rapidly boiling water for 3 to 5 minutes, or until they turn bright green. Drain and place in a dish filled with ice. Melt the butter in a

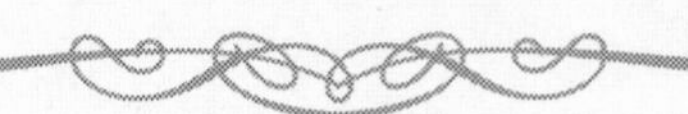

skillet over medium-low heat. Lightly sauté the ginger in the butter 1 minute. Drain the asparagus and add to the skillet. Stir to coat. Serve immediately.

White Ginger Musk

In Hawaii, white ginger flowers are traditionally used in wedding bouquets to give good cheer and health to the bride and groom. Ginger carries creativity, the fire of inspiration, psychic abilities, and powers of good health and success. This is an effective perfume to help you reclaim your life. White ginger (*Hedychium coronarum*) is a species with very sweet-smelling flowers that are reminiscent of honeysuckle, jasmine, and lemon flowers. For this recipe, you will need a test tube or other small round-bottomed glass container with a stopper.

Ginger's roots spread far and wide and are difficult to uproot once they have established themselves. It prefers fertile soil and plenty of watering. Ginger is native to Asia and is cultivated in tropical regions.

3 parts musk oil
2 parts vanilla oil
1 part white ginger oil

Gently swirl all ingredients in a test tube or round-bottomed flask. Cork the container and let it sit in the dark at least 14 days. Use as a body scent or put a few drops in your bath. You can also add the oil to the following bath salt base. Store the container in the refrigerator and use the musk within 2 or 3 years.

Basic Bath Salt Base

This is a basic bath salt recipe that can be varied by adding oils or perfumes to it. The white ginger musk above is an excellent additive or try the honeysuckle or sandalwood perfumes on pages 154 and 233.

3 parts kosher salt or sea salt
2 parts baking soda
2 parts Epsom salts

Mix together all the ingredients. To add scent, mix in an oil or perfume drop by drop until the mixture smells pleasing. Use between 2 tablespoons and ½ cup per bath, as you please. Store bath salts in an air-tight container and use within 1 year.

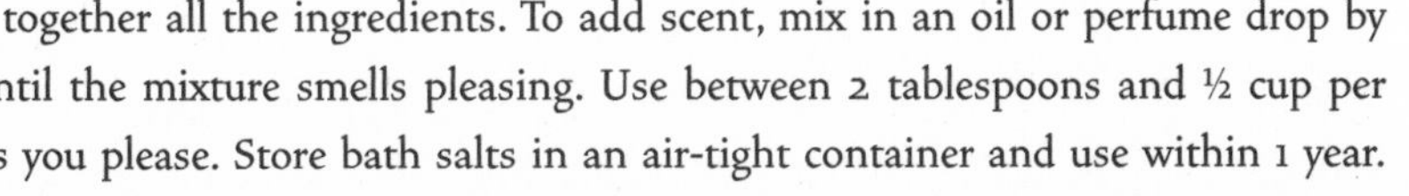

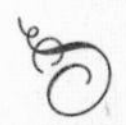

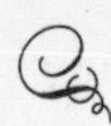

Ginseng

Panax pseudoginseng (Korean), Panax quinquefoliusm (American)

A DOSE OF IMMORTALITY, MAN ROOT, ROOT OF IMMORTALITY, ROOT OF LIFE, SANG

Part Used: root

Ginseng grows in hot and humid climates. The plant's leaves are narrow, glossy, and bright green, with rarely seen yellowish green flowers. Varieties of ginseng have been used for two thousand years from China to North America. Ginseng should not be harvested in the wild, as it takes many years to mature and is becoming endangered. According to history, ginseng promises long life and wisdom. These attributes, combined with ginseng's alleged effect as an aphrodisiac, caused wars all across ginseng territory in historic China. Among its many powers, ginseng is quite beneficial for women. It reduces menstrual problems, relieves exhaustion during childbirth, aids colic, and alleviates the stress and hot flashes associated with menopause. Ginseng has also been known to aid headaches, fever, vomiting, and earaches, to increase sexual desire, and to rejuvenate the fatigued. Ginseng's medicinal properties are believed to treat every human ailment, so it carries with it all possibilities of health and abundant living. Ginseng is associated with the planet and deity Uranus.

Clarity of Wishes

Often, when we desire an outcome or consider prayer or spellwork, we think we know the way to happiness, peace, prosperity, or love. But this is not always true. Messages and guidance we receive from Spirit can be muddled by our perceptions of what we deem acceptable. This ritual declares that the signs leading to fulfillment of your desires be made clear.

1 white candle
Blessing oil

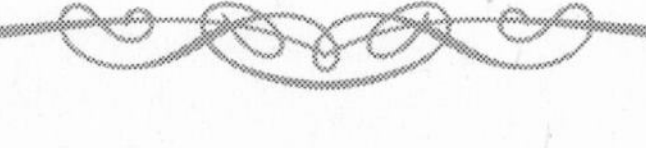

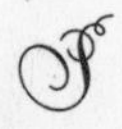

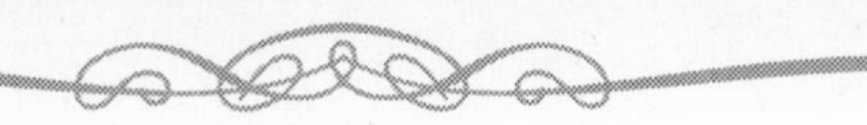

1 teaspoon crushed dried ginseng root
1 teaspoon minced peeled fresh ginger
Small container of salt
1 clear quartz crystal

At the dark of the moon, anoint a white candle with blessing oil. Grind the ginseng root. Sprinkle the ginger and the ginseng over the unlit candle. Hold up a small container of salt in the direction of the north, and bless it by saying,

Element of salt
Pure by nature from all contamination and negativity
I bless thee with my pure intent.

Hold up a small vessel of water in the direction of the west, and bless it by saying,

Element of water
I free thee of contamination and negativity
I bless thee with my pure intent.

Combine the salt and water and sprinkle over a clear quartz crystal. Say,

With holy water, I bless this crystal
With love and light
So that my vision is clear
By my divine right.

Consider the issue that is cloudy for you. Ask for clarity. Light the candle. Hold the crystal close to you and quiet your mind. Focus your attention on your third eye (the area at the center of your forehead) for intelligence and intuitive mental clarity, on your heart center for matters of love and relationships, or on your solar plexus for issues regarding power. When you get a message, write it down. Do not wait for an explosion of words; Spirit often comes quietly.

GINSENG LIKES SHADE AND HEAVY WATER AFTER GROWTH STARTS. IT IS DIFFICULT TO GROW AND IS NOT READY TO USE FOR MANY YEARS. GINSENG IS NATIVE TO CHINA, EASTERN RUSSIA, NORTH KOREA, AND NORTH AMERICA.

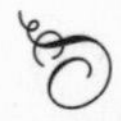

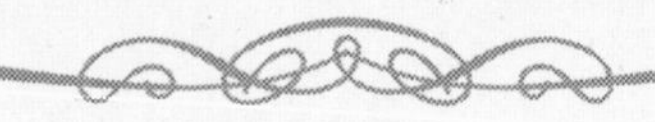

Goldenseal

Hydrastis canadensis

EYE BALM, JAUNDICE ROOT, ORANGEROOT, YELLOW PUCCOON

Part Used: root

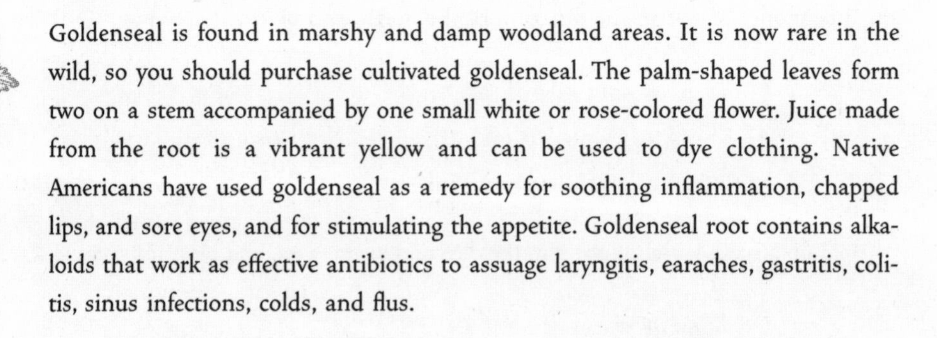

Goldenseal is found in marshy and damp woodland areas. It is now rare in the wild, so you should purchase cultivated goldenseal. The palm-shaped leaves form two on a stem accompanied by one small white or rose-colored flower. Juice made from the root is a vibrant yellow and can be used to dye clothing. Native Americans have used goldenseal as a remedy for soothing inflammation, chapped lips, and sore eyes, and for stimulating the appetite. Goldenseal root contains alkaloids that work as effective antibiotics to assuage laryngitis, earaches, gastritis, colitis, sinus infections, colds, and flus.

THE ALKALOIDS IN GOLDENSEAL ROOT ARE POISONOUS IN LARGE DOSES, SO IT SHOULD NOT BE USED, EVEN EXTERNALLY, WITHOUGH THE APPROVAL OF A HEALTH PRACTITIONER. AVOID USING GOLDENSEAL DURING PREGNANCY.

Goldenseal Salve

This salve helps relieve psoriasis and itchy skin. Allow goldenseal's association with Venus to help you birth a new identity. Skin represents our individuality; it has the ability to touch others and to release negativity.

- ⅓ cup powdered goldenseal root
- ⅓ cup dried burdock leaves
- ⅓ cup myrrh gum
- ¾ cup (180 ml) extra virgin olive oil
- ¼ cup (55 grams) beeswax
- 6 to 8 drops tea tree oil
- 6 to 8 drops essential oil for fragrance, such as lavender or rosemary

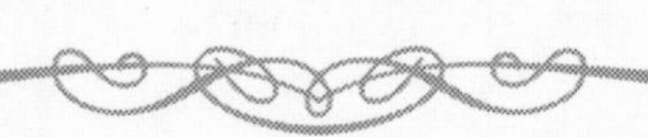

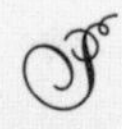

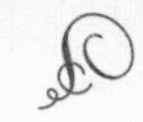

In the top of a double boiler set over simmering water, heat the goldenseal, burdock, myrrh gum, and olive oil 1 hour. Do not allow the mixture to boil. Strain the mixture through muslin or cheesecloth into a stainless steel pot. When just cool enough to handle, wrap the strained herbs in the same fabric and wring out excess oil. Add the beeswax to the oil and heat until melted. Check for desired consistency by placing a tablespoon of the mixture in your freezer for 1 minute. If it's too soft, add more beeswax; if it's too hard, add more oil. Immediately remove the mixture from the heat and add the tea tree and fragrance oils. Pour the salve into small glass jars and store in a cool, dark place. Stored this way, the salve will last for several years.

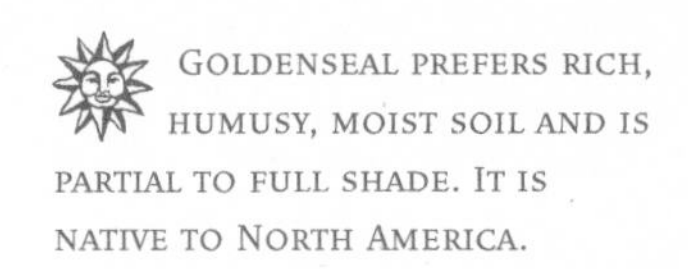

Goldenseal prefers rich, humusy, moist soil and is partial to full shade. It is native to North America.

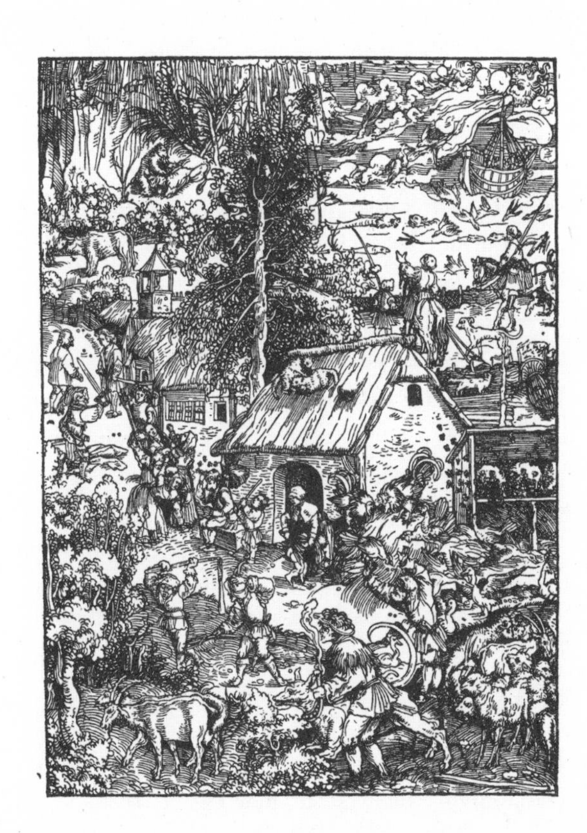

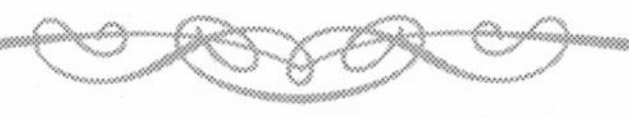

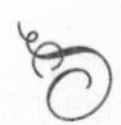

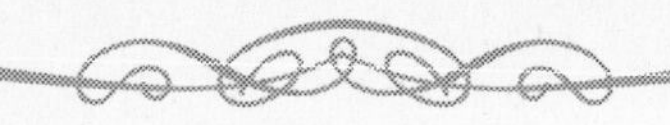

Hawthorn

Crataegus (various species)

FAERIETHORN, HUATH, MAY BLOSSOM, TREE OF CHASTITY, WHITE THORN

Parts Used: berries, flowers, leaves

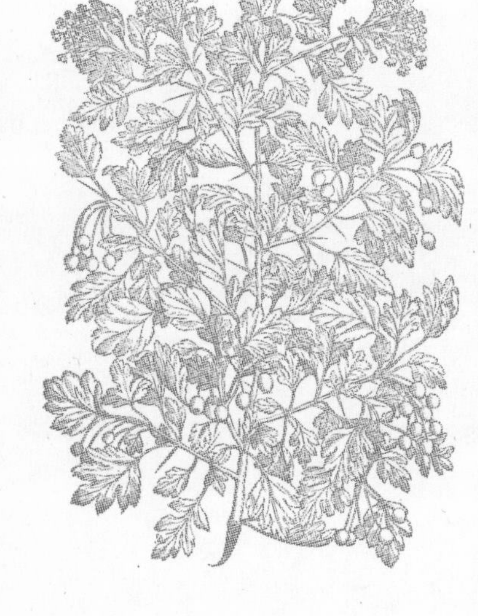

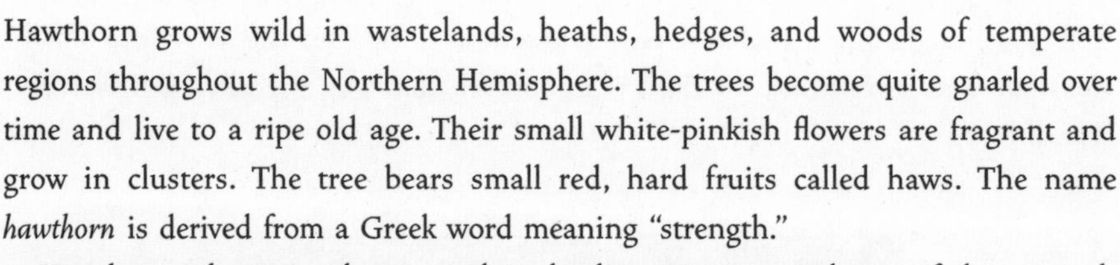

Hawthorn grows wild in wastelands, heaths, hedges, and woods of temperate regions throughout the Northern Hemisphere. The trees become quite gnarled over time and live to a ripe old age. Their small white-pinkish flowers are fragrant and grow in clusters. The tree bears small red, hard fruits called haws. The name *hawthorn* is derived from a Greek word meaning "strength."

Hawthorn takes a gentle approach to healing. It eases weakness of the stomach and cardiovascular system by incremental measures. When the fruit and leaves are used for six months, research shows that they can dilate the arteries, which improves circulation to the extremities, promotes blood circulation, and lowers blood pressure. Taken as a tea or tincture, it has also been recommended to assist irregular heartbeat, regulate high or low blood pressure, and prevent miscarriage.

Hawthorn flowers can be added to a salad, while the fruits make an excellent wine. Hawthorn was an essential plant to early British pagans, who called it *huath* (the ogham name for the letter *h*). It was one of the most important plants for Beltane rituals, as it was thought to stand between the mundane world and the Otherworld of the land of Fey. Hawthorn is used magickally for protection. It is associated with the planet and deity Mars.

TAKEN IN LARGE DOSES, HAWTHORN CAN BE TOXIC. CONSULT A HEALTH PRACTITIONER BEFORE USING MEDICINALLY.

Beltane Soap

MAKES 3 BARS

In early times, Beltane or May Day was a fertility festival, celebrating the promise of the crops and the fecundity of the livestock. May Day festivities were often presided over by the May King and May Queen, who represented the sacred marriage of

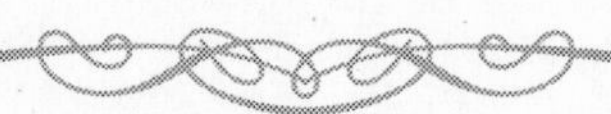

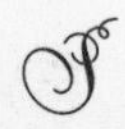

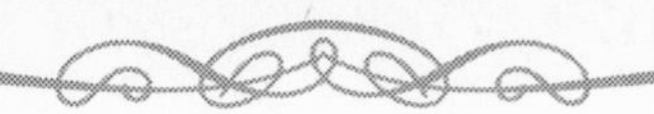
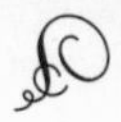

Father Sun and Mother Earth. Hawthorn earned the name "tree of chastity" during a period of English history when the sensuous revelries of May were banned and chastity and purity were enforced. In many areas of northern and western Europe, villages still erect and bedeck maypoles to celebrate the beginning of May. The faeries are known to possess a constant youthfulness, and they love to play. They are especially active during festivities like May Day.

Sunflower oil

1 (4½-ounce) rectangular soap mold

3 small flower soap molds

7 ounces clear glycerin melt-and-pour soap base

Pink mica colorant

Pink gel colorant

8 to 12 drops hawthorn essential oil

This deciduous shrubby tree likes full sun and light watering. Grow it in well-drained soil without too much amendment, or it will produce a lot of disease-prone suckery new growth.

Make this soap during Beltane. As you prepare it, focus on the playfulness and light of youth and say,

A fair maid who, the first of May
Goes to the fields at the break of day
And washes in dew from the hawthorn tree
Will ever after handsome be.

Cover your work surface with waxed paper. Apply a thin, even coat of sunflower oil to the soap molds. Cut 2 ounces of the clear soap base into 1-inch squares and place in a microwave-safe container. Heat in the microwave 40 seconds. Stir. Continue to heat in 10-second intervals until the soap base is completely melted. (You can also choose to melt it on the stove top.) Allow it to cool. Add the desired amount of colorants, stirring constantly until the soap base is evenly coated. Pour the soap into the flower molds and let it set completely. Remove the soaps from the molds and arrange them face down in the rectangular mold. Melt the remaining soap base, and allow it to cool. Stir in the hawthorn oil, 1 drop at a time, until you reach the desired scent strength. Pour the soap into the rectangular mold. Be sure to allow some soap to flow under the flower soaps to keep them from sticking to the mold. When the soap has fully set, approximately 24 hours, remove it from the mold by applying gentle pressure to the back with your thumbs.

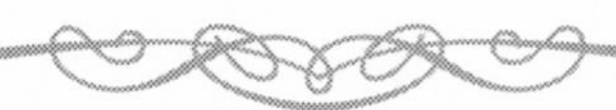

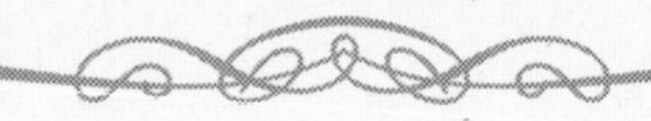

Hazel

Corylus avellana

COLL

Parts Used: nuts, branches

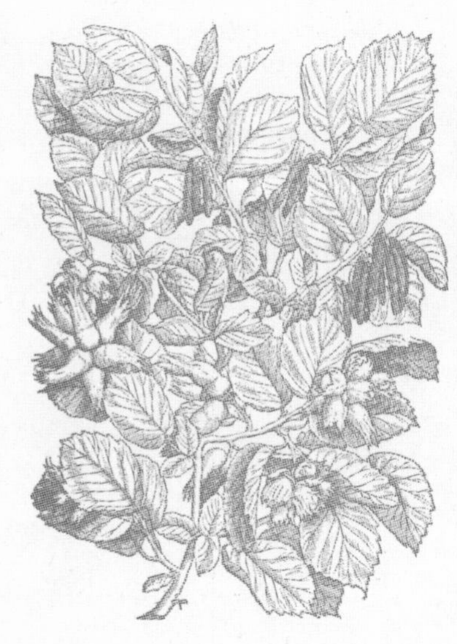

Hazel has wide leaves and is sometimes grown ornamentally. In early Celtic societies, plants played a major role in ceremony and everyday life. The early British alphabet named its letters after the most sacred plants. Hazel was known as *coll* and symbolized the letter *c* or *k*. Hazelnuts were thrown into Brigid's cradle, and Druids often drank mead made from the nuts. According to Celtic folklore, it is believed that nine hazel trees hung over the well of wisdom, dropping their nuts into the water, which flowed into the waterways of the earthly plane. Hazel is associated with Apollo, Artemis, Bel, Diana, Mercury, and Thor.

Mabon Hazelnut–Celery Root Salad

SERVES 6

Hazelnuts are at their peak in the early autumn, ripe for the picking and enjoying at Mabon. Mabon is a time for reaping and harvesting, celebrating life and all its bounty. It is also a holiday to celebrate death, rest, and regeneration. It is known as the feast of Avalon and the festival of the wine harvest. During this sabbat, meditate and explore the inner world, as you slow down and prepare for the winter months.

1½ tablespoons Dijon mustard
2 tablespoons freshly squeezed lemon juice
1 teaspoon organic honey
½ teaspoon salt
¼ cup canola oil
3 tablespoons sour cream
¼ cup hazelnuts
1 medium celery root

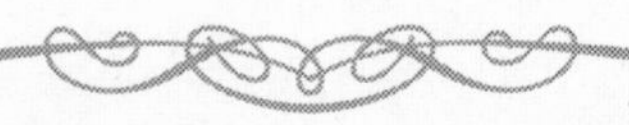

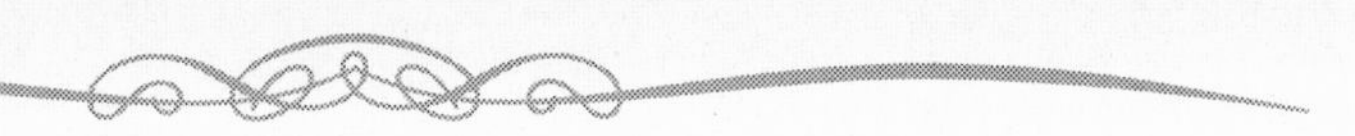

½ firm pear, peeled, grated
2 green onions, thinly sliced
2 teaspoons fresh minced parsley
2 teaspoons fresh minced tarragon

In a small bowl, mix together the mustard, lemon juice, honey, and salt. Add the oil in a thin steady stream, whisking to blend. Stir in the sour cream. Set aside.

Toast the hazelnuts in a dry skillet 5 minutes over medium heat. Rub to remove the skin. Chop the nuts and set aside. Cut off ½ inch of both root and stalk ends of the celery root. Set the root on its end, and using a paring knife, cut the outer layer of flesh from top to bottom, rotating to peel off the entire circumference. Cut the celery root into 1½-inch pieces and then grate. The grated celery root should measure about 2 cups. Place the celery root and the pear in a large bowl; add the dressing, and toss to coat well. Stir in the green onions, parsley, tarragon, and nuts. Season with salt and pepper. Chill 30 minutes and serve.

Hazel does well in full sun to partial shade and likes moderate water. Some areas in the western United States ban the planting of this tree in an effort to stop the spread of eastern filbert blight. Hazel is native to Europe.

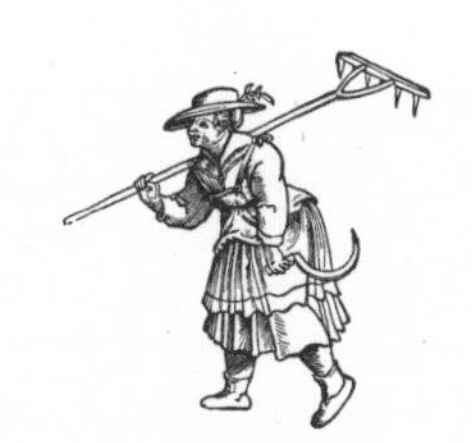

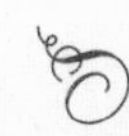

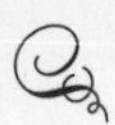

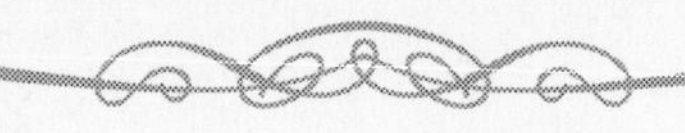

High John the Conqueror

Ipomoea purga

JALAP

Part Used: root

High John the Conqueror prefers sun, light watering, and moderate soil. This herb is native to Mexico and was introduced to Europe in the sixteenth century. Harvest the root during the summer.

High John the Conqueror is an evergreen vine with heart-shaped leaves and trumpetlike purple flowers. It is associated with the sun, and the astrological sign of Leo. High John the Conqueror is used magickally for prosperity, legal and court success, and victory in general.

THIS HERB IS EXTREMELY POISONOUS AND SHOULD NOT BE USED MEDICINALLY UNDER ANY CIRCUMSTANCES.

Free and Clear

This herb works hand in hand with justice. The ritual here is intended to help bring about a proper resolution to court cases. If you are guilty, ask for mercy. Do not ask to get off, because it will only serve to make your penance, once it catches up, even worse. If you are innocent, visualize your freedom from the issue. Try to perform this ritual on a Thursday, as this day is a favorable day for justice and legal matters. But if time does not allow, do not worry about it.

Obtain High John the Conquerer oil and a piece of High John the Conquerer root. Ground, center, and cast a circle. Place 3 drops of the oil in your left hand. Anoint the root with the oil and visualize your wish for your court case. Place the root in a small red bag. Tie the cord in 3 knots. Carry the bag in your left hand when you go to court.

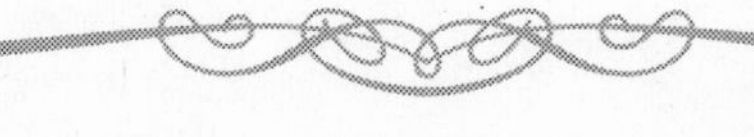

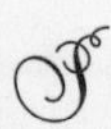

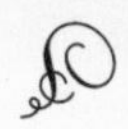

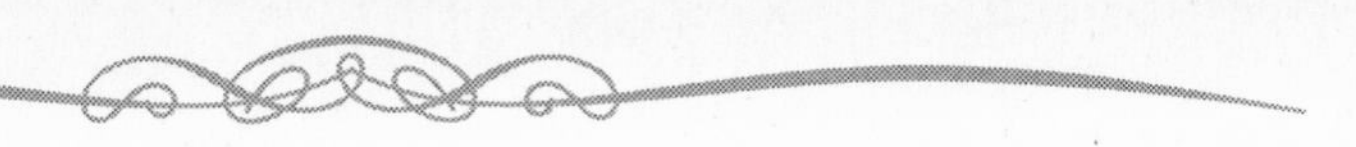

Holly

Ilex aquifolium

TINNE

Part Used: berries

Holly is available in many sizes and varieties. The plants are often found growing in woods or hedges. Its leaves are shiny, usually dark green and toothed, and it bears bright red berries. Holly is closely associated with both Yule (winter solstice) and Litha (summer solstice), as well as the god and planet Saturn.

HOLLY PREFERS FULL SUN TO PARTIAL SHADE AND RICH, SLIGHTLY ACIDIC, GARDEN SOIL WITH GOOD DRAINAGE. IN SOME AREAS WHERE ENGLISH HOLLY (*Ilex aquifolium*) DOES NOT GROW WELL, THE AMERICAN *Ilex opaca* CAN BE SUBSTITUTED. THEY SHOULD BE GROWN IN MALE-FEMALE PAIRS FOR THE PRODUCTION OF BERRIES.

HOLLY BERRIES ARE POISONOUS.

Midwifery Ritual

Both Yule and Litha sabbat celebrations often include an enactment of a battle between two brothers: the Oak King and the Holly King. Litha marks the beginning of the Holly King's reign; he rules the dark half of the year from the summer to the winter, and is thus known as the God of the Waning Year. Yule marks the beginning of the Oak King's reign; he rules the light half of the year, from the winter to the summer, and is thus known as the God of the Waxing Year. The separation of the light and dark halves of the year have nothing to do with good and evil. Light signifies growth and expansion, and dark means withdrawal and rest. Both are necessary. The Holly King reminds us, through his crown of evergreen boughs, that even when all life is apparently gone from the earth in the cold winter months, he holds life in trust for us.

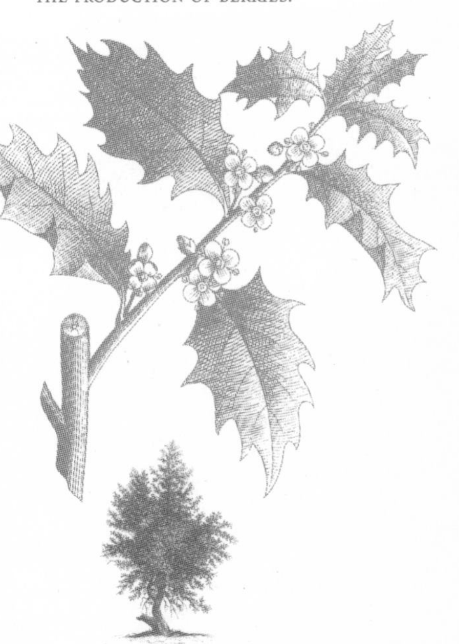

Holly aids us in bringing our abundance and fertility to completion, just like a good friend. A tradition for some pagans is to stay up together all night on the eve of Yule, to be present as a midwife as the Mother births the sun. If you are a night owl, try experiencing part of those wee hours with a telephone and a close yet physically distant friend.

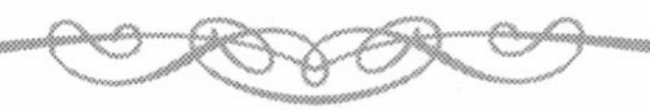

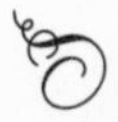

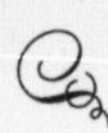

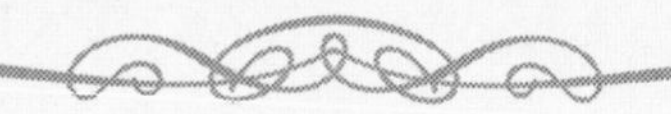

Before Yule eve, gather holly boughs and berries. Sing while you collect them, as this will put you in a good mood and increase the healing potency of the plant. Dry the berries in the sun.

On the eve of Yule, inscribe your astrological sign and any other symbol or name that you associate with yourself on a white candle. Anoint the candle with holly oil. This candle will represent you. You will also need a pink candle for friendship; a gold, green, or red candle for the Yule sabbat; and another candle that represents your intent for the coming year. (For example, use a blue candle for healing, green for prosperity, yellow for bringing in the light.) Place the candles in the four directions, however it makes sense and feels right to you. Position holly boughs between the candles.

At an appointed time, call your friend. Imagine that you are holding hands with your friend. Imagine that you and your friend are two trees, with branches for arms, reaching out for each other. No matter how far apart you are, you both receive strength from the same life-giving soil and sun. Feel energy from your heart center growing roots through your feet into the depths of the earth. Breathe your energy towards your friend's roots. Visualize the space where the two come into contact. Honor and revel in the intermingling of the two energies. The space in which the energies first meet is the child of your unconditional love and support for each another.

Feel the beat of the Mother; your combined energy can dance in celebration. Each is a unique expression. You are drawn together by your similarities as well as your differences. In this separate form, a friend is like the light of the sun: offering opportunities to grow and learn and reminders to celebrate victories, while also acting as a witness to the sadness. Feel the warmth of the sun permeating the soil of Mother Earth. Rise up and feel its radiant glow. The heat warms your soul and encapsulates you with love. Watch the light circle through you, then through your friend, and back again. You have now created a sacred space and both you and your friend are now aware of your identity as channels or conduits for love's power.

Take turns talking. Allow the first part of your conversation to reflect on the events of the past year. Ask yourself what these experiences meant to you and

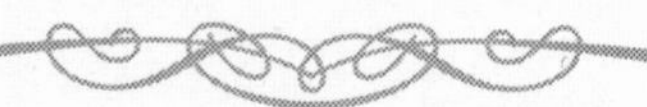

where you can find the presence of Spirit in them. Then talk about wishes and intentions for the new year. Your intentions are declarations and have more force than a wish. Ask yourself how you want the birth of the sun's light to reflect on you. While you talk, string the holly berries on a thick nylon thread. You may choose to string one berry for the event and one for the lesson; or you may choose to make a string of holly berries for your desires.

When you have finished talking, visualize holding hands once more. Focus on the star that you have locked your power onto. On the count of three, unlock your energy from the star. Watch the energy spiral downward in a counterclockwise direction. See it move though the heavens, down through the trees or rooftop, and through the top of your head. As the energy spirals down through your body, keep what you need and let go of the rest. The energy continues to spiral down through your feet and into the earth. The roots that once kept you tied to Mother Earth begin to dissolve. On the count of three, imagine those roots disengaging from the Mother's core.

Yule is a time to honor the coming of the sun, and say good-bye to Mother Moon. Allow the light of your friendship to shine on your lives. True friendship is found when you find joy and respect in each other's life journey.

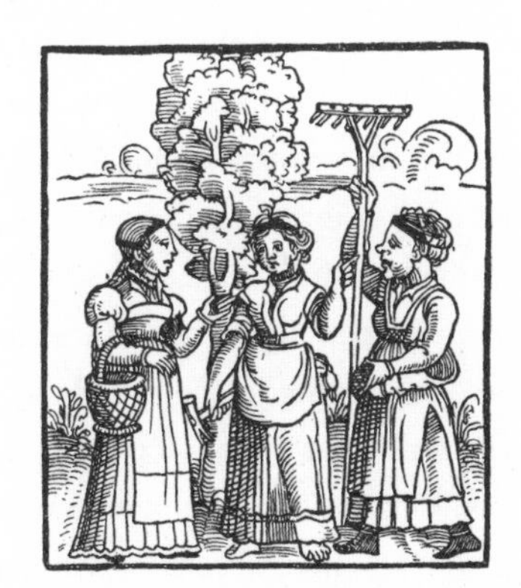

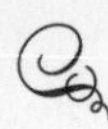

Honeysuckle

Lonicera periclymenum

GOAT'S LEAF, WOODBINE

Parts Used: flowers, leaves, bark

Honeysuckle winds its way through woodlands and hedgerows. It leaves are shiny, grayish, and oval. The herb has a luscious scent emanating from its flowers, which range in color from yellow-cream to pinkish purple and even red. The bark is used as a remedy for swollen glands. The bruised leaves can be applied to wounds, ulcers, and sores. Honeysuckle flowers ease sore throats and can prevent wrinkles. Honeysuckle is known to relieve melancholy and homesickness and is also valued for its ability to increase prosperity and clairvoyance. These two factors bring physical pleasures into harmony with the tranquillity of spiritual awareness. Honeysuckle is associated with the planets and gods of Mercury, Mars, and Jupiter; it resonates with the astrological sign of Cancer.

Heavenly Earth Perfume Meditation

Sometimes those seeking higher vibrations of conscious enlightenment ignore the tactile desires commonly associated with the lower chakras, or energy centers of the body. This does us no good. The chakras all provide illumination within the seven energy vortexes, from the root to the crown. People can be completely ethereal, studying one master after another, and still—because of disowning the importance of the physical realm—find themselves yelling at children, spouses, friends, and strangers. It is important in this earthly existence to bring heaven to earth, to find the beauty and the Divine in the mundane world. It is important to seek beauty in this physical world, not simply for superficial pleasure but in order to demonstrate the beauty that exists in Spirit's divine consciousness. Honey-suckle energy appeals to both earthly and ethereal senses, thereby making it an ideal herb for the following meditation.

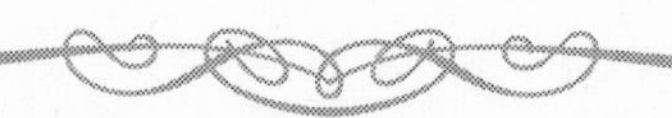

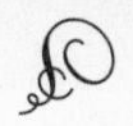
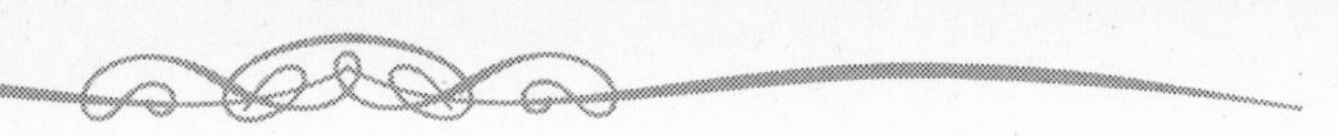

1½ teaspoons beeswax

¼ cup almond essential oil

8 drops honeysuckle essential oil

Gently heat the beeswax and almond oil in a small saucepan until the wax is melted. Remove from the heat and stir in the honeysuckle oil. Let the mixture cool, softening it with your fingers. Pour the mixture into a clean container.

Try a fragrance meditation with this perfume. Apply the perfume to your wrists. Sit down comfortably, with your wrists close to your face. Take five deep breaths. Clear your mind of all clutter. Visualize the crown chakra (at the top of your head) opening and white light streaming into your physical body. Now imagine a moment when your ego and all physical needs and wants are satisfied. See yourself responding to your environment with peace of mind and calmness. Appreciate each thing that comes to you as it passes through. Do not hold on to any one thing. Enjoy each pleasure for what it offers, but when the time comes, allow it to go. Imagine a beautiful feather that has floated down a river. You watch it coming and luxuriate in it for a moment as you hold it or feel it, and then it passes by. To chase the feather downstream would be fruitless and would keep you from knowing the pleasures that are yet to come. For everything there is a time and a season. Now is the time to harmonize the immaterial with the material, the spiritual with the physical, to know heaven on earth.

After you have completed this visualization, you can choose to repeat any of these affirmations that resonate with you:

Spirit wants me to be healthy, wealthy, and wise.

I am a Divine child of Spirit and I now claim my rightful abundance.

I now allow my spirituality and success to become as one.

THIS FLOWERING VINE LIKES SUN OR LIGHT SHADE; IT GROWS BEST INLAND WITH MODERATE WATER. IF YOU CAN'T GROW TRUE WOODBINE, YOU CAN SUBSTITUTE OTHER HONEYSUCKLE (*Lonicera*) SPECIES BETTER ADAPTED TO YOUR AREA. HONEYSUCKLE IS NATIVE TO SOUTHERN EUROPE AND THE CAUCASUS.

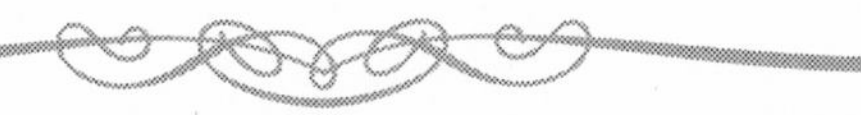

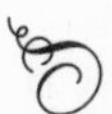

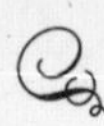

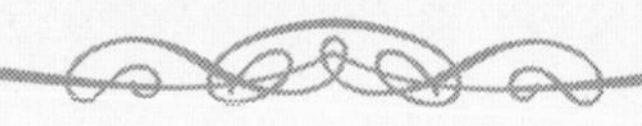

Hop

Humulus lupulus

BEER FLOWER

Parts Used: fruit of female plants, flowers

Hops grow on rich, moist lands. The vine climbs hedgerows and is widely cultivated. Its flowers are yellow-green, and the pale green fruits, called strobiles, are cone-shaped and covered in loose scales. From the strobiles exudes a yellow resinous dust containing lupulin, the source of this herb's medicinal properties. Hop is a bitter herb and is used to aid sleep problems, jittery nerves, earaches, toothaches, and poor appetite. It has been used in England since the seventeenth century to aid digestion, and later it was used to aid menopausal women and increase milk flow in lactating mothers. In the eighteenth century, doctors stuffed hop seeds into pillows to induce sleep for King George III. A poultice of crushed hops, bran, and a bit of water can be applied externally to treat inflammations, sores, swellings, boils, tumors, and cysts.

Hops contain an antispasmodic agent that eases stress-related digestive problems, such as lactose intolerance, peptic ulcers, and irritable bowel syndrome, and aids the body in secreting digestive juices and bile. Hop tea can aid insomnia, headaches, and anxiety. Today it is used as a mild sedative; as a remedy for insomnia, muscle spasms, and cramps; and in shampoos. The herb is believed to contain phytoestrogen, which may help a woman's body use estrogen efficiently. Its curative abilities make it a powerful healing herb in magickal rituals. Hop is associated with the planets and gods Pluto and Mars.

Dream Pillow

Hop invokes the healing element of its associated planets, Pluto and Mars. It is our natural state to be healers and all are in possession of the ability to send the negative and low vibrations of pain to the Divine Source, where they can be

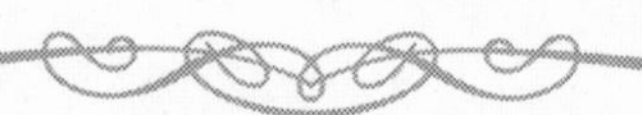

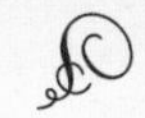

transmuted. If you are having a difficult time claiming the healer within, or if you are in need of healing, make this pillow to create access to radiant health in mind, body, and spirit. Summer solstice, a traditional occasion for gathering herbs for healing, is a perfect time to create this pillow. The sun is at its peak and is believed to possess great curative powers.

1½ cups dried hop flowers
10 to 12 drops lavender essential oil
1 (10- by 6-inch) piece of satin or silk fabric

Hops prefer full sun and water during its growing season. Be sure to ask for a female plant when buying it at a nursery; no male plant is needed to pollinate the female flowers. The plants grow very fast, and will cover an arbor in a single year; cut them down to the ground at the first frost, and they will come back the next year. Fruits will not form until the plant's third year. Hop is native to Europe and Asia.

Pour the hop flowers into a small bowl. Add the essential oil and mix. Iron the fabric. Fold lengthwise, with the outer surface facing inward. Using a small stitch, sew a seam along the bottom and side, ¾ inch from the edge, leaving the top edge open. Sew a second time over the original stitching. Turn the pillow right side out. Fill the pillow with hops mixture until the pillow has reached the desired firmness. Turn down the top so that the outer surface of the material is once again facing inward. Hand-sew or machine-finish the top. As you create this dream pillow, say,

It is now safe to be a healer
Of ailments of body and spirit
I restore myself and others
With love and harmony, I declare it.

Note: Dried lavender or rose petals make a nice addition to the pillow. For a variation, use muslin for one side of the material, and silk or satin on the other. On the muslin, you can draw a power animal or other symbol to create lucid dreams.

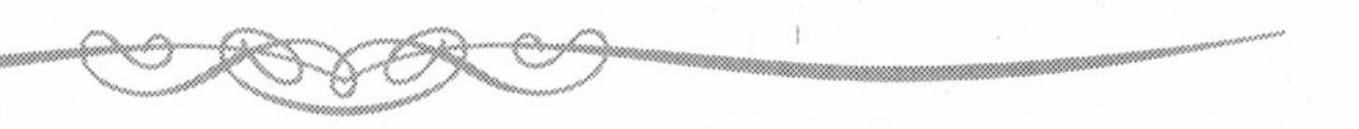

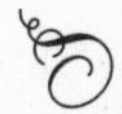

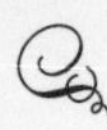

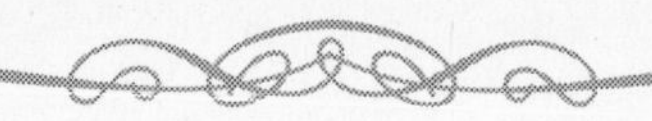

Hyssop

Hyssopus officinalis

ISOPO, YSOPO

Parts used: flowers, leaves, stems

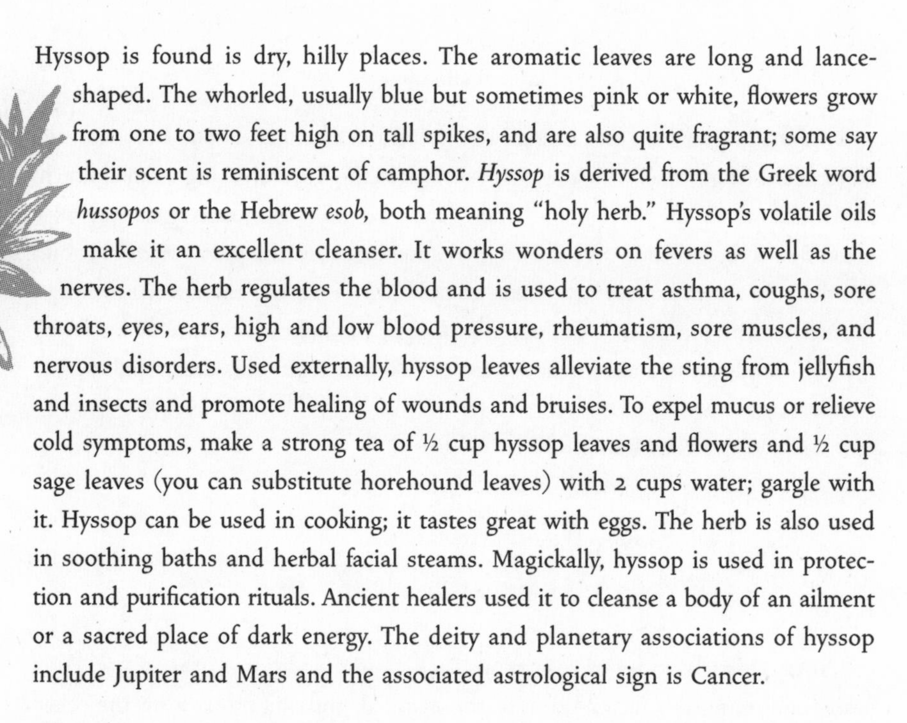

Hyssop is found is dry, hilly places. The aromatic leaves are long and lance-shaped. The whorled, usually blue but sometimes pink or white, flowers grow from one to two feet high on tall spikes, and are also quite fragrant; some say their scent is reminiscent of camphor. *Hyssop* is derived from the Greek word *hussopos* or the Hebrew *esob,* both meaning "holy herb." Hyssop's volatile oils make it an excellent cleanser. It works wonders on fevers as well as the nerves. The herb regulates the blood and is used to treat asthma, coughs, sore throats, eyes, ears, high and low blood pressure, rheumatism, sore muscles, and nervous disorders. Used externally, hyssop leaves alleviate the sting from jellyfish and insects and promote healing of wounds and bruises. To expel mucus or relieve cold symptoms, make a strong tea of ½ cup hyssop leaves and flowers and ½ cup sage leaves (you can substitute horehound leaves) with 2 cups water; gargle with it. Hyssop can be used in cooking; it tastes great with eggs. The herb is also used in soothing baths and herbal facial steams. Magickally, hyssop is used in protection and purification rituals. Ancient healers used it to cleanse a body of an ailment or a sacred place of dark energy. The deity and planetary associations of hyssop include Jupiter and Mars and the associated astrological sign is Cancer.

Children's Aura Cleansing

We are all made of light; as we grow, we accumulate negative thoughts and stories about people, places, and things—like dust blocking sunlight from shining through a window. Children are pure light, without this collection of baggage. They are, however, susceptible to negative energy, akin to amassing dirt on their aura. I successfully practiced this ritual with my youngest son, who became very ill when he picked up the heavy energy of one who lacked any joy in living.

We can heal ourselves of ailments when we change the thought pattern that created them. Children don't necessarily know how to do this for themselves, so we need to cleanse what they have picked up. Visualizing ourselves with radiant health can make it happen. Our bodies are intimately connected to our thoughts. When our emotional bodies store unhealthy thoughts, we must find a way to release them, or they will manifest in physical ways; they can also affect our children's auras. Allow your thoughts to lead you to the light and love of Spirit.

Anoint a pink and blue candle with hyssop oil. Burn hyssop incense. Run a rose quartz through the smoke and set it next to the candle. Stand about 5 feet from your child. Hold your hands out, palms facing toward him or her. Move closer until you feel a change in pressure or tingling sensation, signaling the boundary of his or her aura. Trust your intuition. Gently brush your child's aura by raking your fingers through it. Imagine yourself brushing off the accumulated dirt. Pay close attention to the feet. Tell the child to imagine herself or himself in a pink glowing egg. This affirms that love is all-powerful and can heal. Tell your child that he or she is a perfect child of God or Goddess, Father or Mother God, Spirit, Creator, or whatever terminology works for your family. (In mine, we say God and Mother Earth, like Mom and Dad.) Say,

> God and Mother Earth, loving me [see note]
> Guide my little feet up to thee.

THIS PERENNIAL HERB GROWS IN ALL ZONES AND PREFERS CHALKY, LIGHT, WELL-DRAINED SOIL AND FULL SUN OR LIGHT SHADE; IT NEEDS INFREQUENT WATERING. DO NOT SUBSTITUTE PLANTS OF THE GENUS *Agastache*, COMMONLY CALLED LICORICE HYSSOP. HYSSOP IS NATIVE TO SOUTHERN EUROPE.

Your child may not comprehend that thought guides action, but will probably understand the metaphor of the feet as a guide. You may find that your child winces, similar to the way one does if jostled when feeling racked by the flu. Children are very sensitive to their auras. If this happens, move more slowly or back away a bit—whatever feels right. Do not concentrate on the illusion of your child's sickness or repeat that he or she is sick. Allow the child to concentrate on her or himself as whole and complete. (It helps to understand that it was your child's aura, not thoughts, that attracted the illness.)

Note: You can also substitute your child's name for "me."

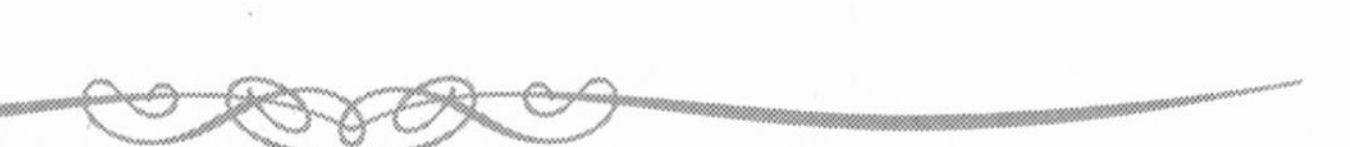

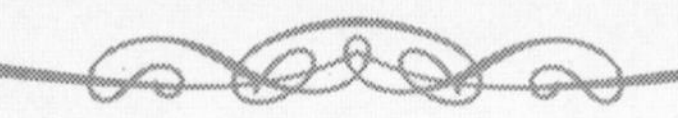

Jasmine

Jasminum (various species)

JESSAMIN, MOONLIGHT ON THE GROVE

Part Used: flower

Jasmine grows in different zones, depending on the species. The strongly scented flowers are often white and the leaves are dark green. Jasmine increases self-confidence, self-love, spiritual love, prophetic dreams, and prosperity. It is associated with the goddess Diana, the god and planet Jupiter, and the moon.

Jasmine Lip Balm

The essence of jasmine is particularly appropriate for application on one of the thinnest layers of skin protecting our bodies: our lips. Lips are quite responsive to touch, one of the key erogenous zones, and a focal point for those of the opposite sex. Regularly hydrating this sensitive area prevents cracking and drying. This lip balm will create a sexy, glossy look that will turn heads; and the jasmine, which has been used for centuries to create love and induce passion, will increase your libido and help you feel more glamorous.

¼ cup jojoba oil
1 tablespoon vitamin E oil
1 tablespoon beeswax
10 drops jasmine essential oil

Combine the joboba oil, vitamin E, and beeswax in a small saucepan over low heat and warm until the wax is melted. Remove from the heat. Add the jasmine essential oil and blend the mixture thoroughly, saying,

It's glamorous and sexy that I want to feel
Beautiful inside and outside will appeal

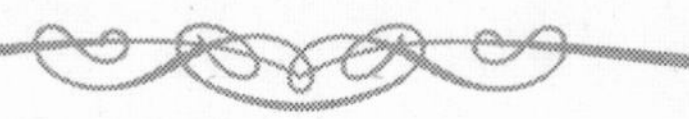

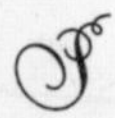

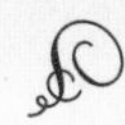

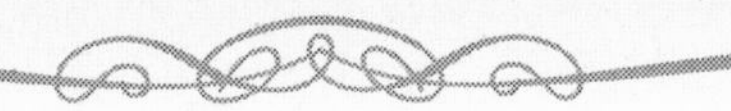

For I am true beauty as you now can see
Alluring and lovely and natural as can be.

Pour the mixture into ¼-ounce or ½-ounce tins or cosmetic jars while still warm. The lip balm will keep for up to 1 year or longer if refrigerated.

Note: Other herbs that work as aphrodisiacs include patchouli, cinnamon, ylang-ylang, rose, geranium, vanilla, and red clover.

Jasmine species are either evergreen or deciduous shrubs or vines. In general, they prefer frequent watering and full to partial sun. Jasmine is native to northern India, Pakistan, and the northwestern Himalayas.

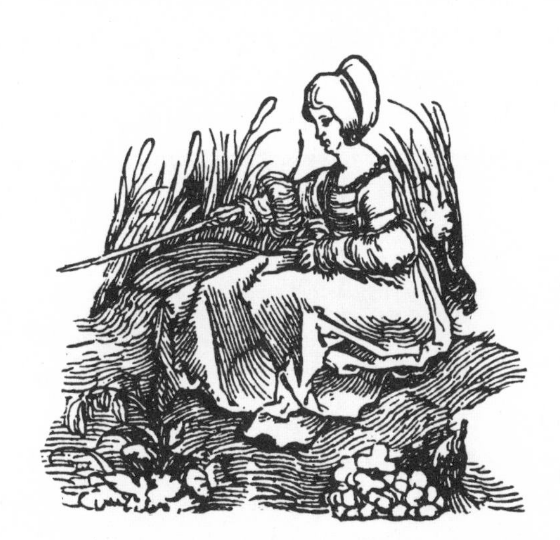

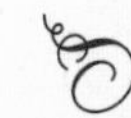

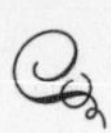
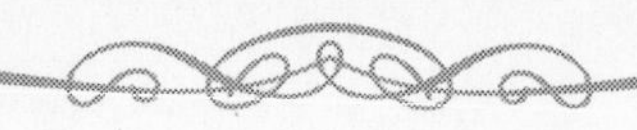

Juniper

Juniperus (various species)

ENEBRO, GIN BERRY, JENEVER

Part Used: berries

Juniper is an evergreen shrub or tree; the genus contains more than seventy species, which grow in all climate zones. Juniper destroys fungus and aids in combating kidney, urinary, and bladder infections; juniper carries protection, success, antitheft, and love powers. Juniper corresponds to the planet Jupiter, which rules over the development of vitality and confidence, the maintenance of faith, and the lifting of spirits. It is also associated with Mars, the sun, and the astrological sign of Aries. Juniper will expand the concepts or physicality with which you are working. Juniper is highly rejuvenating, energizing, and invigorating. In aromatherapy, juniper acts as an astringent, reducing water retention and eliminating toxins.

JUNIPER IS GENERALLY CONSIDERED SAFE IN SMALL DOSES, BUT CAN BE TOXIC IF OVERUSED. JUNIPER SHOULD BE AVOIDED BY PEOPLE WITH KIDNEY DISEASE AND BY PREGNANT WOMEN.

Magickal Mosquito Net

Because juniper carries the ability to protect, this spell can be used either to safeguard a circle for magick or for more mundane purposes, such as camping in a damp area. Try this ritual if you find yourself beset by insects and other pests. (This spell was developed by Dawn Marie, a witch born and bred in Southern California, who has been practicing an eclectic form of Wicca for more than a decade.)

Light juniper incense in a cauldron and carry a wand. Walk thrice widdershins (counterclockwise) around the area from which the insects are to be banished. After completing the three circuits, throw glitter around inside the circle to solidify the magick of intention and establish it as holy ground or sacred space. Say,

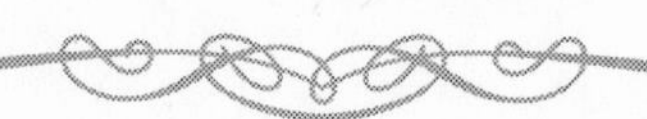

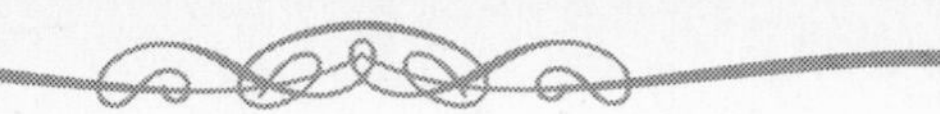

Winged insects, now hear me
From this circle we banish thee
Until the morrow, when the sun does rise,
Creatures be gone; any bug that flies.

By the Powers of the west,
Here there shall be no pest.
By the Powers of the south,
This repellent comes from my mouth.
By the Powers of the east,
On us you'll not feast.
By the Powers of the north,
This shall come forth.

By the power of three
So mote it be!

JUNIPER PREFERS FULL SUN ALONG THE COAST AND FULL TO PARTIAL SUN INLAND. WATER NEEDS DEPEND ON THE VARIETY. JUNIPER IS FOUND IN EUROPE, SOUTHWESTERN ASIA, AND NORTH AMERICA.

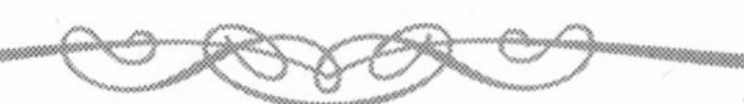

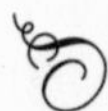

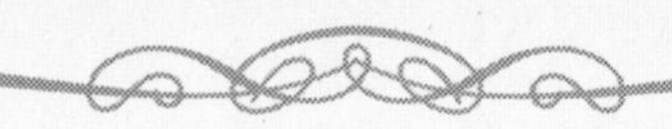

Kava

Piper methysticum

INTOXICATING PEPPER, KAVA-KAVA

Part Used: rhizome

Indigenous to Polynesia, the Sandwich Islands, and South Sea islands, kava is a tall shrub with large green leaves and very short flower spikes. Every Polynesian ceremony begins with a round of kava. A fermented liquor is made by chewing the roots; then the root and saliva are mixed with pure water or coconut water. The mixture looks like dirty dishwater, and its taste is one that, for many, requires getting used to. But if you like it, you really like it.

Kava treats sleep problems, anxiety, endometriosis, tension headaches, gout, rheumatism, arthritis, and many heart diseases. Do not combine it with alcohol, take more than the prescribed amount, or use while pregnant or nursing. It is often used to reduce stress, because while it is an effective relaxant, it also helps maintain alertness. Kava is known as an aphrodisiac.

DO NOT TAKE KAVA IF YOU HAVE OR SUSPECT LIVER PROBLEMS.

Finding Earth

Kava is often used to help reach the astral realms. It stimulates the second (sacral) chakra and the sixth chakra, also known as the third eye. The herb allows one's brain waves to move into theta rhythm, where all healing, meditation, and spellwork take place. When the third eye is activated, new insights or viewpoints can be perceived—the real magick. Meanwhile, one is kept grounded in the earthly world of mutating physicality, duality, creativity, and emotions centered in the second chakra (located in the lower abdomen).

In addition to accessing the astral realms of your spirituality, kava's earthiness helps connect you with the primal energy of the earth. Kava will help you feel earth's pulsating aura—above the soil and resonating through it.

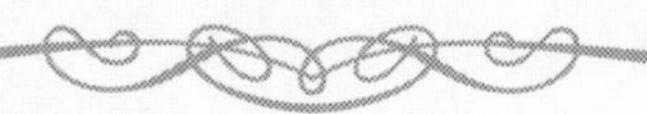

If possible, conduct this ritual outside. Light a gray advent candle with a glass covering to protect the flame from the wind. Mix kava extract with 1 cup of water, according to the following formula: ¼ teaspoon if you weigh between 90 and 130 pounds; ½ teaspoon if between 130 and 175; ¾ teaspoon if between 175 and 225; 1 teaspoon if between 225 and 300.

Sit very still, with the palms of your hands facing up and resting on your thighs. Look into the candle's flame and take ten deep breaths. Close your eyes and imagine a silver light of energy vibrating around you and under the ground below you. This is the primitive, original energy that has existed since the birth of our planet earth. This energy mostly pulsates horizontally, but any direction is possible. Slightly sway with the light. You are one with this energy. Visualize the earth being formed. Witness the birth and evolution of life on earth.

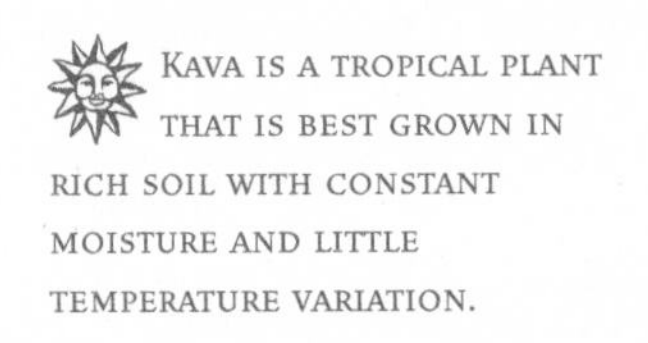

Kava is a tropical plant that is best grown in rich soil with constant moisture and little temperature variation.

Breathe in the silver light of the earth's aura. Take from it and give to it. Sip the kava, and imagine a life in which you understand the seasons as fluctuations of your own body. Imagine the first people to walk the land upon which you are currently sitting. If you know how they dressed or lived, imagine yourself dressed as they were and doing the daily activities they did. Imagine tasting their food, be it acorn meal, corn, wild fruits or flowers, or kava. (If you do not know what the indigenous people ate or wore, go with the first image that comes to mind or see yourself surrounded in a natural scene without any buildings.)

Once you tap into the way people lived upon the land you now walk, you call up their energy, and are able to more deeply explore the earth's energy field, and feel the divine rhythms of life. With these rhythms fully embedded, you will feel more compassion and love.

When you are done, visualize the energy moving in a diagonal line from your third eye (the center of your forehead) through your heart and down to your second chakra. See the energy loop around and move back up to your third eye in a figure eight. Feel the power of bringing earth's energy to your inner sight and center of creativity. Imagine the silver light swirling into you from earth and then out of you through your breath ten times. Douse the flame.

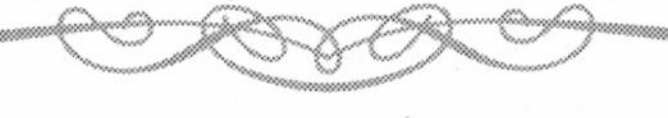

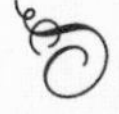

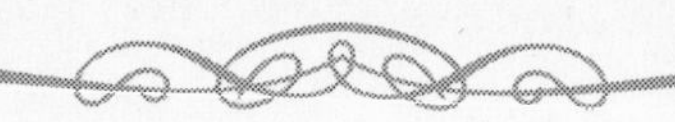

Lavender

Lavandula angustifolia

ELF LEAF, GARDEN LAVENDER, SPIKE, TRUE LAVENDER

Part Used: flower

Lavender originates from Europe and is mostly found on dry, sandy land or in rocky places. It is widely cultivated, especially on mountainsides and in coastal regions. Spikes of bluish-purple fragrant flowers float atop tall stems above mounds of gray leaves. Magickal powers most often attributed to lavender are love, protection, and purification. Its associated deities and planets are Adonis and Venus (the Roman Aphrodite).

Lavender derives its name from the Latin *lavare*, which means "to wash." The pure, fresh scent of lavender is widely used in baths, linen closets, perfumes, and soaps. An infusion of lavender, applied topically, works wonders as a remedy for insect bites, cuts, bruises, and aches. Dried lavender bunches are often hung in the corners of rooms to repel flies and mosquitoes.

Lavender's calming properties have been known to help insomnia, jittery nerves, stomach problems, and depression; to regenerate skin cells; to protect against skin infections; and to relieve headaches. As a nerve tonic, it can treat fainting, sunstroke, vomiting, hysteria, and swelling limbs. An infusion of the flowers can be used as a gargle for sore throats and colds, in a bath to relieve tension, or as a compress to relieve cold symptoms and congestion. Lavender works to calm and relax nervous or excited animals. A bottle of essential oil can be waved under the animal's nose for a few seconds, or a lavender sachet or pillow can be placed where the animal sleeps. Lavender is associated with the planets and deities Saturn, Mercury, and Hecate. Its astrological affiliation is Virgo. In magick, the herb is used for clairvoyance, stability, prosperity, blessing, and calming.

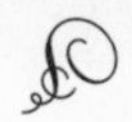

Lovely Lavender Cookies

MAKES 5 DOZEN

Lavender has a delicate flavor that not only attracts bees, but calls to young and old alike. To flavor teas or lemonade, mix equal parts dried lavender leaves and sugar. Grind in a blender or food processor and let sit for at least a week.

- ½ pound (2 sticks) unsalted butter, room temperature
- ½ cup sugar
- 2 teaspoons minced lemon zest
- 1½ cups all-purpose flour
- 2 tablespoons dried lavender flowers, finely chopped

Preheat the oven to 350°F. In a bowl, beat the butter and sugar until light and fluffy. Add the lemon zest, flour, and lavender, and stir until a soft dough forms. Drop the dough by teaspoonfuls onto lightly greased baking sheets. Flatten the cookies with the bottom of a glass dipped in flour. Bake 15 to 18 minutes, until the edges are golden brown. Cool on wire racks before storing.

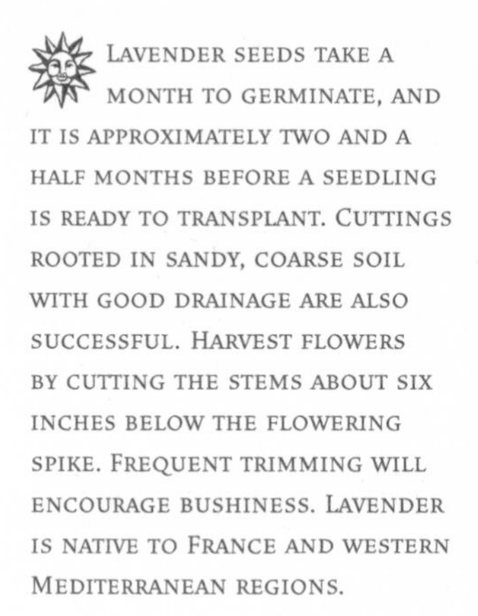

LAVENDER SEEDS TAKE A MONTH TO GERMINATE, AND IT IS APPROXIMATELY TWO AND A HALF MONTHS BEFORE A SEEDLING IS READY TO TRANSPLANT. CUTTINGS ROOTED IN SANDY, COARSE SOIL WITH GOOD DRAINAGE ARE ALSO SUCCESSFUL. HARVEST FLOWERS BY CUTTING THE STEMS ABOUT SIX INCHES BELOW THE FLOWERING SPIKE. FREQUENT TRIMMING WILL ENCOURAGE BUSHINESS. LAVENDER IS NATIVE TO FRANCE AND WESTERN MEDITERRANEAN REGIONS.

Maypole Decoration

The rising of the constellation Pleiades on the dawn horizon heralds Beltane. The first and most beautiful of the Pleiades (also known as the Seven Sisters) is Mai, for whom the month of May is named. The Beltane festival is the time of her wedding to the God. Beltane signifies an important stage in the relationship between the Goddess and God. God is represented by the sun and growing light in winter months, as well as the seed of creation embodied by the new vegetation growing upon the Goddess. The masculine energy—often referred to as the Horned Man, Cerrnunos, or Pan—matures, assuming the place as lover and mate of the Goddess. The God's virile force helps the Goddess bloom and give life across the land.

Beltane celebrations traditionally begin at sundown on April 30, when young people search the woods for the perfect Maypole. Throughout the night, the revelers sing, dance, and indulge in the joyous coupling that brings in harvest and abundance. At dawn, they return, bearing with them a living tree. This tree is then erected in the center of town, in the hope that the Tree Spirit will come forth to

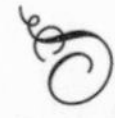

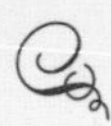

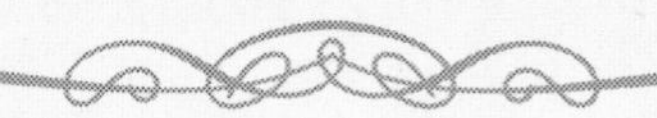

make fertile the women and animals. The revelers then join hands and dance around the tree to call upon its spirit of fertility. The pole is a phallic symbol of God, and the flowing ribbons and flowers adorning the top represent the Goddess. Once the ribbons are wrapped completely around, it is representative of the child.

When my children and I made this Maypole, we bought unfinished wooden children and wings from the craft store and created our own people to decorate with. You can use any little people you have.

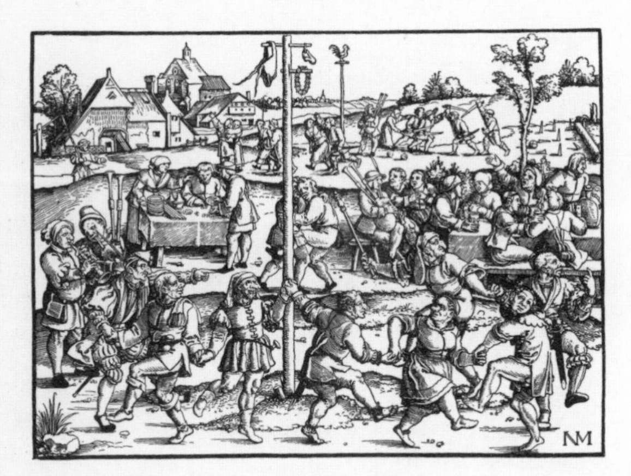

1 (12-inch) dowel with a ½-inch diameter
Acrylic paint
10 dried lavender stalks, flowers intact
Craft wire
4 to 6 ribbons, 18 inches long
Spanish moss or decorative moss
Dry foam disk, at least 1½ inches thick and 6 inches in diameter
Faery figurines or other character figurines
Silk flowers

Paint the dowel green or brown or the traditional Maypole colors of striped red and white. Cut the lavender stems to 1½ inches below the flowers. Using the wire, bind the lavender stems around the top of the dowel, flowers facing up. Secure one ribbon to cover the wire. Secure another ribbon to the wire, next to the first, about ¼ inch away. Repeat this process until all the ribbons are dangling from just underneath the top of the dowel. Cut a 2-inch square piece of moss. Poke a hole through the center of moss and stick base of the dowel through the hole. Pull the moss up to the flowers so that it hides the wire on the dowel; the ribbons will drape over the moss. Plant the dowel in the dry foam. Use additional moss to cover the foam. Fan the ribbons out to about 6 inches from the center of the dowel. Place four to six faery figurines on each place where the ribbons fall; it will look as if the figurines are holding the ribbon. Decorate the moss with flowers. Place the decoration on a family Beltane altar, the dinner table, or wherever you like.

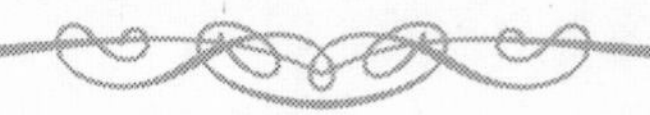

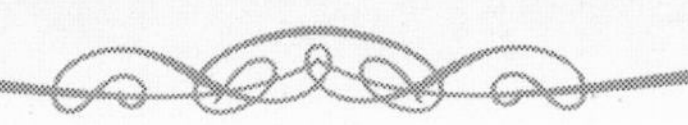

Lily

Lilium (various species)

FLOWER OF DEATH

Part Used: flower

Lilies are often found wild in woodlands and shady places. There are many kinds of lily, mostly grown for their ornamental flowers. Lilies have been used to aid nervous ailments, dizziness, lymph irregularities, and high blood pressure. Because many varieties bloom in spring, the lily is symbolically associated with death and rebirth. Lily is associated with the moon, a perfect representation of the transcendence from death to birth.

LILIES PREFER DEEP, LOOSE, WELL-DRAINED SOIL, AMPLE WATERING, AND SHADE AT THE BASE WITH SUN ON THE FLOWERS. LILIES GROW WILD IN ASIA, EUROPE, AND NORTH AMERICA.

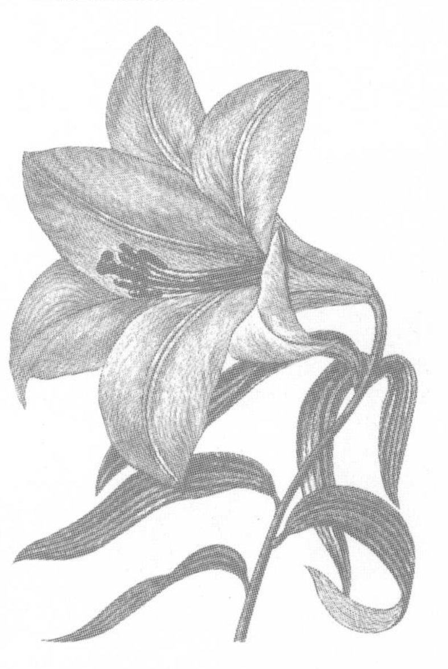

LILY RHIZOMES ARE POISONOUS.

Past Life

We are souls on simultaneous journeys into the past and future. Time was created so that we can experience each moment in its entirety. There are occasions when our memories of a past life are so strong that they adversely affect our current lives. If the pain or joy of a past life is constantly interrupting the present moment, then we are not truly experiencing life. Ostara is a perfect opportunity to birth a new you, and try this meditation.

To perform this meditation, place three lilies in a vase. Anoint a white candle with lily oil. Light the candle. Sit quietly and concentrate on your third eye, the place just above your eyebrows in the middle of your forehead. When you are ready, look into the flame. Be still for at least fifteen minutes. Allow thoughts to come to your awareness and then gently guide them out of your mind. At the end of the time, write down any symbols or messages that came to you, especially those that do not make logical sense. Often the heart is the first to understand what needs to be done. Some time may pass before all the symbols and messages are clarified for you.

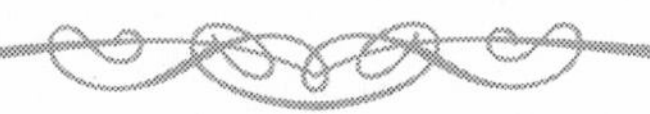

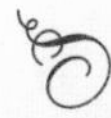

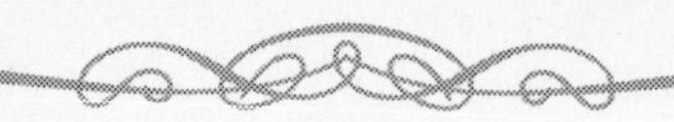

Lovage

Levisticum officinale

CHINESE LOVAGE, LAVOSE, LOVE ROOT, SEA PARSLEY

Parts Used: root, seeds, leaves, stems

Lovage has glossy, deep green leaves and flat clusters of small, yellowish green flowers. It tastes like celery. Lovage treats fevers, rheumatism, jaundice, malaria, sore throats, and kidney stones. In the early eighteenth century, lovage was used to treat all manner of ailments. Lovage is used as a mild diuretic, as a digestive aid, and as a face wash for freckles. It is known as a purifier. Lovage is commonly used in love spells and to attract romantic liaisons. Lovage is associated with the sun and the astrological sign of Taurus. Taurus is associated with self-ease and people born under this sign are an open book with no hidden agenda: what you see is what you get. Therefore, lovage is used to attract a lover who will accept you as you are.

Pasta Fagioli

SERVES 2 AS A MAIN COURSE

Lovage can attract love into your life. This recipe is great for a first dinner with a new love. You can also serve it to rekindle a waning romance. As you stir everything together, light a red and pink candle and think thoughts of passion, love, and romance. Set the table with red candles and fresh flowers. Serve with a nice red wine and crusty Italian bread to sop up the sauce. (This recipe was donated by Johanna Karlin, a first-rate kitchen witch.)

2 cups dried beans (such as cannellini beans)
1 pound bowtie pasta
1 bunch lovage
2 tablespoons olive oil
1 onion, chopped
4 cloves garlic, minced

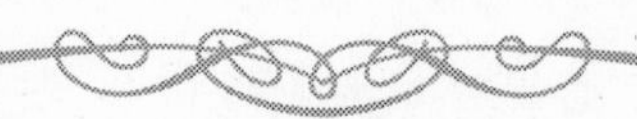

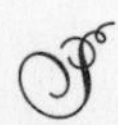

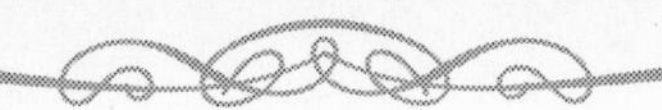

Soak the beans in cold water for 3 hours. Drain, place in a large pot, and cover with fresh water. Simmer until tender, about 2 hours. Boil a large pot of water, and then cook the pasta according to the directions on the package. Meanwhile, chop the lovage. When the pasta is done, drain it, reserving 2 cups of the cooking water. Add the oil to the pasta pot over medium heat. Add the onion and cook until translucent, about 7 minutes. Add the garlic and lovage. Sauté 1 minute. Add the beans, pasta, and reserved pasta water. Simmer until well blended. Season with salt and pepper to taste.

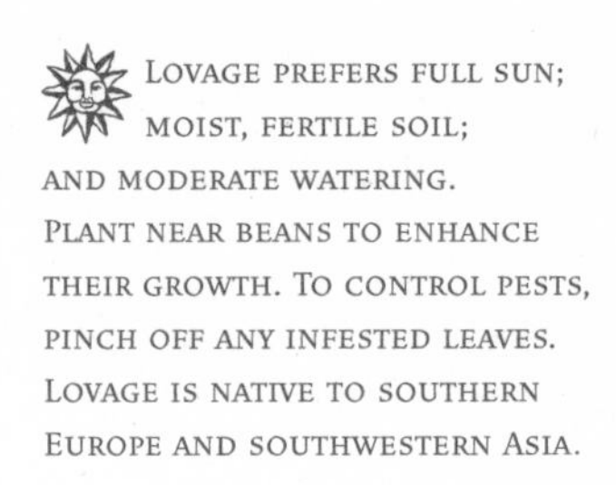

LOVAGE PREFERS FULL SUN; MOIST, FERTILE SOIL; AND MODERATE WATERING. PLANT NEAR BEANS TO ENHANCE THEIR GROWTH. TO CONTROL PESTS, PINCH OFF ANY INFESTED LEAVES. LOVAGE IS NATIVE TO SOUTHERN EUROPE AND SOUTHWESTERN ASIA.

Lovage Oil

MAKES 1½ CUPS

Use this oil in sautés, marinades, and salad dressings.

- 1 cup extra virgin olive oil
- 3 (2-inch-long) lovage sprigs
- 1 clove garlic, sliced
- 3 large celery leaves

Gently heat oil over medium-low heat 3 to 5 minutes; do not boil. Place the lovage, garlic, and celery leaves in a glass jar. Pour the warmed oil over the herbs. Let the oil cool. Strain the herbs out. Cover and store the mixture in a cool, dry place up to 6 months.

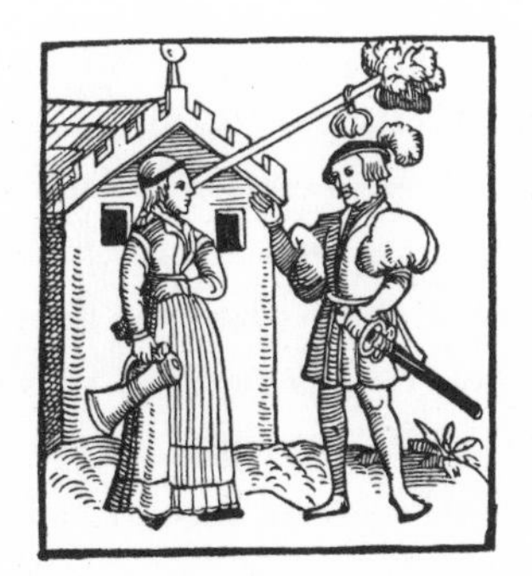

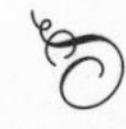

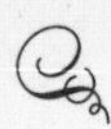
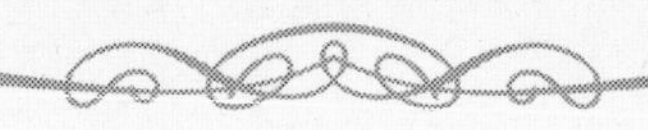

Marigold

Tagetes patula

GOLDEN FLOWER OF DEATH, ZEMPASÚCHIL

Part Used: flower

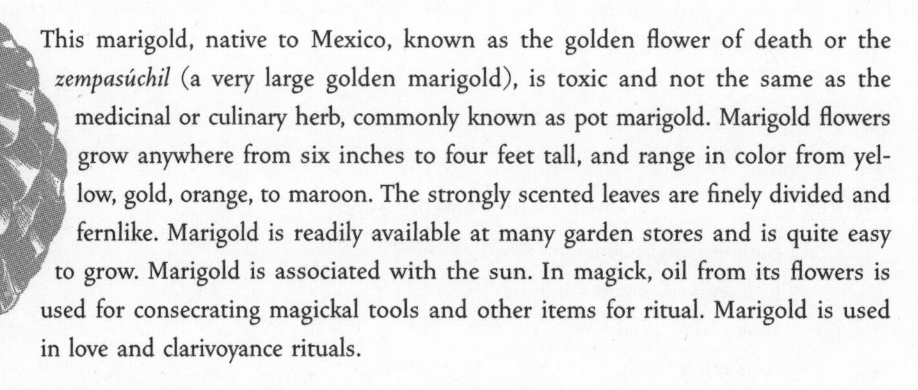

This marigold, native to Mexico, known as the golden flower of death or the *zempasúchil* (a very large golden marigold), is toxic and not the same as the medicinal or culinary herb, commonly known as pot marigold. Marigold flowers grow anywhere from six inches to four feet tall, and range in color from yellow, gold, orange, to maroon. The strongly scented leaves are finely divided and fernlike. Marigold is readily available at many garden stores and is quite easy to grow. Marigold is associated with the sun. In magick, oil from its flowers is used for consecrating magickal tools and other items for ritual. Marigold is used in love and clarivoyance rituals.

Dia de los Muertos Celebration

Zempasúchil adorns pathways and altars for Dia de los Muertos (Day of the Dead), celebrated from October 31 to November 2. These yellow-orange trails from cemeteries to homes are lovingly made for people who have crossed over, so that their spirits can find the way home to visit their families. This holiday, originating with the Aztecs, and formerly observed in August, honors and remembers the dead with reverence and mirth. Instead of fearing death, the celebrants embrace it. Male and female skeleton dolls are found everywhere; candy skulls sport names of all origins. Each family builds and decorates a personal altar (*ofrenda*) every year.

In Mexican tradition, the devil doesn't have the same meaning that he does in Western Christianity. People of Aztec background consider the devil a fool, with no power over people other than what is given to him freely by people living in fear of him. In fact, the devil did not even exist in Aztec culture before their conversion to Christianity. When the Spaniards attempted to convert the indigenous people of Mexico, they merely incorporated the symbols of the crucifix and devil

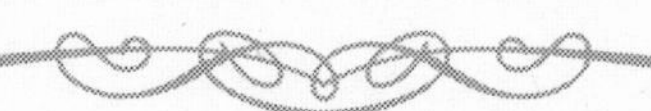

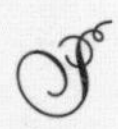

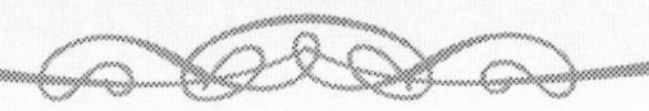

into the preexisting celebration, which the Spaniards moved to November 2 to coincide with All Saints' Day.

For your celebration, decorate your Dia de los Muertos altar with skeletons, boxes to represent coffins, candles, a bowl of water for the visitors from the other side to wash their hands, bowls of treats (like excess Halloween candy), and lots of marigolds. Traditionally, long stalks of sugarcane are tied to the front legs of the table and formed into a large arch over the altar. Invite guests to bring a picture of a loved one to place on the altar. In the center of the altar, place two vessels, bowls or cauldrons. One will be filled with marigold seeds, and the other will have small blank sheets of paper and a few pencils. Invite your guests to write a message to the deceased, a loved one on the threshold of death, or a blessing for themselves or another person. Fold up the sheet and place it back in the bowl. After this, they can take a few marigold seeds to plant at home.

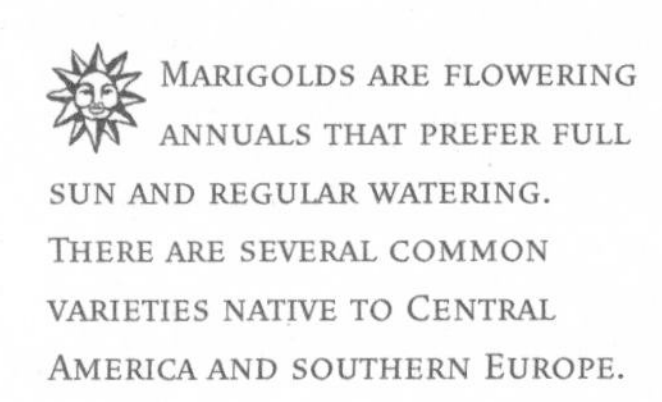

Marigolds are flowering annuals that prefer full sun and regular watering. There are several common varieties native to Central America and southern Europe.

Ask your guests to bring a favorite food of their deceased one. Make sure you make a communal dish, such as tamales, cookies, or anise *pan de los muertos* (page 58). If you cast a circle before the celebration, the notes to the dead can be burned so that Spirit and wind can carry the messages to the loved ones.

Another fun celebration activity is communication with the other side. Use fifteen marigold flowers to weave a lei (fishing line works well for this). Prepare a special room or chair. Invite one guest at a time to sit in the chair and wear the lei. Ask a friend skilled in the psychic arts to interpret or channel messages from the deceased to the person wearing the lei.

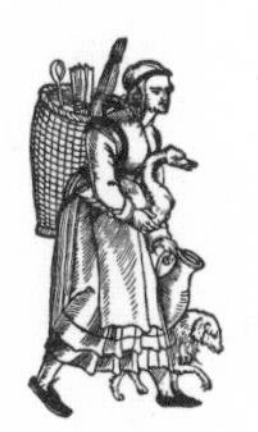

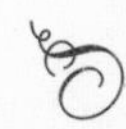

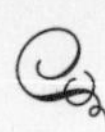

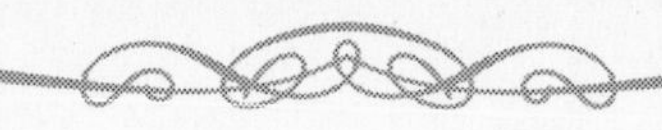

Marjoram

Origanum majorana

JOY OF THE MOUNTAINS, KNOTTED MARJORAM, MOUNTAIN MINT, SWEET MARJORAM

Parts Used: flowers, leaves

The marjoram that is found growing wild on hill slopes (*Origanum vulgare*), does not have scented leaves, so be sure to get sweet marjoram. Its gray-green leaves are slightly downy and highly aromatic. The herb's pale pink to sometimes white flowers are honey-sweet. Marjoram treats digestive complaints, halitosis, colds, inflammation of the mouth and throat, morning sickness, nightmares, fear, depression, shaky nerves, fevers, jaundice, aches and pains, rheumatism, earaches, toothaches, headaches, infected cuts, stings, and bug bites. It is effective when used in a protection amulet. Sprigs of the herb can adorn doorways, can add greenery to cut flowers, or can be placed in rooms to increase the safe, positive vibrations of a space. An infusion of marjoram in vodka, apple cider vinegar, or olive oil can be sprinkled to cleanse magickal objects or the altar. Marjoram is associated with the goddess Aphrodite and the godddess and planet Venus. It is a powerful herb to use in a love spell as it represents an undying love; it is also common in handfastings, weddings, and funerals. In ancient Greece, wreaths of marjoram were worn by couples newly joined in matrimony. Marjoram invokes Thor and Jupiter and their protection from thunder and lightning.

Marjoram Stir-Fry

SERVES 4

When used in culinary dishes, marjoram can draw happiness and love into the lives of those who eat it. Serve this over Chinese noodles or basmati white or brown rice.

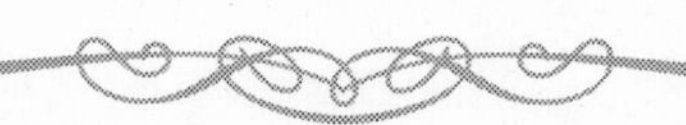

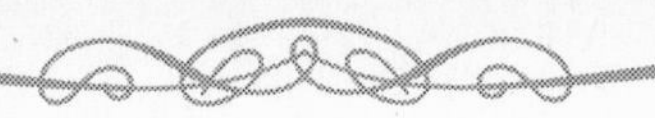

- 2 tablespoons butter
- ½ medium onion, chopped
- 1 cup halved mushrooms
- 3 tablespoons olive oil
- ½ cup broccoli florets and diced stems
- ½ red bell pepper, julienned
- ½ yellow bell pepper, julienned
- 3 cloves garlic, chopped
- 1 cup extra-firm tofu, cubed
- ¼ cup chopped fresh marjoram leaves
- 1 tablespoon cornstarch
- 1 teaspoon sugar
- ½ teaspoon salt
- 1 tablespoon grated fresh ginger
- 1 tablespoon soy sauce
- 1 tablespoon dry vegetable bouillon
- 1 cup boiling water

THIS HERB PREFERS FULL SUN, LIGHT WATER, AND SANDY SOIL. MARJORAM IS NATIVE TO THE MEDITERRANEAN REGION.

Melt the butter in a wok or large skillet and add the onion. Sauté 2 minutes. Add the mushrooms and sauté 5 minutes. Transfer the vegetables to a bowl. In the same wok, heat the oil and add the broccoli and bell peppers. Stir-fry 3 minutes. Add the garlic, tofu, and marjoram and stir-fry 2 minutes longer. In a small bowl, whisk together the cornstarch, sugar, salt, ginger, and soy sauce. Dissolve the bouillon in the boiling water. Add to the cornstarch mixture. Pour into the wok. Cook and stir until the mixture boils and thickens. Decrease the heat to medium-low and simmer, covered, just until vegetables are crisp-tender, about 5 minutes. Stir in the mushrooms and onions. Serve immediately.

Marjoram Butter

MAKES ¼ POUND

In Spain, marjoram is sprinkled on salads. I like to make this butter and then use it to sauté veggies; or I spread it over crusty bread for a special treat.

- 1 tablespoon minced fresh marjoram leaves
- 1 clove garlic, pressed
- ½ cup (1 stick) unsalted butter, room temperature

Combine all the ingredients in a small bowl, then shape into a log. Enclose in plastic wrap or an airtight container. It will keep in the refrigerator for 1 month or in the freezer for 3 months.

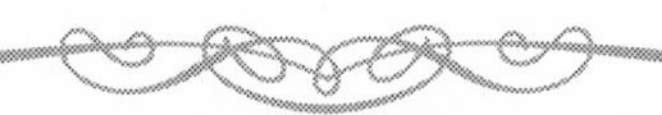

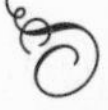

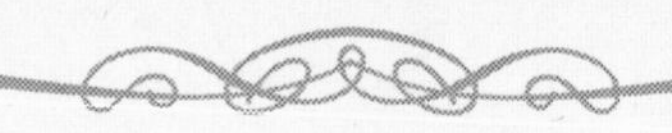

Milk Thistle

Silybum marianum

BLESSED THISTLE, LADY'S THISTLE, MARY THISTLE, WILD ARTICHOKE

Parts Used: seeds, fruit, leaves, stems

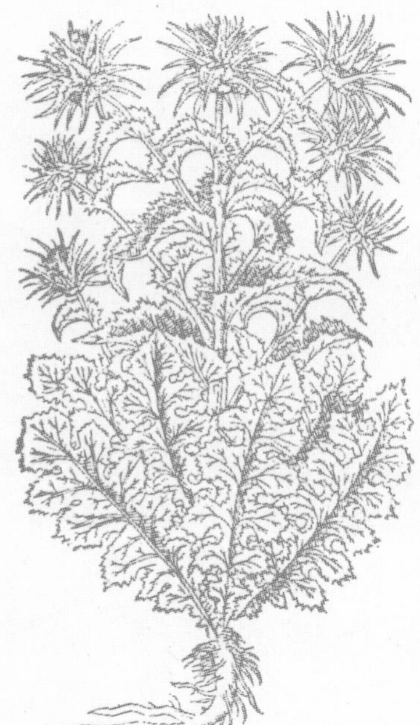

Milk thistle is found in pastures and wastelands. Its leaves are large and gray with silver-white veins and prickly edges. The herb's purple flowers are large and surrounded by spines. It is believed that milk thistle received its medicinal powers and the name *marianum* because a drop of milk from the Virgin Mary's breast fell on the plant as she cut thistle fodder for her donkey. For centuries, milk thistle has been used to aid all manner of problems associated with the liver. It enhances liver detoxification with its active ingredient, silymarin, which binds to liver membranes, preventing damage from toxic chemicals and free radicals. Milk thistle increases milk production in lactating women.

Release Anger

When working properly, the liver processes and releases bile to break down and digest our food. This destructive process is necessary for a healthy body. When we hold on to primitive negative emotions, they get stored in the liver. Anger corrodes the vessel that contains it. In our society, anger in most forms is not always an acceptable emotion for people, especially women, to express. Anger can be healthy when it is managed. Yet we often run from this emotion, keeping busy, shopping, overeating, drinking, and other addictions to avoid facing the feeling. This serves only to separate ourselves from our emotions, perpetuating the anger because we are buying into the fear and belief in the unworthiness of "ugly" emotions.

When we allow angry feelings to control us in this way, we are out of homeostasis or balance. Homeostasis is often thought to come about when opposite forces are in equal proportion; but in fact, it exists when contrary states of being work in harmony. The next time you are feeling exceptionally angry, try this meditation. The milk thistle in it cleanses hate and supports love.

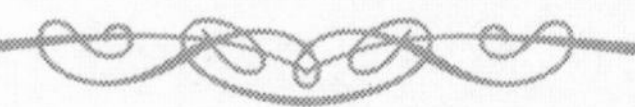

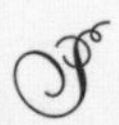

Add ¼ cup milk thistle seeds to 2 cups water. Bring to a boil. Steep 15 minutes. Strain the herbs from the tea.

Light a white candle and begin to sip the tea. Write down everything you are angry about. Circle the words that trigger the strongest reaction. Make a list of these words. For each word, ask yourself what are the benefits and rewards for holding on to this state of being. Recognize the damage caused by holding on to these hurtful feelings.

Now write down all the circled trigger words on a separate piece of paper. Sprinkle a small pinch of milk thistle seeds on the paper. Fold the paper away from you. Write,

I no longer attract these hurtful feelings into my life.

It is okay to be angry. It can activate change. But once change has been motivated, let go of the anger. You have drawn every experience and person into your life for your highest good, not your human comfort. Fold the paper again and write,

I no longer see these hurtful feelings in my life.

When you choose to act from a place of true power and birthright to receive love, you do not need anger to protect you. Turn the paper so that when you fold it again, you fold it away from you. Fold it again and write in red marker or dragon's blood ink,

I see only love
I attract only love
I am love.

Keep the paper on your altar, burn it safely, or bury it. The ending that resonates with you is the right one to do.

Milk thistle prefers rich soil and ample sunlight. It is native to the Mediterranean and has naturalized in California and Australia.

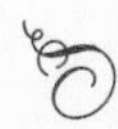

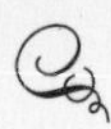

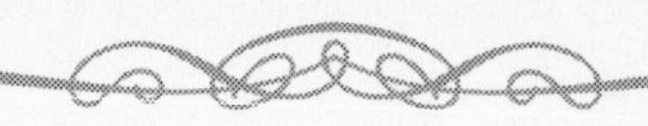

Mint

Mentha (various species)

BRANDY MINT, GARDEN MINT, LAMMIT, OUR LADY'S MINT

Part Used: leaves

Mint is found in moist places and among rocks. Its rough, narrow leaves are very fragrant. The thin flowers are pale mauve and strongly scented. The species most commonly used medicinally are peppermint (*Mentha piperite*) and spearmint (*Mentha spicata*). The herb treats headaches, poor appetite, digestive disorders, infertility, and low sexual desire. Mint can be added to fruit, tuna, and green salads, to fresh yogurt, and to vinegars. According to legend, when Persephone discovered that Pluto was in love with the beautiful nymph Minthe, she went into a rage and turned Minthe into a lowly plant. Although Pluto could not undo Persephone's magic, he was able to alter it. Whenever Minthe was trod upon, her scent became sweeter and more fragrant. Her name changed to Mentha, which became her botanical name.

Magickally, mint is used for purification and prophetic dreams, and in love, prosperity, legal, and success rituals. Mint remedies include aiding flatulence, flus or colds, insomnia, fevers in children, menstrual cramps, toothaches, halitosis, chapped hands, sore mouth or throat, and insect bites. If steeped with vinegar and rosemary, it can relieve dandruff. A bath made from any variety of mint can be invigorating.

MINT IS BELIEVED TO DIMINISH MILK SUPPLY AND SHOULD BE AVOIDED BY LACTATING MOTHERS. EATING TOO MUCH EUROPEAN PENNYROYAL (*Mentha pulegium*) MAY CAUSE CONVULSIONS, LIVER DAMAGE, AND COMA.

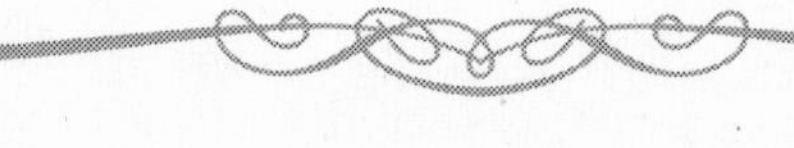

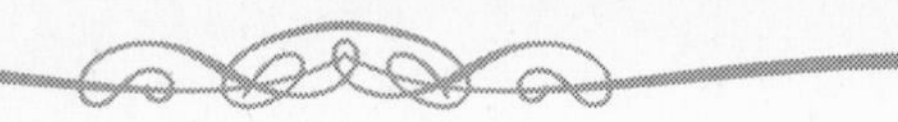

Tantalizing Tabbouleh

SERVES 4 AS AN APPETIZER

Tabbouleh is a very popular dish in the Middle East. It is served cold as an appetizer accompanied by crisp bread or crackers, or as a summertime salad. Mint, associated with Venus, can bring peace and balance. Let peace begin with you. Venus can bring you to a place of balance where serenity and calmness live and breathe in you.

If you are feeling nervous about your state of peace, begin by smudging yourself with smoldering sage leaves. The simple act of allowing the sage smoke to filter through your house has an amazingly calming effect. Next, light several candles. As you prepare the tabbouleh, play soft music that is ethereal and uplifting. Working at a slow pace may feel uncomfortable at first, but it can be safe. Know that while you may feel chaotic, it is the nature of the universe to find order in chaos. Breathe in peace and begin to feel the order and balance.

MAKE SURE MINT HAS PLENTY OF ROOM TO GROW, AS IT IS AN INVASIVE PLANT, ABLE TO SEND UP NEW PLANTS FROM ITS SPREADING ROOTS. IT PREFERS RICH, MOIST, WELL-DRAINED SOIL AND FULL SUN TO PARTIAL SHADE. IT IS A GOOD COMPANION PLANT FOR CABBAGE AND TOMATOES, AS IT WILL REPEL APHIDS, FLEA BEETLES, AND VARIOUS CABBAGE PESTS. MINTS ARE NATIVE TO EUROPE, ASIA, AND NORTH AMERICA.

2 cups fine bulgur cracked wheat
1½ cups chopped, seeded tomatoes
1½ cups minced fresh parsley
2 teaspoons salt
½ cup minced fresh mint
½ cup freshly squeezed lemon juice
½ cup virgin olive oil
2 cups cooked or canned garbanzo beans (chickpeas)

Place the bulgur in a saucepan or bowl and add enough boiling water to cover. Cover the pan and let stand until fluffy, about 2 hours. Drain well, squeezing out extra liquid. Add all remaining ingredients and stir. Chill 1 hour.

Note: If you are using canned garbanzo beans, rinse before adding to the tabbouleh.

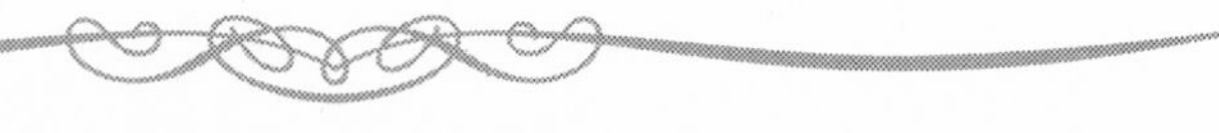

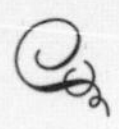

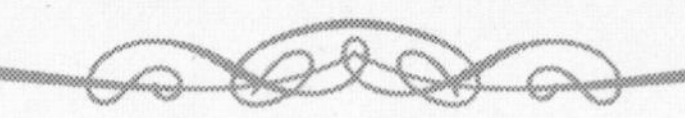

Mint Vinegar

Makes 1 cup

Mint is named after the nymph Mentha. According to Greek myth, a nymph is a young and beautiful female spirit who serves as a guardian of trees, water, and other parts of nature. Nymphs are considered lesser deities; they are neither human nor immortal. They are named for either the location in which they dwell or for a particular function of nature. Many nymphs are represented as musical, amorous, and gentle, but some are associated with wilder aspects of nature and are akin to satyrs. Still others are vengeful and capable of destruction.

As guardians of nature, nymphs implore us to remember that we, too, are stewards of land and sea. As you make this vinegar, reflect on the fact that no matter how trivial your life may seem, you are indeed a hero or heroine finding his or her way back home to the caretaker of our Mother, the earth. Use this vinegar as a dressing for spring salads, or drizzle it over tender meat.

1 cup white wine vinegar
1 teaspoon honey
3 (2-inch-long) sprigs mint
¼ teaspoon cardamom seeds

In a small saucepan, heat the vinegar and honey over medium heat 3 to 5 minutes; do not boil. Place the mint and the cardamom seeds in a glass jar. Pour the vinegar mixture over the herbs. Let the vinegar cool, then cover it and store in a cool, dark place for up to a year.

Brigid's Flame

Peppermint is an invigorating scent used to uplift and awaken the senses. Its healing and purification properties make it an herb of Imbolc, also known as Brigid's Day. Brigid is the goddess of fire, healing, craftsmanship, and creativity. She symbolizes the bride and is central to the Imbolc sabbat.

When Ireland was Christianized, the pagan goddess Brigid was transformed into the human Brigid, the daughter of a Druid. The story is that St. Patrick con-

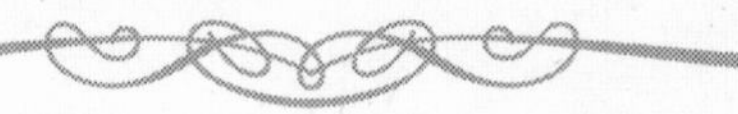

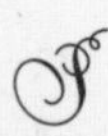

verted and baptized her. After her death, she was canonized. She retained many of the attributes that were associated with the pagan goddess, including performing miracles, promoting fertility, inventing whistling and the healing art of keening, and possessing the power to appoint bishops, who must be goldsmiths. All the way into the eighteenth century, nineteen nuns tended her continually burning sacred flame at a women-only shrine in the Church of the Oak in Kildare, Ireland. There, an ancient song was sung to her: "Brigid, excellent woman, sudden flame, may the bright fiery sun take us to the lasting kingdom."

Imbolc is a late-winter holy day honoring the return of the light and the inspiration of new ideas that will be birthed in the spring. Even though the first light has come, there are several weeks left of winter; this is the time to review what has been learned during the quiet time of the year. It is an opportunity to see the silver lining on all the work you have done.

As you make these candles, meditate on peppermint's innate ability to heal and purify. Ask that Brigid help you focus on healing and forgiving, to create a new you that will be birthed in spring.

2 gold beeswax sheets
2 red beeswax sheets
4 candle wicks
10 to 12 drops of peppermint essential oil

Cut each beeswax sheet in half diagonally. Using 1 red piece and 1 gold piece for each candle, place 1 triangular piece atop another, overlapping but slightly offset. Press the wick into the bottom sheet so that it is embedded in the wax. Roll the 2 pieces up together; double-colored spirals will appear as you roll. Repeat to make 4 candles. Dab each candle with peppermint oil. Press firmly but gently with both palms, using a cradling motion to feel for any uneven areas. Roll back and forth to compress the wax. Snip the wicks off, leaving half an inch at the top.

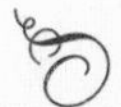

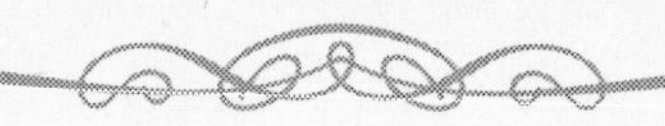

Mistletoe

Viscum album

ALL HEAL, GOLDEN BOUGH, THUNDER BESOM

Parts Used: berries, leaves

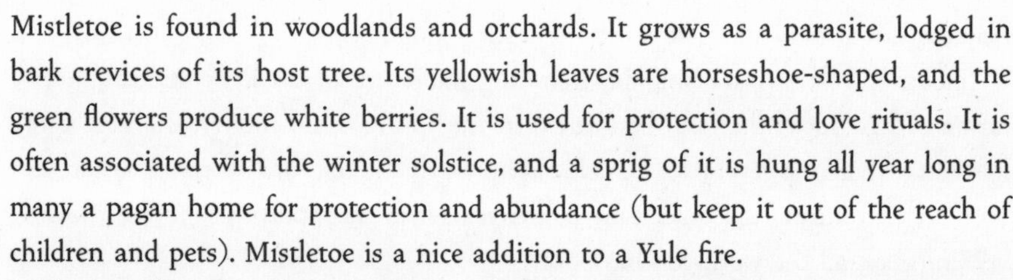

Mistletoe is found in woodlands and orchards. It grows as a parasite, lodged in bark crevices of its host tree. Its yellowish leaves are horseshoe-shaped, and the green flowers produce white berries. It is used for protection and love rituals. It is often associated with the winter solstice, and a sprig of it is hung all year long in many a pagan home for protection and abundance (but keep it out of the reach of children and pets). Mistletoe is a nice addition to a Yule fire.

The Druids gathered this "golden bough" on midsummer's eve and at the winter solstice, cutting it with a golden scythe and catching it in a cloth, so that it never touched the ground. They believed mistletoe could open all locks, treat all ills, and conduct lightning. "All heal" is the name most commonly used for mistletoe by modern Druids. In magick, mistletoe represents immortality, rebirth, protection, harmony, blessings, and good fortune. It is used to invoke Odin and Aphrodite.

BOTH AMERICAN AND EUROPEAN MISTLETOE CAN BE TOXIC,
AND SHOULD NOT BE TAKEN INTERNALLY.

Passage to Manhood

This ritual is designed for a boy of about thirteen about to embark on the passage to manhood, using the venerated and holy mistletoe for guidance. The ceremonoy symbolizes the process of first embracing, and then transcending, man's animal nature.

On midsummer's eve, stay up all night listening to bardic stories about the noble heroes of the past told by older men (or reading them, if you are alone). At first light on midsummer's day (Litha), go outside—skyclad (naked) if you prefer, or simply clothed—and pick vervain, gathering it with your left hand and cutting it

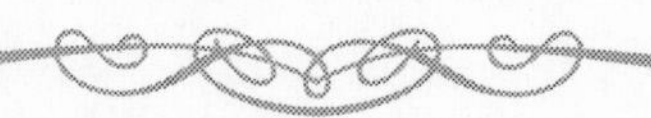

with your right. Bless the plant, and leave it an offering of pure water. (If you have no access to fresh vervain, then buy some and leave it outside overnight to gather on Litha.) Draw yourself a bath and, while the tub is filling, make yourself a cup of tea from a little of the vervain; hang the rest to dry. Skip breakfast if you can; immerse yourself in the warm clean water and then sip the tea. Soak for a few minutes, until you feel purified within and without.

Dry off, and in a quiet, somewhat darkened place, light some charcoal on a brazier. Sit cross-legged with the brazier in front of you, and sprinkle a few leaves of dried mistletoe gathered from the previous winter solstice (Yule) on the charcoal. Continue to feed the charcoal bits of mistletoe as you allow the sweet resinous scent of the burning herb to envelop you, body and spirit. When you feel ready, lift your arms out to your sides, elbows bent so that your hands point straight up on either side of your head. Close your eyes, and silently call on Cernunnos, the Horned One, the ancient, antlered European god of masculine energy, whose real name is lost in antiquity. Ask him for guidance on your journey into manhood. Walk with him, if he will take you at this time, through the cycle of death and rebirth, which we all must take.

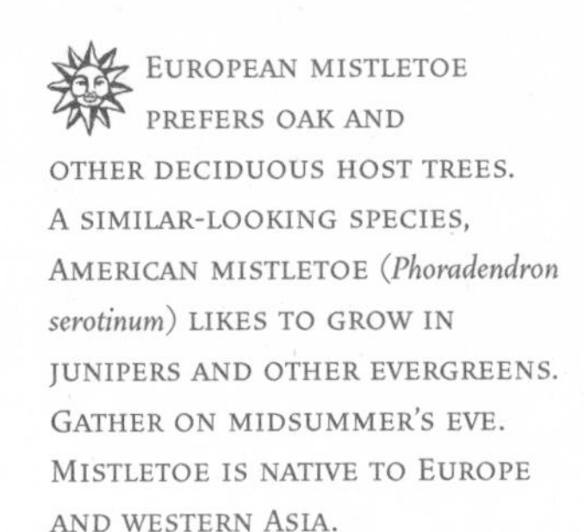

European mistletoe prefers oak and other deciduous host trees. A similar-looking species, American mistletoe (*Phoradendron serotinum*) likes to grow in junipers and other evergreens. Gather on midsummer's eve. Mistletoe is native to Europe and western Asia.

When it is time for your meditation to end, he will bid you farewell. Thank him, arise, and dress in practical clothes, but wear a white shirt of some sort. You may eat something light at this time, if necessary.

Now, travel with your friends to someplace where mistletoe grows and can be cut. It is best to have picked out your spot in advance, so that you can be sure to arrive a bit before midday. When you arrive, take a moment to clear your head, and call on Cernunnos for his blessing. Make an offering to the tree; an ample amount of water with a little plant food added is appropriate. After making your offering, you may take the mistletoe. Take the bough in your left hand and cut it with your right; or simply snap it off. If possible, climb the tree, or if you must, use a ladder.

Wrap the bough in white cloth for the journey, return home, and hang it up to dry. Eat a good meal in the company of your friends. The cutting of the mistletoe at noon on midsummer symbolizes the sacrifice of masculine energy at the height of masculine power. But by the same token, only by being cut down and dried does this inconspicuous green herb, incapable of growing on its own, become the

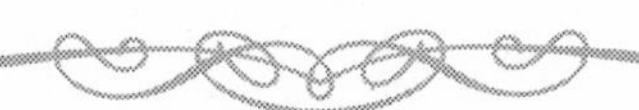

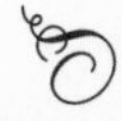

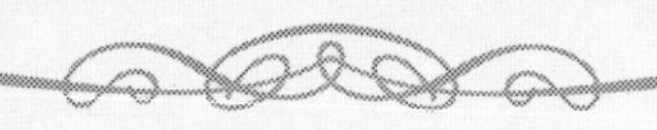

Motherwort

Leonurus cardiaca

HEART HEAL, LION'S EAR, LION'S TAIL, MOTHER HERB

Parts Used: leaves, flowers, stems

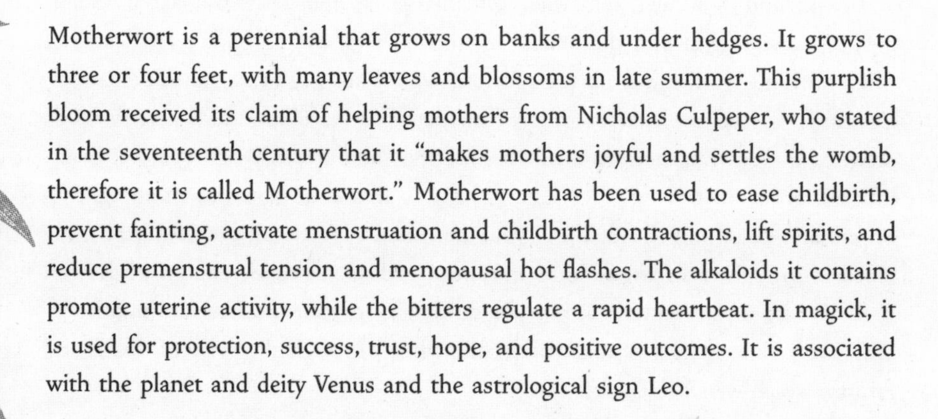

Motherwort is a perennial that grows on banks and under hedges. It grows to three or four feet, with many leaves and blossoms in late summer. This purplish bloom received its claim of helping mothers from Nicholas Culpeper, who stated in the seventeenth century that it "makes mothers joyful and settles the womb, therefore it is called Motherwort." Motherwort has been used to ease childbirth, prevent fainting, activate menstruation and childbirth contractions, lift spirits, and reduce premenstrual tension and menopausal hot flashes. The alkaloids it contains promote uterine activity, while the bitters regulate a rapid heartbeat. In magick, it is used for protection, success, trust, hope, and positive outcomes. It is associated with the planet and deity Venus and the astrological sign Leo.

IF YOU HAVE SENSITIVE SKIN, YOU SHOULD AVOID HANDLING MOTHERWORT.

Mama's Little Helper

Parenting requires on-the-job understanding, for which we often have no formal experience. It takes faith in oneself, flexibility, steadfastness, and courage. There is a tenacity that comes with motherhood and pushes her through sleep-deprived days and colic-ridden nights. Parents must invoke the courage to accept the situation as is, turning the reins over to Spirit. The Purple Heart of courage is manifest in this flower's bloom. (This ritual was donated by Cathi Martinez Budd, an aficionado of folklore, faery tales, and eclectic education.)

Dry motherwort flowers and glue them to a headband or wreath. Alternatively, you can mix the blooms with dried lavender and rose petals and place in a muslin bag for calming and courage. Host a tea party a few months after a babe is born.

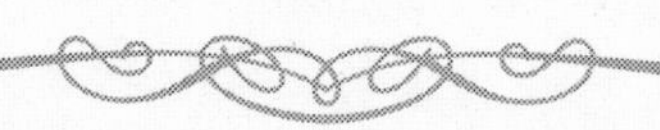

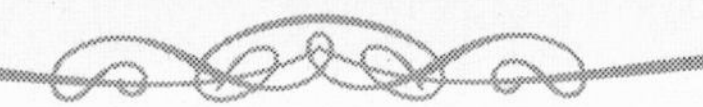

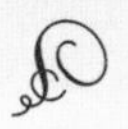

This celebration can be an observance of the new joy for both the mother and father. When you mail out invitations, include a blank sheet of paper on which the guests can write a wish for the new parents and their child as he/she begins his/her life journey. During the party the guests can read their blessings aloud. Take a picture of each guest reading their wish and then affix the wish next to the photograph in a Faery Godparents scrapbook.

At the party, you can offer a clove spice pillow (page 100) to honor the father (protector) and the motherwort wreath or bag to honor the mother (nurturer).

Attach to the gift of the pillow, wreath, or bag the following poem, to be repeated for a new mother (or father)—especially during particularly difficult days of impatience, fatigue, loneliness, and sadness:

I am a Mother/Father
    I am not perfect
A heart of courage sustains me
    Even though I cannot see
Low days, medium, and high I will have
    And I accept all three.

Start from seed, planting in full sun with some extra space. The plant should spread rapidly on its own in a climate that suits its needs, though it does not flourish in much of the West. A native of Europe, motherwort has colonized large areas of the eastern United States, populating vacant lots and the edges of highways.

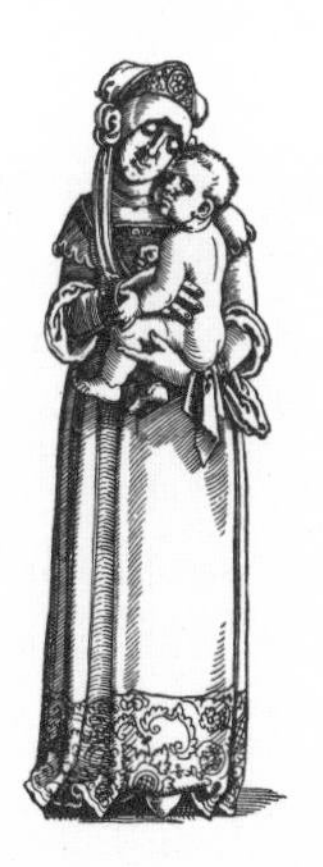

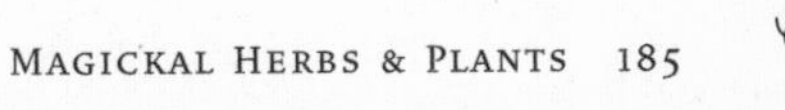

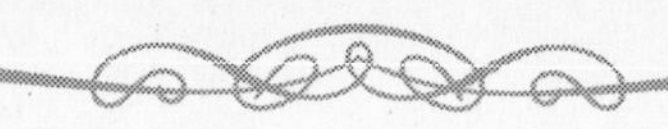

Mugwort

Artemisia vulgaris

ARTEMIS HERB, FELON HERB, OLD UNCLE HARRY, SAILOR'S TOBACCO, WITCH HERB

Parts Used: leaves, root

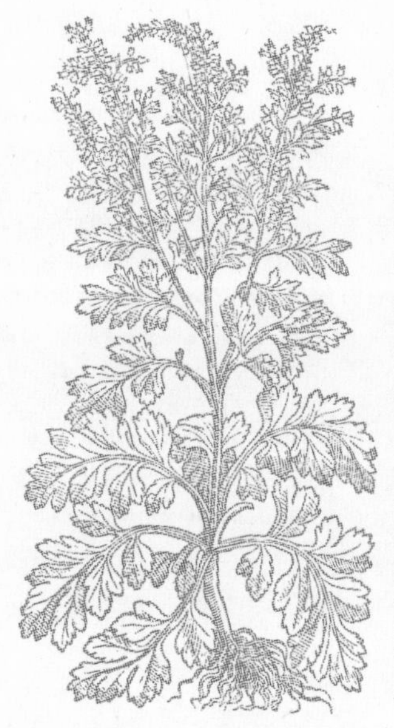

Mugwort is a perennial shrub with dark green leaves and clusters of reddish or yellow flowers. Native Californians have used a decoction of mugwort leaves for headaches, colic, bronchitis, and rheumatism. After childbirth it is taken to promote blood circulation and it makes a successful moth repellent. In China, mugwort was hung to protect the bearer from evil spirits on Dragon Festival, held on the fifth day of the fifth moon. In the Middle Ages it was believed that a crown of mugwort worn on St. John's Eve would protect the wearer from evil possession. Mugwort is used extensively for protection and banishing and has been for centuries. The herb was once stuffed in pillows to induce happy, prophetic dreams. Mixed with chamomile it makes an excellent muscle-relaxing bath. Mugwort is the herb for clairvoyance, traveling, protection, and consecration. It is associated with Artemis and Diana.

Banishment Incense

This powerful incense was prepared for a dear friend who was suffering a psychic attack against her home and spirit. The friend designed her own ritual, but this incense cleared out all resident unwanted entities and energies. It placed an impenetrable shell of protection around her property and her being. This incense is best prepared on the full moon and used on a waning moon in Pisces. (This recipe is from Rue Founder of Moonshadow Sanctuary; Rue is a practicing Witch and an intuitive healer.)

2 tablespoons dried angelica root
2 tablespoons dried marshmallow root
2 tablespoons dried red clover blossoms and leaves

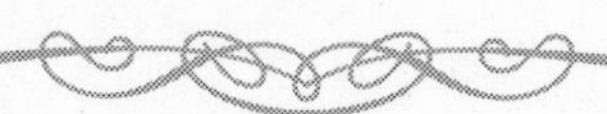

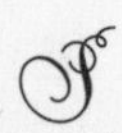

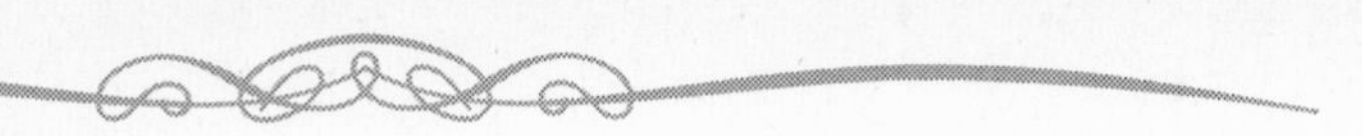

1 tablespoon dried yarrow flowers

1 tablespoon dried mugwort leaves

1 teaspoon dried sandalwood powder

Place the angelica and marshmallow in a coffee grinder or spice grinder and process to the consistency of coarse coffee grounds. (I realize that some may scorn the use of an electrical appliance, but roots can be stubborn and using a combination of the fire and air energies—electricity—works really well.) Scrape the mixture into a mortar, and add the red clover, yarrow, mugwort, and sandalwood. Crush the mixture together with the pestle, always blending in a widdershins (counterclockwise) direction. Press your intention for banishment and protection into the blend. Pour the mixture into the storage container you have chosen. Seal the container tightly and allow the powers of the herbs to integrate for a few days.

Burn this incense on a charcoal round at the beginning of your ritual to chase away the unwanted and again at the end of your ritual to seal the protection. You may want to use this incense in conjunction with a Witch's Ladder-Binding Cord spell (see page 191).

Mugwort prefers average to poor soil and full sun. Gather it during a full moon in late summer. Mugwort grows in temperate regions of the Northern Hemisphere.

Moon Scry

Try this ritual on a full moon near Samhain, when the boundary between the Otherworld and the mundane is easily crossed. You will be able to receive messages or symbols that will light your path with clear thinking and a sense of peace. Scrying—the divinatory act of gazing at an object until prophetic visions, symbols, or messages appear—has been used for centuries by cultures both indigenous and transplanted. A visionary focal point, such as calm water, a black mirror, or a crystal ball, is used as a portal to discern answers from the highest vibrations of consciousness. While methods of scrying differ, they all require concentration and patience. After concentrating, mental images, visions, and impressions appear. However, if you try too hard to see images, nothing will form; if you are impatient, the answer will be inaccurate or unclear. It is best to relax and be calm, trusting that you have the ability to tap into the highest truth and good for all.

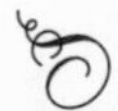

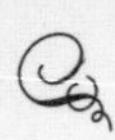

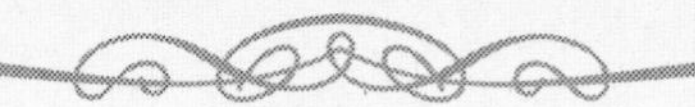

Once you have set a sacred space, allow the physical eyes to relax, letting the third eye (in the middle of your forehead) open and receive needed information. Realize that this focal point is a doorway into the astral plane, allowing for communication with higher realms and the subconscious. Scrying develops your clairvoyant abilities and is especially helpful for strengthening your third eye.

3 teaspoons dried mugwort leaves
3 teaspoons dried wormwood leaves
Fresh spring water

Ground yourself by taking some time to become fully aware of your surroundings. Bring yourself to the present and try not to allow your thoughts to become distracted. Imagine a rainbow-colored ray of light—the energy that runs in front of your spine—known as your kundalini, or chakra alignment. Mix the herbs in a mortar with a pestle. Fill a cauldron with fresh spring water. Place the herbs in the cauldron.

Close your eyes and take three deep breaths. Think of a question that you desire to have answered. Stare into the water with unfocused eyes. Make a mental note of any images or words that appear to you. Do not discard anything that percolates to the surface of your awareness, even when it seems unrelated. Symbols have a way of communicating volumes of insights that our consciousness would block. When you have finished, write down all the information that you received. Place your hands over the notes and say,

Dear God and Goddess, thank you for this gift
I pray that it brings the desired shift
I promise to use this information in love and light
That I may reflect your goodness and might.

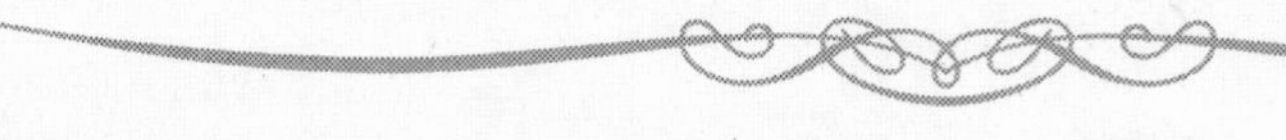

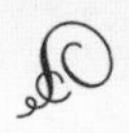

Mullein

Verbascum (various species)

BLANKET LEAF, CANDLEWICK PLANT, HAG'S TAPER, JUPITER'S STAFF, LADY'S FOXGLOVE

Parts Used: leaves, flowers

Mullein is found along waysides. Its downy leaves form a broad, gray mat, which is how it received the nickname "blanket leaf." The yellow, roselike flowers grow on tall spikes and have a honey scent. Mullein contains tannins, which act as an astringent to reduce bleeding and constrict tissue. The herb also has high concentrations of mucilage, flavonoids, saponins, and volatile oils. Mullein treats coughs, pneumonia, bronchitis, tuberculosis, asthma, bowel disorders, poor sleep, headaches, sinus troubles, and earaches. In magick circles, mullein is used for protection and courage. It is associated with women and the planet and god Saturn.

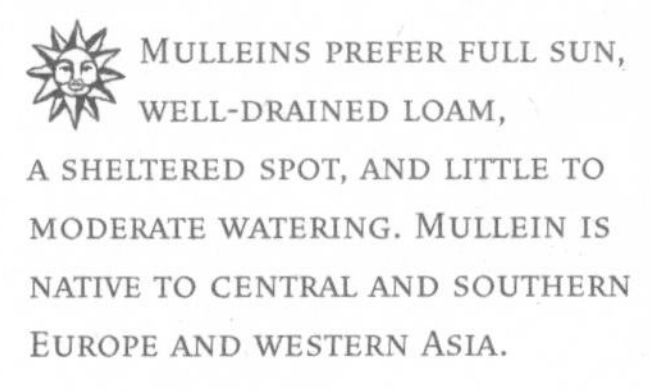
MULLEINS PREFER FULL SUN, WELL-DRAINED LOAM, A SHELTERED SPOT, AND LITTLE TO MODERATE WATERING. MULLEIN IS NATIVE TO CENTRAL AND SOUTHERN EUROPE AND WESTERN ASIA.

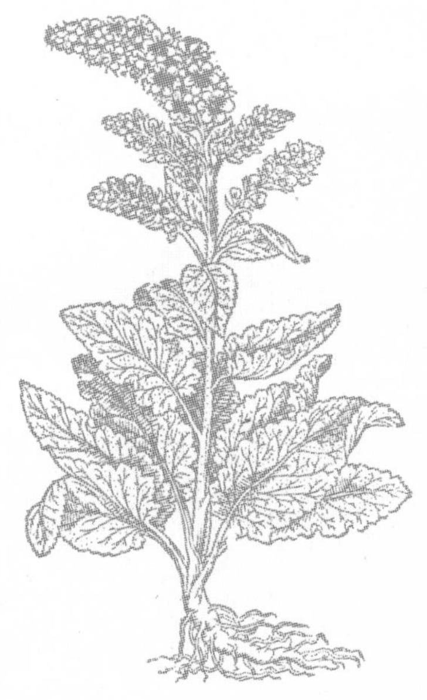

True Listening

This is a healing recipe that focuses on restoring health, not destroying or abolishing pain. Too often we disregard our pain and push it away. Our hurts and pains are like children that need to be embraced, brought into our bosom, and acknowledged. Whenever you are hurting, pay close attention to the location of your ailment and consider the message being offered by the discomfort. When pain has lodged in the ear, often something is happening in our immediate environment that we do not want to hear (it can also be a sign of lactose intolerance). Consider whether there is fighting or disharmony around you. Are people gossiping? Are you sending yourself negative messages?

Holding a space of true listening means that you are opening yourself to acceptance and nonjudgmentalism. Things are perfect just the way they are because they are happening. Listen with an open heart. Do not attach hurtful meanings to the messages you receive. See yourself in perfect alignment with Spirit—living and listening in harmony and love. For this ritual, you will need an ear cone, available

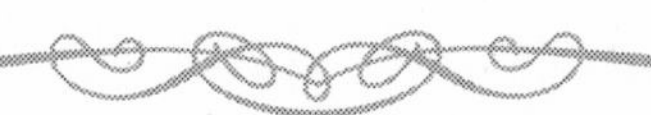

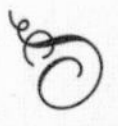

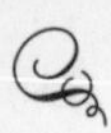

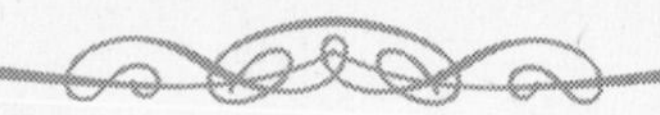

at whole food markets, New Age and occult stores. This is a good ritual to repeat at each of the equinoxes and solstices. Light a candle appropriate to the season: such as orange for autumn, red for winter, green for spring, or yellow for summer; the color choice depends upon your intention of embracing the holiday. Consult the directions on the ear cone package and begin the ear coning. After the ear coning, allow a few drops of slightly warmed garlic- and mullein-infused oil to drip into your ear. Be very careful to not overheat the oil. Test on your wrist to be sure it is lukewarm, not hot. This process will enable you to hear new messages at the turn of each new season.

½ cup garlic cloves

½ cup mullein flowers

1 cup olive oil

½ teaspoon vitamin E oil

Fill a small jar with the garlic and mullein. Cover with the olive oil, and screw on a tight-fitting lid. Let sit for 6 weeks in a dark, cool place. Strain out the herbs. Add the vitamin E oil to the oil and store in a dark place until you are ready to use it. It will keep for 1 year.

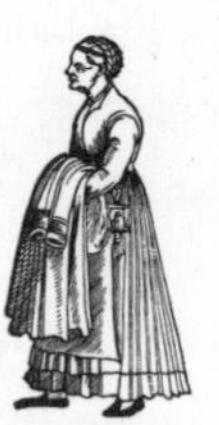

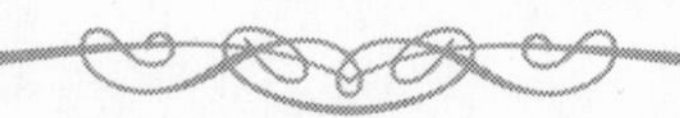

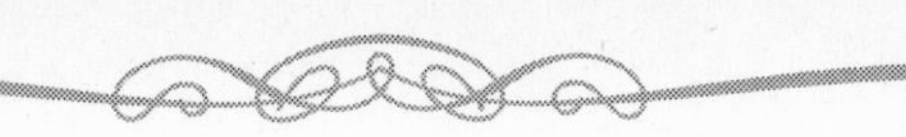

Myrrh

Commiphora myrrha

GUM MYRRH TREE, KARAN

Part Used: gum

Myrrh is usually used to protect and purify and is often combined with frankincense. It can be utilized in attraction spells, or anytime your work needs a little push; it purifies and protects both the magician and his work. Myrrh is antibiotic and antiseptic and was used by the Egyptians in preparing the body for the afterlife. The Queen of Sheba used myrrh oil in her seduction of Solomon. According to Greek myth, Myrrha, daughter of the king of Syria, escaped Aphrodite's jealousy and coercion to commit incest with her father, Thesis, when the gods turned her into a myrrh tree. It is said that the drops of gum resin are Myrrha's tears. According to biblical legend, gold, frankincense, and myrrh were the gifts of the three wise men.

Myrrh is both antifungal and astringent, and good for oral ulcers and gum inflammation or infections as well as chapped skin. Burning myrrh repels mosquitoes. Combine 1 cup of warm water, ½ teaspoon myrrh tincture, 1 drop of mint essential oil, 1 drop of orange essential oil, and 1 drop of tea tree oil for a breath-freshening antiseptic gargle. Myrrh invokes the goddesses Cybele, Demeter, Isis, Hecate, and Rhea and the gods Jupiter, Adonis, and Saturn.

Witch's Ladder-Binding Cord

This spell will help you to attract positive energy into your life; negative energy will be bound into the cord.

At sunrise or sunset, anoint a three-foot piece of black cord with myrrh oil. Use crow feathers or other objects to represent the negative energy you are locking into the cord. Tie one object into each knot and breathe your intentions into the knot. Repeat for a total of nine knots; as you tie, say,

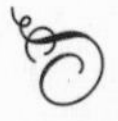

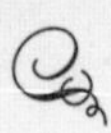

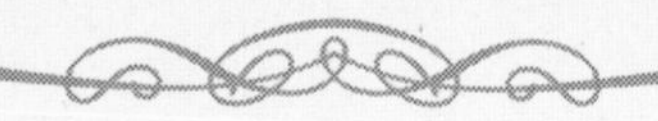

Tie one, the spell's begun

Tie two, no power undo

Tie three, so mote it be

Tie four, forever more

Tie five, this charm's alive

Tie six, its magick fix

Tie seven, now under heaven

Tie eight, work winds of fate

Tie nine, to my design.

Hang the cord on your front door to affirm your intention to keep negative energy away. (For different types of spells, you may place the knotted cord on your altar or a mirror, or burn and bury it with other items.)

Saturn's Potpourri

You can purchase myrrh and sandalwood by the ounce at most magickal shops. Myrrh is used to heighten spiritual connection during rituals and holidays. Allow the awareness and knowledge of the many deities associated with myrrh to flow through you. Every story of a god or goddess is an amplified parable of your life—expanded and turned into myth. When you align yourself with the unstoppable immortality of a deity, you can do the great work of the cosmos and fill your divine purpose.

Myrrh's connection to Saturn can help you relax into the understanding of your life's pattern. When you are about 26½ years of age, Saturn returns into your astrological chart, motivating you to develop self-discipline, self-respect, and faith in your destiny. Once Saturn returns, the next 3 to 5 years will be a time for you to focus on intention, process, and progress in your life. It is a time of the death of your old self. During this period, your faith will be challenged, as all former beliefs and crutches disappear and you must stand alone.

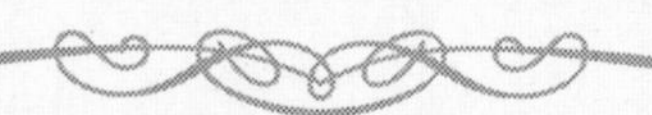

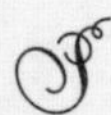

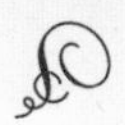

When you reach the end of this period, you will have come through a powerful yet difficult time. You now have intimate knowledge of your deepest passions and greatest fears. This is the time when you have the opportunity to become your own best friend. Make this potpourri in perfect love and the perfect trust of who you are.

¼ cup myrrh gum
¼ cup sandalwood chips
¼ cup dried rose petals
¼ cup dried fir needles
5 dried eucalyptus leaves, crushed
Sláinte cologne (page 233)

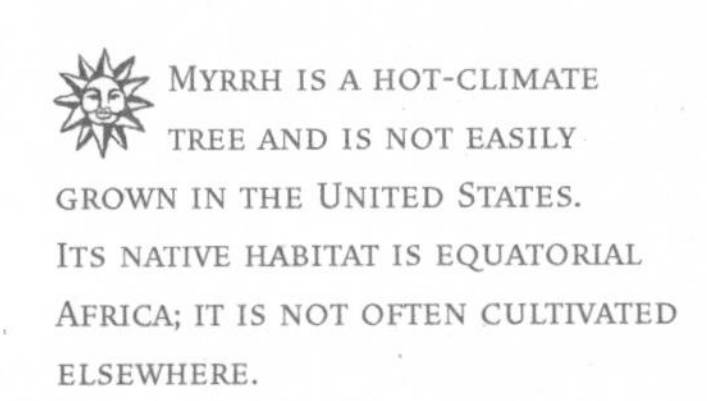

Myrrh is a hot-climate tree and is not easily grown in the United States. Its native habitat is equatorial Africa; it is not often cultivated elsewhere.

Mix together the myrrh, sandalwood, rose, fir, and eucalyptus. Add sláinte cologne 1 drop at a time until you reach a pleasing scent. Store potpourri in a basket, glass jar, or ceramic container; keep it as long as the scent pleases you.

Variation: You may also want to add 6 to 10 drops of either fir or balsam essential oil, which will intensify the scent and make it last longer.

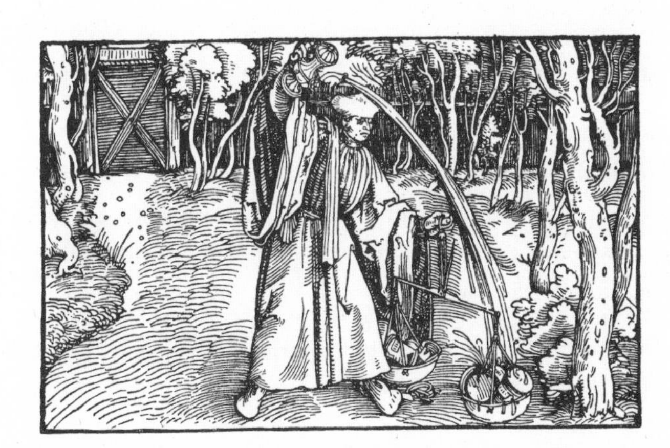

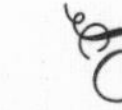

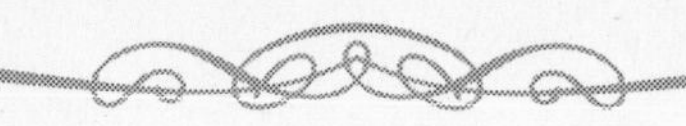

Nettle

Urtica dioica

STINGING NETTLE, WILD SPINACH

Parts Used: leaves, roots, seeds, flowers, stalks

NETTLE PREFERS RICH, MOIST SOIL AND FULL SUN TO PARTIAL SHADE; IT GROWS IN TEMPERATE REGIONS WORLDWIDE. HANDLE STINGING NETTLE WITH CARE; WEAR PROTECTIVE GLOVES.

Nettle is found growing over wastelands and in hedgerows. The serrated leaves are hairy and dull green, and they possess formic acid, which burns the human skin. Native Americans used nettle as a tonic after childbirth to prevent hemorrhaging and encourage milk production. They also used it to treat colds, gout, stomachaches, and hair loss. In Europe, nettle tea was gargled to expel kidney stones, ease sore throats, and reduce water retention. Nettle has the ability to stem bleeding, including nosebleeds, heavy menstrual flow, and wounds. Those lacking sufficient iron find nettle an effective cure for anemia. Nettle is one of the most chlorophyll-rich plants in the world, containing very high levels of minerals and vitamins. The leaves can be boiled for several minutes to remove the formic acid and eaten as a vegetable. Nettle is used to protect and banish in magickal work. Nettle is associated with the planet and god Mars.

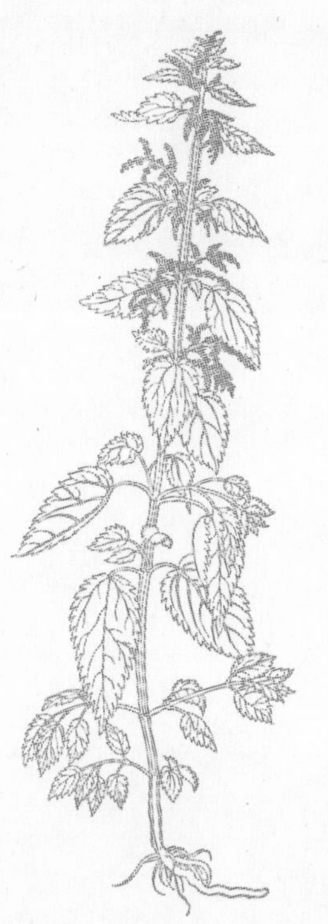

Nettle Hair Rinse

Nettle is an astringent, which restricts oil production. It will improve hair texture and color, and relieve dandruff. This rinse is great to use when you are camping or plan to be outdoors for a few days where you don't have the means or desire for a daily shower. You can pour half a cup over your hair to eliminate the greasy, grimy feeling of dirty hair.

- 2 cups water
- ¼ cup chopped fresh nettle leaves
- ¼ cup fresh sage leaves

Bring the water to a boil. Place the nettle and sage in a bowl and pour the boiling water over. Steep the mixture 15 minutes. Strain out the herbs and pour the rinse into a bottle. Cover and store in a cool place. This rinse will keep for 2 days.

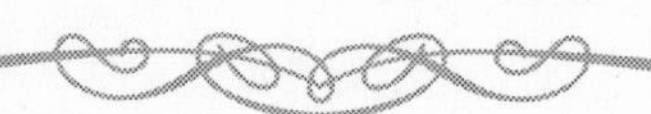

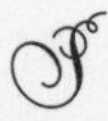

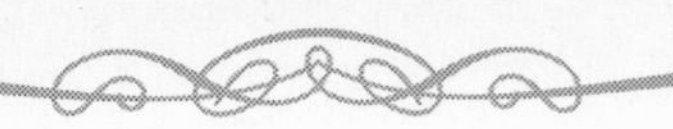

Nutmeg

Myristica fragrans

NUX MOSCHATA

Part Used: seeds

Nutmeg is propogated from seed and sown when ripe. It will yield fruit after eight years and up to sixty years. Nutmeg relieves muscle spasms, prevents vomiting, and is used as a stimulant. In India, nutmeg is considered an aphrodisiac and believed to increase sexual stamina. Grated nutmeg can be made into a paste to treat eczema. Taken internally, it relieves digestive problems. Nutmeg carries the magickal powers of clairvoyance and divination. It is used in spells that work with earth energies, or enhance joy, love, money, luck, and health.

NUTMEG IS A LARGE TROPICAL TREE, GROWN MAINLY IN INDONESIA AND THE WEST INDIES.

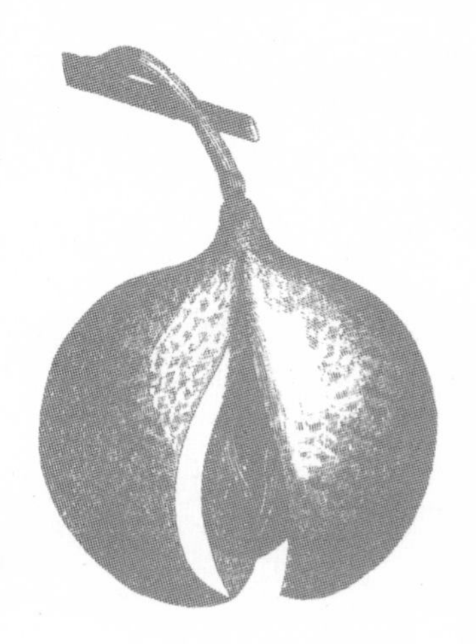

LOW DOSES OF NUTMEG ARE RECOMMENDED AS THE HERB IS A HALLUCINOGEN. IT HAS BEEN REPORTED THAT EATING JUST TWO WHOLE NUTMEG SEEDS CAN CAUSE DEATH.

Rebellious Peppers

SERVES 6

Nutmeg is associated with the planets Jupiter and Uranus. Jupiter aids us in success, victory, and luck. It does not recognize the possibility of defeat. Using Jupiter's energy, try to imagine a life without defeat. This does not mean that you get whatever you want, but that you are present in every moment, accepting it as it appears, not wishing it could be different. This acceptance allows you to find the beauty and grace in all things. With these attributes there is no defeat, only experience. Uranus derives its name from the Greek god of heaven. The god Uranus was a person-ification of the sky and was also believed to be the youngest son of Gaia. The planet Uranus is the first of the invisible planets, and its discovery in 1781 was a surprise; up to that time only seven planets had been identified. At that time, the number seven symbolized death. With the discovery of the eighth planet, the possibility of additional worlds and life after death became

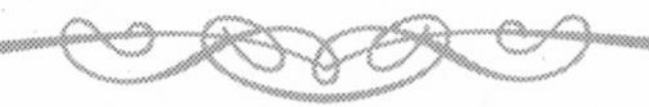

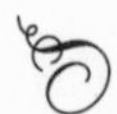

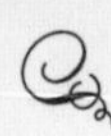

more real. Hence, Uranus came to symbolize the transcendence of the known self to greater illimitable realities.

The function of Uranus is to develop the individual without an adherence to social rules. Uranus represents an opportunity to grow in expanding ways, constantly birthing a new self. As you cook these peppers, tap in to the grand, unfathomable nature of yourself. Be aware that there are no walls, rules, or lines that can hold you back as you develop the freedom of your individuality. As you allow for full expression, invite true intimacy with yourself and others. Only when you can allow yourself or another to be without judgment will you be free.

Uranus is the planet of rebellion and mutiny. If you feel trapped in mores that no longer work for you, light a candle that represents autonomy and freedom. Know that you do not have defend your right to be free; you must just affirm and claim it. Say,

I am safe and supported to be expansive and free
I now let go of ties that bind me
And embrace the individuality of my enlarged nature
With conscious choice beyond stagnant rules of culture.

2 yellow bell peppers
2 orange bell peppers
1 cup orange juice
1½ teaspoons grated nutmeg
1 teaspoon cinnamon
1 teaspoon minced fresh thyme

Roast the peppers by either holding them over a high gas flame until blackened, or placing them in the broiler until blackened. Wrap them in a paper towel and then place them in a plastic bag; let sit for 15 minutes. Remove the peppers from the bag and rub the blackened skin off with a paper towel. Julienne the peppers, discarding the seeds and ribs, and transfer to a serving bowl. Whisk together the juice, nutmeg, cinnamon, and them in a small bowl. Pour the blend over the peppers and serve.

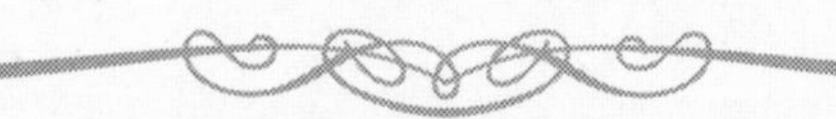

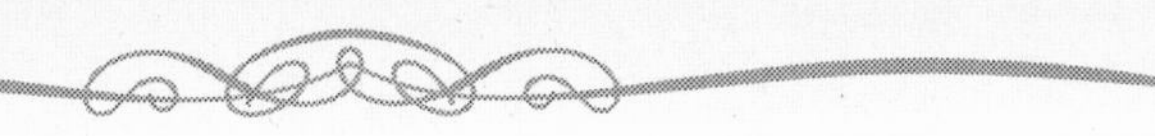

Oak

Quercus (various species)

DUIR, JOVE'S NUTS

Parts Used: leaves, nuts, branches

For Wiccans, oak is the most royal and holy of all trees and has a long history in mythology. Messages from the gods at the oak grove at Dodona in Greece were interpreted from the sound of the wind in the oak leaves. A crown of oak leaves was awarded in Greco-Roman times for saving a life and for victory in the Pythian games. The Norse gods Odin and Thor and Greco-Roman Zeus/Jupiter, along with other thunder gods, are connected to the oak.

Faeries are believed to live in the oaks. Oak is one of the longest-living trees, spanning generation after generation, and thus was venerated by the Druids. Very often, an acorn was carved at the end of a Druid's wand, and oak leaves were worn or carried for protection. Oaks were planted to mark boundaries for important meetings and ceremonies. One possible derivation of the word *Druid* is *dru-wid*, meaning "knower of oak trees," though *deru* also means "truth" or "troth"; therefore an alternate meaning could be "knower of the truth." In the ancient Celtic, the oak is called *duir*, which originated from the Gaelic and Sanskrit words meaning "door." This door can represent a portal to other worlds, new levels of spirituality, or inner strength. Oak is usually the fuel for the midsummer fires and the log for the Yule fire, since the oak virtually stands at the doorway of the great turning points of the year.

An oak tree will take seventy to eighty years to produce its first acorn. The fallen branches make excellent wands. Oak is used for fertility, protection, attraction, and longevity and is associated with truth, growth, kings, and understanding. Sit with an oak tree to bring a sense of calm and to build upon your inner strength. The oak will help you call up your courage and restore your faith. Today, powerful rituals are conducted in stands of oak trees.

OAK TREES PREFER FULL SUN. DO NOT WATER NATIVE TREES, THOUGH THE PLANTED ONES DO LIKE OCCASIONAL WATERING. OAK TREES GROW VIGOROUSLY AND QUICKLY. OAKS CAN BENEFIT FROM PERIODIC GROOMING BUT LARGE BRANCHES SHOULD NOT BE CUT. OAK TREES GROW IN EUROPE AND NORTH AMERICA.

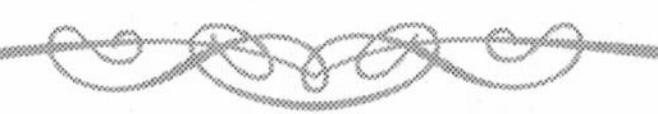

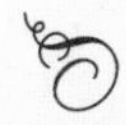

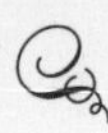

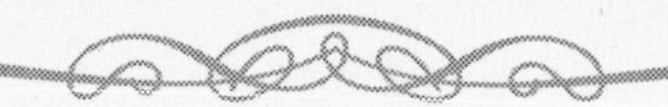

The juice from crushed oak leaves can be applied directly to cuts or wounds. An infusion of the leaves relieves tired and inflamed eyes, cuts and burns, bleeding gums, hemorrhoids, varicose veins, and sore throats.

Solstice Oak Candle

The oak is virile and is representative of the Young God. He battles his brother, Holly, at Yule and Litha. The oak is known as king of midwinter and rules during the months the sun is waxing, from December to June. At Yule the Oak King takes his throne from the Holly King, known as the king of midsummer, who rules during the months the sun is waning, from June to December.

Light this candle and a log for your Yule fire. Throw some holly into the fire as you release the old and bring in the new. Allow the oak to represent all that you want to manifest in the coming year. Our modern-day New Year's resolutions originated with the Yuletide tradition of liberation from the past to pave the way for a better future.

Candle-painting medium
Acrylic paint, brown and green
Oak leaf and acorn rubber stamps
1 cream or white pillar candle, any size
Hemp rope
3 cinnamon sticks
2 or 3 oak leaves on small branches, preferably with acorns attached

Mix together the candle-painting medium and each acrylic paint individually. Paint the rubber stamps with the paint mixture. Carefully press 1 stamp at a time onto the candle while slowly rotating the candle to ensure an even image. Place the stamp marks in any arrangement you desire. Tie the rope around the candle as you would a present. Tie in the cinnamon sticks and oak leaves. Burn as desired.

Note: You can obtain candle-painting medium at craft supply stores.

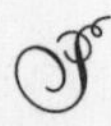

Oregano

Origanum vulgare

ORIGANO, ORGANY

Part Used: leaves

Oregano is an herbaceous perennial with hairy, erect square stems, two-lipped flowers that range in color from white to purple, and oval, pointed leaves. Traditionally oregano was primarily used for medicinal purposes, but today is often used in cooking. (*Origanum vulgare* variety *hirtum* is best for cooking.) Oregano poultices alleviate sore and tired muscles and insect bites. The herb treats coughs, asthma, toothaches, rheumatism, irregular menstruation, and headaches. Place fresh leaves in a muslin bag and dampen with warm water. Place the poultice over body aches and stiff joints.

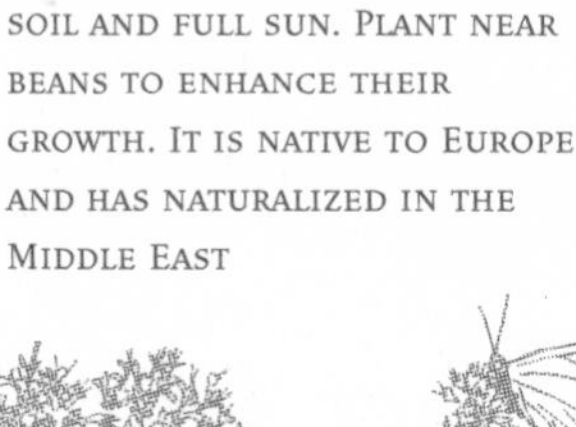
OREGANO DOES WELL IN ORDINARY, WELL-DRAINED SOIL AND FULL SUN. PLANT NEAR BEANS TO ENHANCE THEIR GROWTH. IT IS NATIVE TO EUROPE AND HAS NATURALIZED IN THE MIDDLE EAST

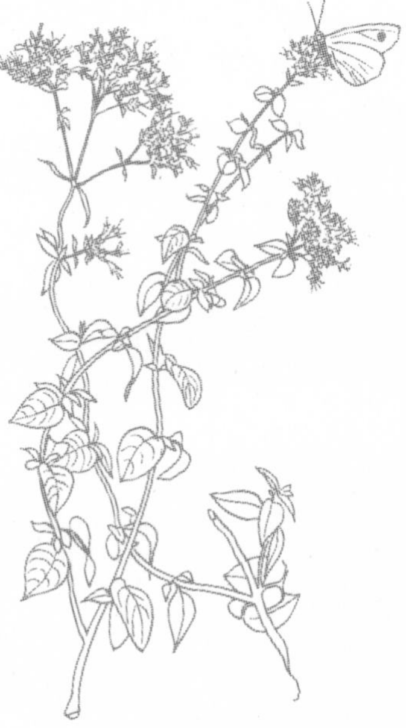

Oaxacan Summer Dish

SERVES 6

Oregano is associated with Mars, whose function is to catapult us into adventure. Under the guidance of this fierce planet, you will find courage and act on it. Combined with the summer holiday, the intent of this dish and herb asks you to find an area in your life in which you have become dormant (excluding parts of yourself that need the regeneration of calm) and bring it out into the sunshine. Employ the enthusiasm of Mars to seek opportunities and quests of all kinds.

- 2 small red potatoes
- 6 ears corn
- 2 tablespoons butter
- ½ medium white onion, chopped
- 1 medium acorn squash, peeled, chopped into small pieces
- 2 poblano peppers, roasted, seeded, julienned
- 6 cloves garlic, minced
- ½ cup thyme vegetable stock (see page 239)

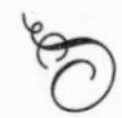

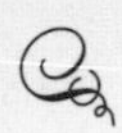

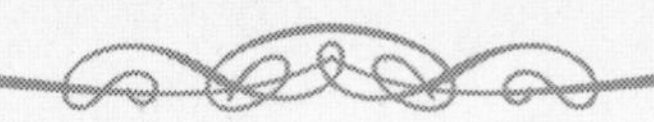

½ cup fresh oregano, chopped

1 tablespoon fresh epazote leaf

½ cup sour cream

6 ounces mild feta cheese

Organic corn tortillas, warmed

Bring a large pot of water to boil on the stove top. Add the potatoes and cook 10 to 12 minutes. Add the corn and cook an additional 6 minutes, or until the corn is just tender. Drain. Remove kernels from the cobs and set aside. In a large skillet, heat the butter over medium-high heat; add the onions and sauté 5 minutes, until translucent. Add the potatoes, corn, acorn squash, poblanos, and garlic. Cook 10 minutes. Add the vegetable stock, oregano, and epazote. Bring to simmer, then stir in the sour cream and top with the cheese. Cover, decrease heat to low, and cook 5 to 10 minutes longer, or until the cheese melts. Serve with warm tortillas.

Note: Epazote can be found at specialty and gourmet markets.

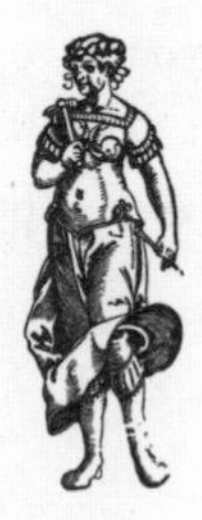

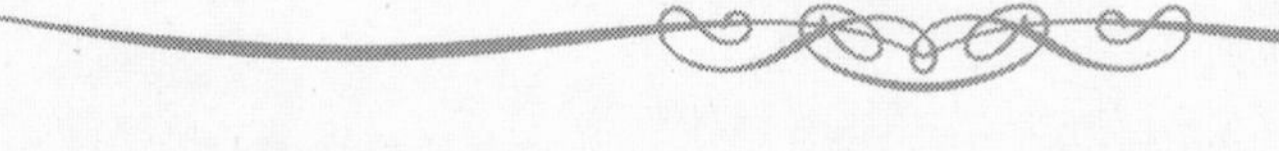

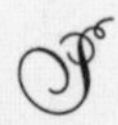

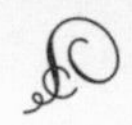

Orrisroot

Iris germanica var. florentina

FLORENTINE IRIS, QUEEN ELIZABETH ROOT

Part Used: rhizome

Orrisroot is primarily used for love and new beginnings. You can make sachets of orrisroot powder mixed with rose petals as gifts for new friends or for a loved one. Burn orrisroot incense during the beginning of a relationship. Dried for two years and then powdered, the rhizome makes an original and beautiful perfume base. It is used to honor spring, the moon, and the maiden form of the Goddess.

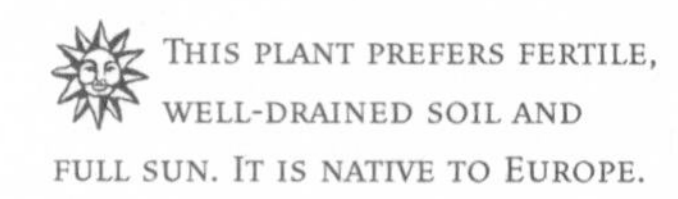

THIS PLANT PREFERS FERTILE, WELL-DRAINED SOIL AND FULL SUN. IT IS NATIVE TO EUROPE.

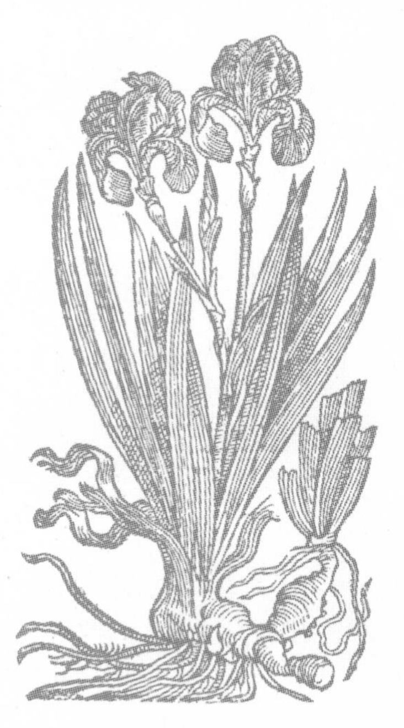

Sweet Love Spell

This love spell is designed to bring love into your life. It is not intended to be cast over any particular individual other than yourself.

Begin this spell on a Friday, and work over a span of three days. On the first night, place two human-figure-shaped, pink candles about a foot apart. Anoint them with orrisroot oil and rose oil. As you light the candles, call on self-love. Sprinkle rose petals around the base of the candles. Imagine all the gifts that have been bestowed on you and make you who you are. Honor yourself, for then it is easier to find the beauty in others. Douse the flames. On the second night, draw the candles a few inches closer. Anoint again with oils. Light the candles and visualize the feeling of being loved. What does it sound, taste, or smell like? Sit and meditate on this for a moment and then douse the flames. On the third night, bring the candles close enough to touch. On a lace doily, place an apple. Imagine a companionship that honors the joyful dance of two open spaces or beings of energy. Light the candles, and as the flames burn the candles all the way down, eat the apple. This symbolizes bringing love into your being. Bury the core. Put the doily, rose petals, and the wax drippings in a paper bag. Place the sack under your mattress until the spell has manifested.

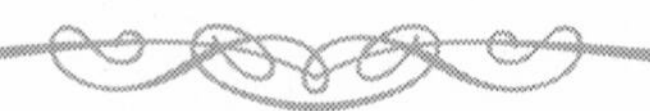

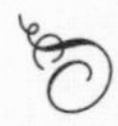

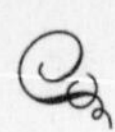

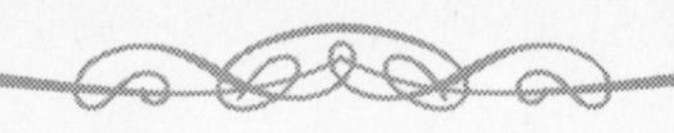

Parsley

Petroseliinum crispum

DEVIL'S OATMEAL, MERRY PARSLEY

Parts Used: seeds, leaves

Parsley is widely cultivated; in the wild it is found on dry rocky slopes. The intense green leaves can be either curly or flat. The Romans used parsley during their orgies to remove the rancid smell of liquor. The Greeks associated the herb with Hercules, fed it to their racehorses, and awarded victors crowns of parsley, as they believed the herb to represent and possess great power and strength. They even went so far as to wear chaplets of parsley at banquets to keep them sober. The herb was also associated with death, and sprinkled on the deceased to deodorize them.

Parsley is recommended as cancer prevention if the disease is prevalent in the family. The herb is used to treat all disorders of the urinary tract, as well as jaundice, kidney stones, anemia, arthritis, and sciatica. Steep bruised leaves in vinegar and apply to swollen breasts to dry up milk production. A tea made of the seeds will clear away head lice, stimulate hair growth, remove dandruff, and soothe insect stings. Parsley pulp or juice fed to an animal on an empty stomach will help relieve gastric upset. The herb contains a good amount of vitamin C.

Parsley is used in prosperity and forgiveness spells. It is believed to have been included in some ancient flying ointments. Parsley is most powerful when gathered on a Friday—to coincide with Venus—during a waxing moon. According to Greek mythology, parsley sprung from the god Archemorus, the forerunner of death. Folktales say that only the wicked grow parsley and that if parsley grows well at your home, the woman is powerful. Planetary and deity associations of parsley are Mercury, Venus, and Persephone. Parsley is also associated with the Mother aspect of the Goddess.

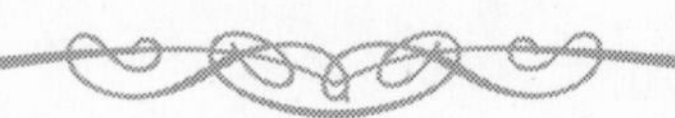

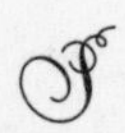

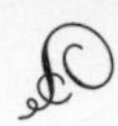

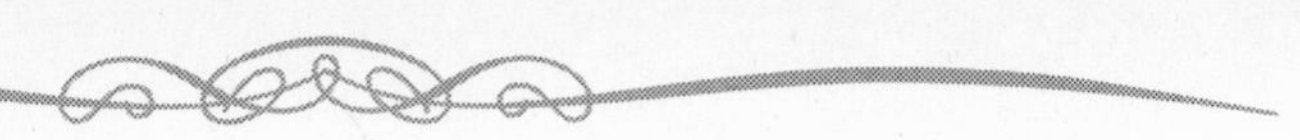

Parsley Stuffing

SERVES 8 TO 10

This dish is excellent as a stuffing for a holiday turkey or a side dish. As you prepare it, consider the Mother (or Father) aspect of your being. Remember a particularly difficult time in your life, when you did not act with the highest vibration. While the stuffing bakes, write a letter to yourself from the parent within. Give yourself permission to have made a mistake, and grow from the situation. There are no mistakes in life, only opportunities for learning. Do not judge; digest the situation and let it pass. When you are done with your letter, throw it into the Mabon or Yule fire. Allow the gentleness of the Mother or Father to caress you.

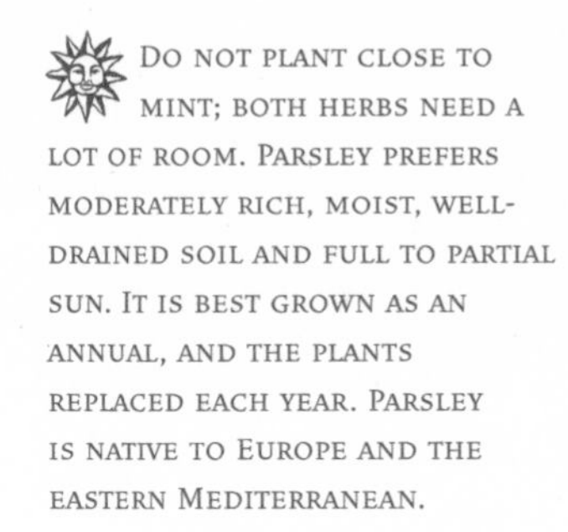

DO NOT PLANT CLOSE TO MINT; BOTH HERBS NEED A LOT OF ROOM. PARSLEY PREFERS MODERATELY RICH, MOIST, WELL-DRAINED SOIL AND FULL TO PARTIAL SUN. IT IS BEST GROWN AS AN ANNUAL, AND THE PLANTS REPLACED EACH YEAR. PARSLEY IS NATIVE TO EUROPE AND THE EASTERN MEDITERRANEAN.

½ cup (1 stick) unsalted butter
1½ cups chopped white onion
1½ cups chopped celery
½ cup minced fresh parsley
2 teaspoons minced fresh sage
2 teaspoons minced fresh thyme
½ teaspoon freshly ground black pepper
12 cups stale challah bread (approximately 2 loaves), cut into ½-inch cubes
2 cups chicken or vegetable broth
3 large eggs, lightly beaten
1½ teaspoons salt

Preheat the oven to 350°F. Butter a 13 by 9-inch glass baking dish. In a large skillet, melt the butter over medium heat. Reserve 2 tablespoons of the melted butter. Return the skillet to the heat; add the onion and celery and sauté until translucent, 7 to 9 minutes. Stir in the parsley, sage, thyme, and pepper; cook for 1 minute longer. Transfer to a large mixing bowl. Add the bread cubes, broth, eggs, and salt. Toss gently. Transfer the mixture to the prepared baking dish and drizzle with the reserved melted butter. Cover tightly with foil and bake 30 minutes. Remove the foil and bake until a golden-brown crust forms, 15 to 20 minutes longer.

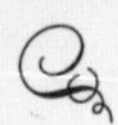

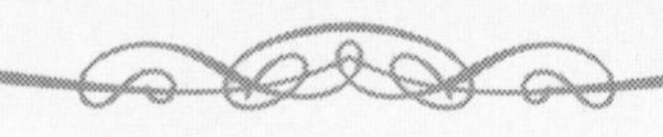

Passionflower

Passiflora incarnata

HOLY TRINITY FLOWER, MAYPOP, PASSION VINE

Parts Used: flowers, leaves, woody vines, fruit

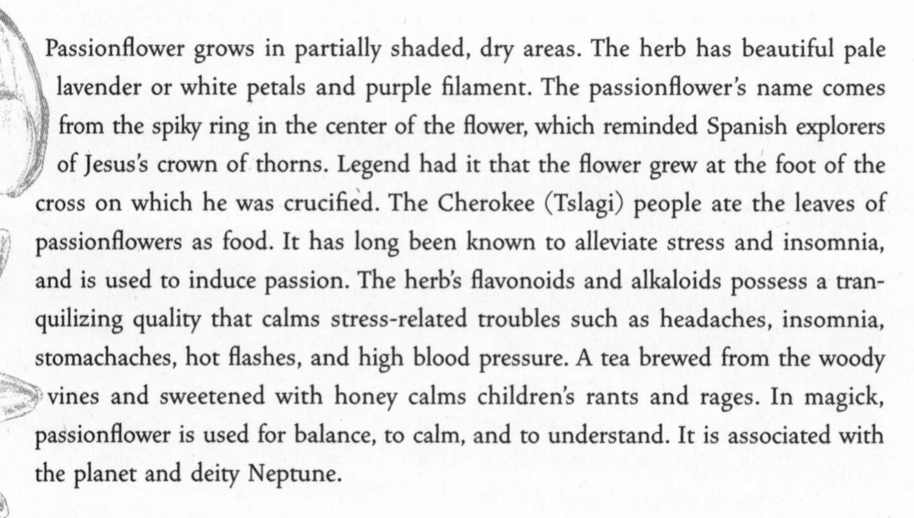

Passionflower grows in partially shaded, dry areas. The herb has beautiful pale lavender or white petals and purple filament. The passionflower's name comes from the spiky ring in the center of the flower, which reminded Spanish explorers of Jesus's crown of thorns. Legend had it that the flower grew at the foot of the cross on which he was crucified. The Cherokee (Tslagi) people ate the leaves of passionflowers as food. It has long been known to alleviate stress and insomnia, and is used to induce passion. The herb's flavonoids and alkaloids possess a tranquilizing quality that calms stress-related troubles such as headaches, insomnia, stomachaches, hot flashes, and high blood pressure. A tea brewed from the woody vines and sweetened with honey calms children's rants and rages. In magick, passionflower is used for balance, to calm, and to understand. It is associated with the planet and deity Neptune.

Midsummer Passionflower Punch

SERVES 8 TO 10

Family is important all year round, and is celebrated with much intent during Litha. Serve this punch during a family celebration at midsummer. The number six is associated with finding the balance between spirituality and love. It represents the cosmic Mother and all qualities and occupations that minister to or care for others. The number six relates to accepting your responsibilities and sharing with joy. It also symbolizes the ability to bring about justice, truth, and peace.

You may either buy the passion fruit juice or extract it yourself. Slice a ripe passion fruit in half. Scoop out the flesh and place it in a fine-meshed sieve over a bowl. Squeeze out the juice by pressing with a wooden spoon. Discard the seeds and pulp. (Jennifer Carmel Knowles, artist and organic chef, donated this recipe.)

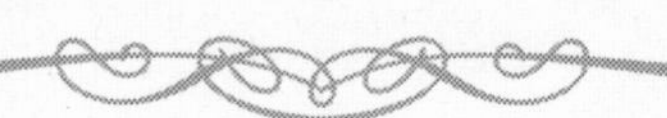

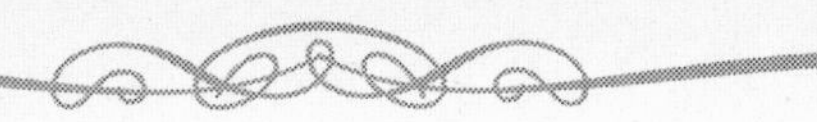

Leaves from 4 sprigs mint

¼ cup sugar

4 cups seltzer water

6 cups passion fruit juice

1 lime

Ice cubes

6 passionflowers

Bruise the mint leaves with the sugar in a mortar and pestle. Transfer the mixture to a serving bowl. Pour the seltzer water and passion fruit juice over the leaves. Squeeze in the juice of the lime. Add ice cubes and garnish with the passionflowers.

Variation: You can substitute club soda or sparkling water for the seltzer water.

Passionflower is an apt climber and prone to dominating other plants; it should be pruned regularly to keep it from getting out of control. It prefers partial shade and deep, well-drained, fertile soil, and is easy to grow from seed. It is native to the southern United States and Central and South America.

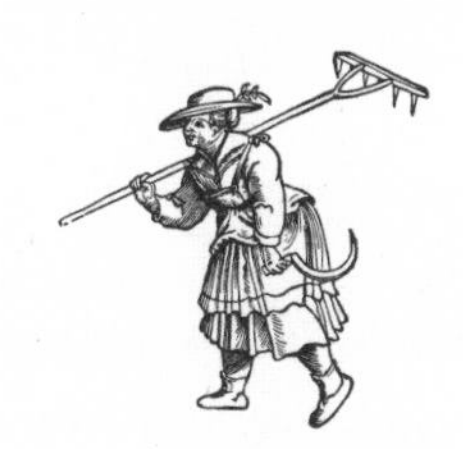

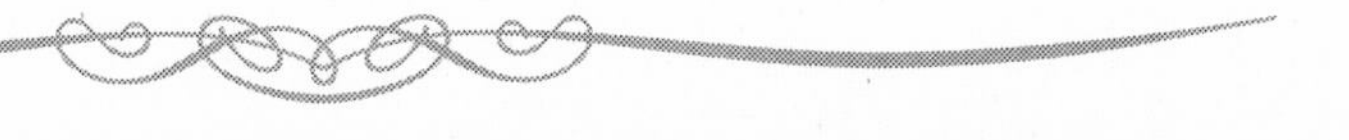

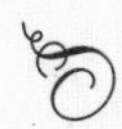

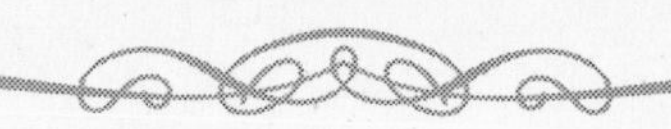

Patchouli

Pogostemon cablin

PUCHA-POT

Part Used: leaves

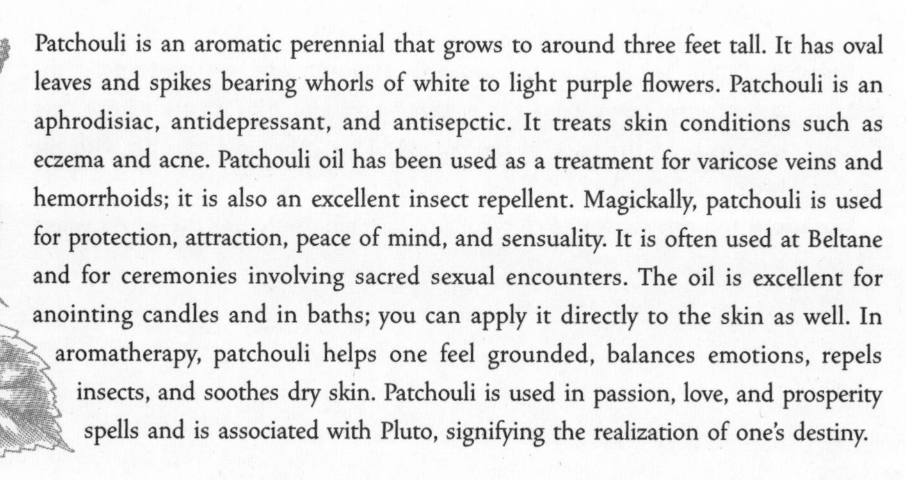

Patchouli is an aromatic perennial that grows to around three feet tall. It has oval leaves and spikes bearing whorls of white to light purple flowers. Patchouli is an aphrodisiac, antidepressant, and antisepctic. It treats skin conditions such as eczema and acne. Patchouli oil has been used as a treatment for varicose veins and hemorrhoids; it is also an excellent insect repellent. Magickally, patchouli is used for protection, attraction, peace of mind, and sensuality. It is often used at Beltane and for ceremonies involving sacred sexual encounters. The oil is excellent for anointing candles and in baths; you can apply it directly to the skin as well. In aromatherapy, patchouli helps one feel grounded, balances emotions, repels insects, and soothes dry skin. Patchouli is used in passion, love, and prosperity spells and is associated with Pluto, signifying the realization of one's destiny.

I've Got the Power

We often ignore pain, sadness, anger, and fear. But we cannot embrace our power until we acknowledge these feelings and befriend our human fragility. Patchouli is also commonly used in prosperity spells. Begin a money-drawing spell on a Thursday during a waxing moon.

This spell focuses on empowering the light within. Concentrate on using all energy to feel your gifts from Spirit. Patchouli represents both the feminine and masculine sides of our nature. Sandalwood represents the desire to bring our power to the earthly level. Frankincense is used for manifestation; your hair is a representation of your power.

The power of three is used to create harmony, manifestation, creativity, progression, receptivity, abundance, and new opportunities. It represents the emotions and the combined energy or divine union of the Father, Mother, and Child.

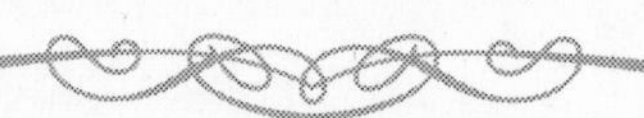

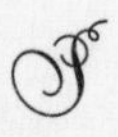

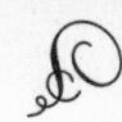

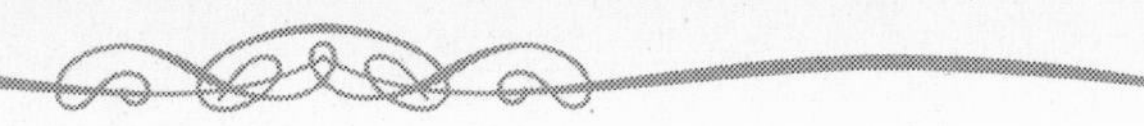

3 drops patchouli essential oil
3 drops sandalwood essential oil
3 drops frankincense essential oil

Combine the patchouli and sandalwood oils in the palm of your hand and apply the mixture under your arms and at the wrists. Dab the frankincense oil behind your ears and knees. Rub your hands together and rub them through your hair. Tease your hair from the scalp through to the ends. Say,

I now invoke my pain, sadness, anger, and fear
To transform to light to be used here
I call upon my power to rise from within me
To shine forth as power good and free
By my will, so mote it be
Three times three times three.

Alternately, you can anoint the same oil over a green candle and say,

Oils, work for prosperity
Bringing abundance to me
I ask this in love and light
By my will and by my right.

PATCHOULI IS NATIVE TO EAST INDIA, MALAYSIA, AND THE PHILIPPINES. IT IS CULTIVATED IN TROPICAL AND SUBTROPICAL REGIONS.

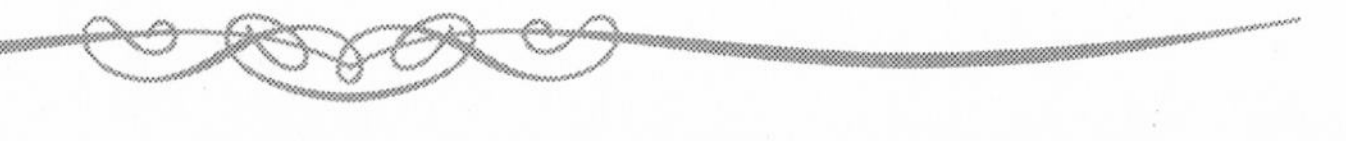

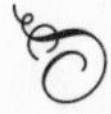

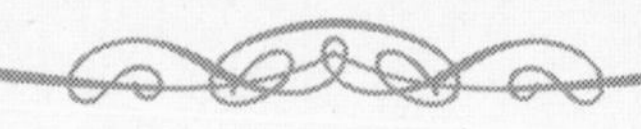

Pine

Pinus (various species)

OIL OF TURPENTINE TREE

Parts Used: cones, needles, nuts

Pine trees usually grow on rocky slopes and sandy barrens. There are about ninety different types of pine trees. They are all highly sensitive to air pollution. The inner bark of white pine (*Pinus strobus*) is used in cough medicine; Native Americans also used this bark as an astringent. Scotch pine (*Pinus sylvestris*) was used by Native Americans as a diuretic and to help break a fever. Pine is used to cleanse a house or outside circle of negative energies. It can be combined with sandalwood as an incense to create a magickal night of passion. Pine's associated gods are Poseidon and Thor.

Abundance Bath

The nuts and cones of a pine tree truly represent its strongest vibration: abundance. A full moon close to midwinter is the best time to perform this ritual. This season holds the promise of the boundless possibilities of the beginning of the calendar year, the phase of the moon represents fullness and wealth, and the pine symbolizes fertility. Combining these three prosperous elements reinforces your ability to manifest from the universe's limitless resources. *Prosperity, abundance*, and *wealth* can refer to more than material possessions and security; they are whatever enriches and sustains you in life.

Light a green candle. Place pine nuts, cones, and needles on a gold scarf or cloth. Play the music of nature, especially forest sounds. Pour ⅛ cup of pine needles into a muslin bag and place it in a warm bath. Soak for at least 15 minutes. Allow yourself to imagine what it would feel like if your every need were met. Be at peace without the drama of struggle. See it, smell it, taste it. Repeat the following chant three times:

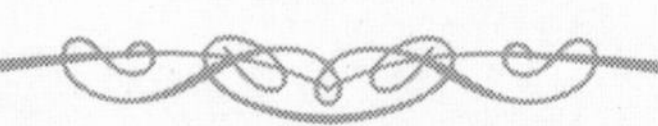

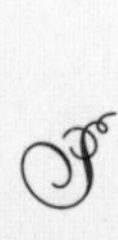

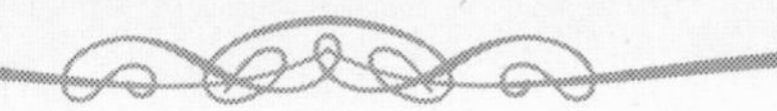

I call upon the universe to provide for me
A state of comfort with my forthcoming prosperity
Abundance is mine for I wish it so
Blessings upon all as my wealth grows.

After you are done bathing, write down any images or words that appeared to you. Glue or affix pine needles into your journal, diary, or book of shadows.

Most pine trees require full sun, well-drained soil, and a little watering.

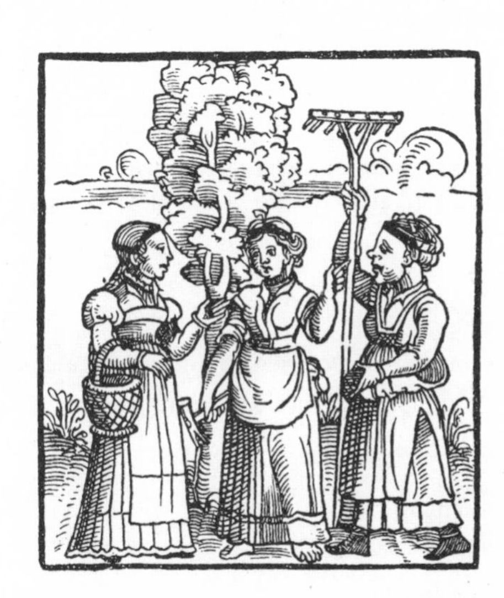

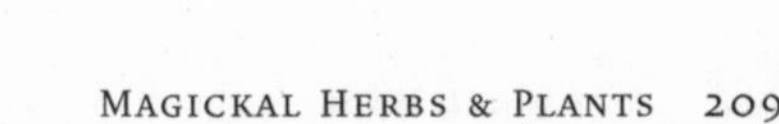

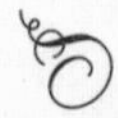

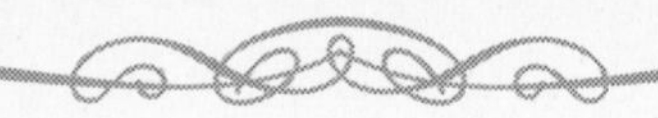

Poppy

Papaver

Blind buff, bread-seed poppy, head waak

Parts Used: leaves, flowers, seeds

Poppy is found in waste places, cornfields, and gardens. The leaves are silvery green, hairy, and fernlike. The petals range from orange to red, often with blue-black bases. The herb's leaves and flowers are used to treat asthma, hay fever, coughs, and pneumonia. The seeds are a nervine, and are used to promote sleep, soothe excitability, and relieve aches, headaches, pinkeye, and ulcers. Poppy is associated with the planets and gods Saturn and Neptune.

THE SAP OF THE FLOWERS CONTAINS A VARIETY OF ALKALOIDS, SOME OF THEM DANGEROUS; BUT BY THE TIME THE FRUIT HAS RIPENED AND THE SEEDS ARE READY TO HARVEST, NO TRACE OF THESE ALKALOIDS REMAINS.

Fertility Salad

Serves 4

Poppy is ruled by the moon, so it carries strong feminine as well as fertility, prosperity, and creative powers. Strawberries, also in this salad, are associated with love and its powerful force because of their red color.

- 2 tablespoons sunflower oil
- 2 tablespoons freshly squeezed orange juice
- 2 tablespoons organic honey
- 1 tablespoon rice vinegar
- 2 teaspoons Dijon mustard
- 1 teaspoon poppy seeds
- 2 cups arugula, torn into bite-size pieces
- 2 cups butter lettuce, torn into bite-size pieces

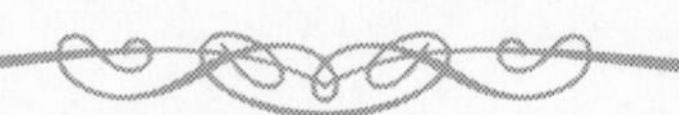

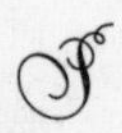

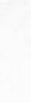

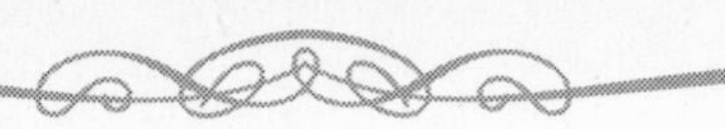

2 cups red leaf lettuce, torn into bite-size pieces

1 cup sliced strawberries

¾ cup sunflower sprouts

¾ cup (1 by 1¼-inch) pieces jicama

2 kiwi fruit, peeled, halved lengthwise, sliced

1 tablespoon sunflower seeds

Place the oil, juice, honey, vinegar, mustard, and poppy seeds in a tightly covered container and shake well. Mix the arugula, butter lettuce, and red leaf lettuce in a deep bowl. Arrange the strawberries, sprouts, jicama, and kiwis in rows atop the lettuces. Sprinkle sunflower seeds on top.

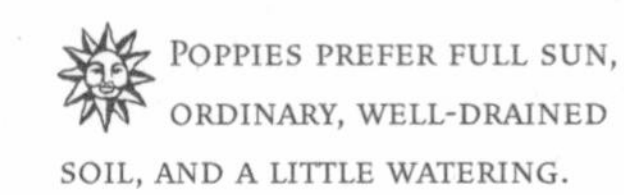

POPPIES PREFER FULL SUN, ORDINARY, WELL-DRAINED SOIL, AND A LITTLE WATERING.

Poppy Seed Scrub

Poppy is associated with Neptune, the planet that epitomizes the observer, the witness, and consciousness itself. By working with this planet, we realize the interconnectedness of all things and come to know ourselves as Divinity. With the help of poppy and Neptune, step beyond the limitations of the mind. Shed your ego as you scrub your face and come to see your place in the global community.

1 cup rolled oats

¼ cup poppy seeds

2 cups kaolin clay

2 tablespoons fresh calendula flowers

Separately grind oats and poppy seeds to a fine powder (you can use a mortar and pestle, food processor, or coffee grinder). Combine the oats and seeds with the clay and flowers. Transfer the mixture to a jar with a tight-fitting lid. It will keep for up to 1 year.

To use, mix 2 tablespoons of the scrub with enough water to form a thin paste. Rub on your face using gentle circular motions. Rinse off with warm water. Follow with the revitalizing comfrey toner on page 103.

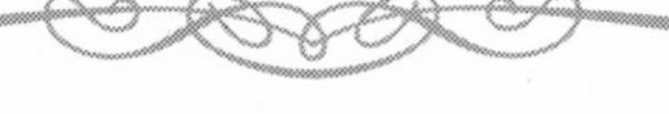

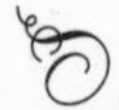

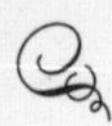
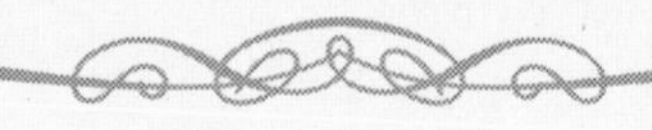

Red Clover

Trifolium pratense

BEE BREAD, COW CLOVER, HONEYSTALKS, PRIZE HERB, THREE-LEAVED GRASS, TREFOIL

Parts Used: flowers, leaves

Red Clover is found in pastures and gardens. The dark purple-pink flowers are globe-shaped and smell richly like honey. The leaves are grouped in threes and often mottled. Many herbalists value red clover; it is known to treat the young and old, cleanse blood, treat colds and coughs, restore fertility, soothe nerves, and induce sleep. It is beneficial for all types of cancer. Red clover is fed to horses to speed recovery from viral infections. Protection rituals often incorporate red clover. It is believed that if you gather dew from its petals or leaves on May Day, before the sunrise, the herb will help you look younger. Magickally, it is used for protection, banishing, clear sight, and love.

Women's Brew

This tea is naturally sweet, nurturing, nourishing, and strengthening, just like women. It includes oatstraw, which has the ability to calm nerves and increase strength; it is also beneficial to your skin, hair, and nails. Nettle is a tonic herb with blood-cleansing properties. Nettle is also used to treat urinary complaints, stones, hair growth, women's health issues, arthritis, asthma, and mucus. Damiana is a powerful aphrodisiac; it is often mixed with St. John's wort to form an anti-depressant. In magick it is used for love, lust, and healing. Stevia is a natural sweetener.

This weed brew can be made for any gathering that honors the female trinity of maiden, mother, and crone, sipped throughout the day, or drunk on any occasion you deem appropriate. (This recipe was donated by Jacquie DuBois, who sells herbs, oils, and homeopathy and vintage goods; you can visit her website at www.themoonmother.com.)

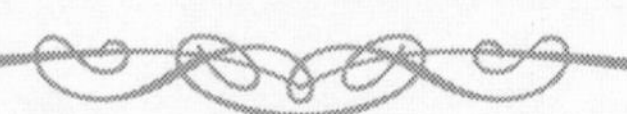

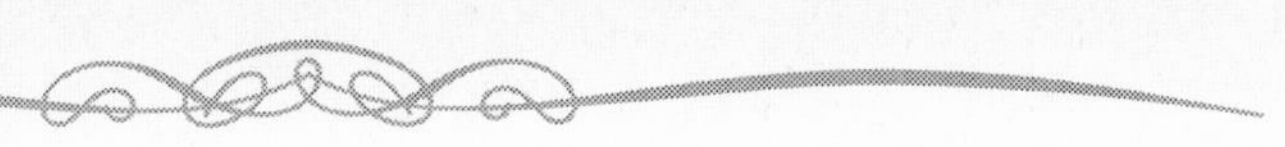

¼ cup dried red clover flowers
¼ cup dried oatstraw stems and husks
¼ cup dried nettle leaves
1 tablespoon dried stevia leaves
¼ cup dried damiana leaves

Mix all the ingredients together, all the while concentrating on all aspects of your womanhood. Use 1 teaspoon of the mixture per cup of water, or increase the quantity to suit your preference. Pour hot water over the herbs and let steep 15 minutes. Strain the herbs before drinking the warm tea.

Red clover prefers full sun to partial shade. It requires deep watering until established. It is often grown as a cover crop on fallow fields, because it restores nitrogen to the soil—so if it volunteers in your garden, don't treat it like a weed! Red clover is native to Europe and Asia; it has naturalized in North America and Australia.

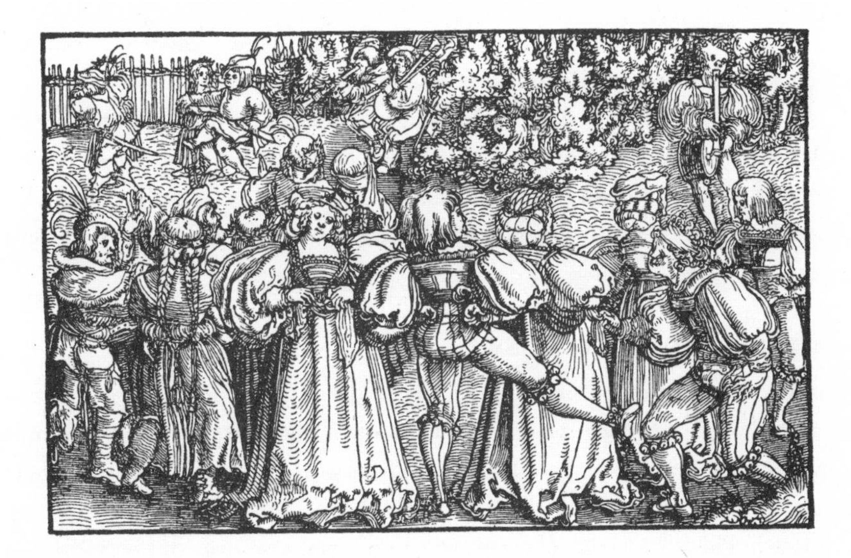

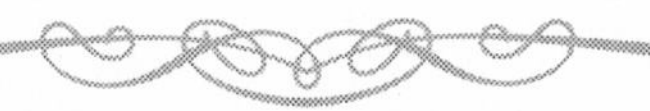

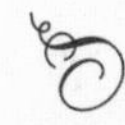

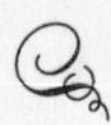

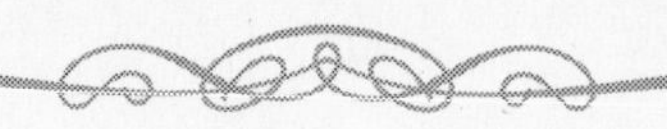

Red Raspberry

Rubus idaeus

BRAMBLE

Part Used: leaves

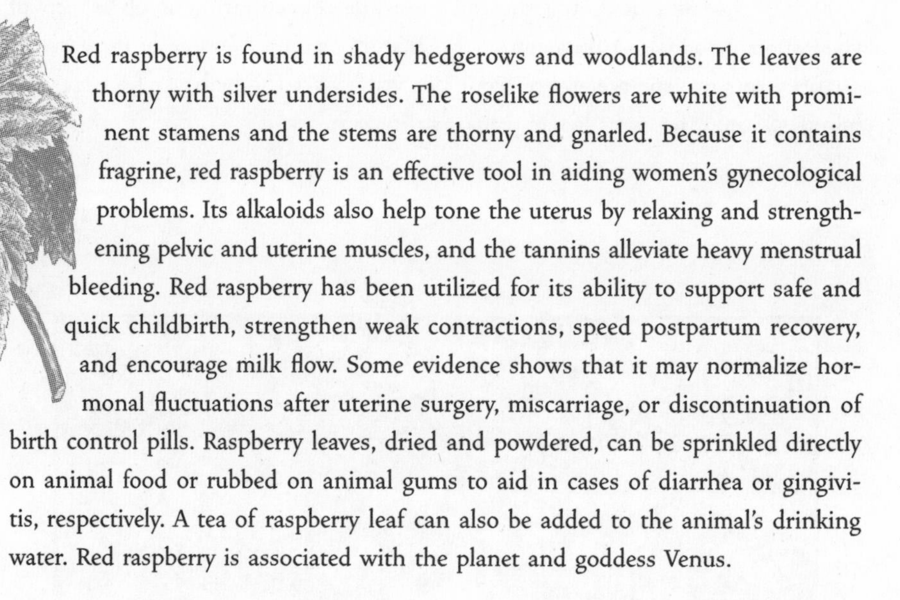

Red raspberry is found in shady hedgerows and woodlands. The leaves are thorny with silver undersides. The roselike flowers are white with prominent stamens and the stems are thorny and gnarled. Because it contains fragrine, red raspberry is an effective tool in aiding women's gynecological problems. Its alkaloids also help tone the uterus by relaxing and strengthening pelvic and uterine muscles, and the tannins alleviate heavy menstrual bleeding. Red raspberry has been utilized for its ability to support safe and quick childbirth, strengthen weak contractions, speed postpartum recovery, and encourage milk flow. Some evidence shows that it may normalize hormonal fluctuations after uterine surgery, miscarriage, or discontinuation of birth control pills. Raspberry leaves, dried and powdered, can be sprinkled directly on animal food or rubbed on animal gums to aid in cases of diarrhea or gingivitis, respectively. A tea of raspberry leaf can also be added to the animal's drinking water. Red raspberry is associated with the planet and goddess Venus.

Maiden Moon Incense

This incense and ritual were designed for my niece, Olivia, in honor of her first moon cycle. Whenever we create a menarche ritual that celebrates the burgeoning growth of a young woman, we take a stand for peace. Historically, women have discarded their menstrual blood as if it were shameful and a sin to be a woman. Any witch will tell you that the most powerful spell a woman can perform uses her own blood. When we are strong and honor all aspects of woman, we will not need to snipe or be bitchy. Our power will come from self-love. Women are most powerful during their menses. Channel this extraordinary energy and remember to honor yourself. Our spirits cannot be broken.

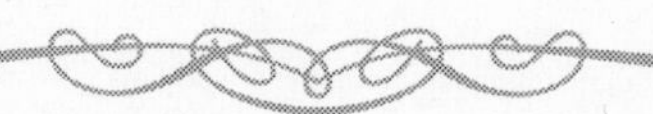

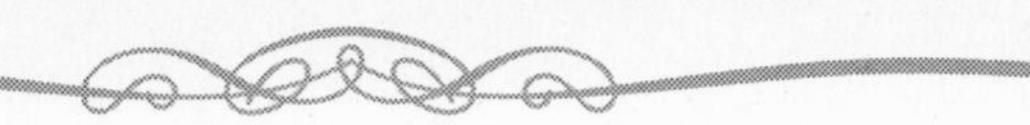

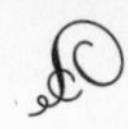

2 tablespoons dried red raspberry leaves
2 tablespoons dried dandelion leaves
2 tablespoons dried jasmine flowers

Combine all the herbs in a small bowl. Stir 3 times in a clockwise direction.

After the first moon of a young maiden, invite her to participate in a circle. Light a charcoal in a fire-retardent container. Sprinkle the incense mixture over the hot charcoal. When the incense begins to smoke, bless the elements of fire and air by saying,

Red raspberry for the cauldron of our womb
Dandelion to recognize seeds in bloom
Jasmine for safety in beauty and power
We call upon the three this red hour.

This plant likes a lot of water and full sun to light shade. It is native to Europe and Asia.

At the time of cakes and ale, use the maiden tea and blessing on page 112 for the ale and serve cakes. During the time for the circle's work, pass a basketful of red beads and leather cord. Invite each woman to string a bead on a cord. As she does, she can choose to tell the story of her first menses or what it means to her to be a woman, or both. Lastly, allow the maiden to ask any questions. Close the circle.

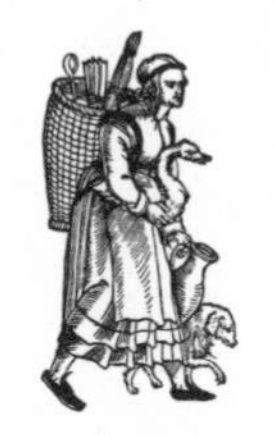

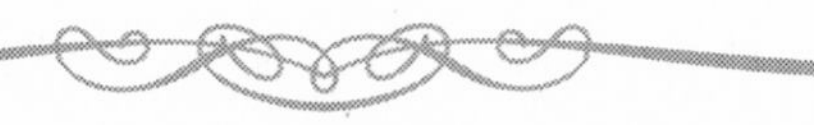

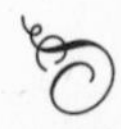

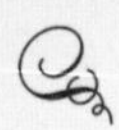

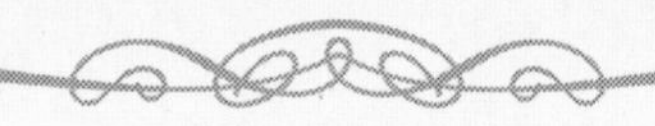

Rose

Rosa (various species)

FIELD ROSE, HUNDRED-LEAVED ROSE, RED ROSE, QUEEN OF THE GARDEN

Parts Used: flowers, hips

Roses are found in hedgerows, woodlands, and gardens. The leaves are thin and the stems carry thorns. The flowers range widely in color, each with a different meaning. Red symbolizes passion and desire; pink, simplicity and happy love; white, innocence and purity; yellow, friendship. The fruits, called hips, are hard and usually red. Rose is a gentle astringent, slight laxative, and general tonic. When rose petals or rose essential oil are added to a base oil such as almond, avocado, grape seed, olive, or hazelnut oil, the mixture can be used for a variety of healing purposes, including cell rejuvenation, infection fighting, a cure for insomnia, and to heal broken capillaries and eczema. Rose makes a good antiseptic. Heated in a diffuser, rose oil increases love, sensuality, clairvoyance, fertility, and compassion, and helps to release anger or guilt. Add one to two tablespoons of fresh rose petals or ten to twelve drops of rose essential oil to four ounces of base oil to make a rejuvenating massage oil or an aid for depression, jet lag, labor pains, stretch marks, or sunburns. Rose-leaf tea can be used as a skin rinse for contact dermatitis and flea bites. Rose is associated with Aphrodite and purification.

Rose Petal–Oatmeal Bath

Rose's combined associations of Aphrodite and purification invoke love in its purest form: tender, determined, uninhibited, desirous, and rare. It is the love that flings itself to the four directions in lustful search for more and the love that caresses the child. It is love in its totality. Before you bathe, light rose incense and a rose-scented or pink candle. As you bathe, circle your heart center and call this love to your human existence. You are already love in your spirit form, but as a human it is easy to forget the luminescent light and omnipresent love from which you originate; remember this as you bathe.

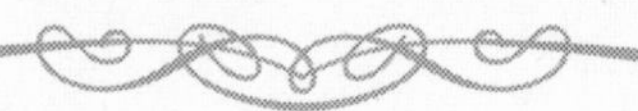

⅓ cup old-fashioned oats	¼ cup fresh or ⅛ cup dried crushed rose petals
⅓ cup powdered milk	1 tablespoon dried lavender flowers

Combine all the ingredients and let sit for at least a week in a glass jar. When ready to use, put about 2 or 3 tablespoons in a muslin bag, tying tightly at the top. Tie the bag to the faucet when running the bath. While in the bath, rub the bag over your skin for extra benefits.

MOST ROSES DO WELL IN WELL-DRAINED, CLAY-BASED SOIL AND FULL SUN TO PARTIAL SHADE (DEPENDING ON THE SPECIES). THEY LIKE TO BE FED WELL AND OFTEN, AND ALL BUT THE VINING TYPES NEED TO BE PRUNED BACK SEVERELY ONCE A YEAR, SO THEY CAN REST.

Rose Herbal Mask

It is particularly important for us to create self-love. All too often we associate our acceptance and love of self with our appearance. This body you wear is like a mask, and you can choose to hide behind the illusion or use the mask as a way to practice taking care of yourself, ridding yourself of old ways of being, and valuing regeneration and rebirth.

Masks deep-clean pores, soften dry skin, boost circulation, and peel away dead skin cells. As you wait for the mask to dry, relax. The actual act of just sitting and being allows and creates a space for silence. In silence, all manner of information can come through to you. You do not have to hold on to any of your thoughts—they are not you. You are true light, merely reflecting life's experience through your unique prism.

- ½ cup almonds, ground to a fine powder
- 1 cup (250 ml) old-fashioned oats, ground to a fine powder
- ½ cup finely ground dried rose petals
- ¼ cup powdered kelp
- 1½ cups green clay
- 1 tablespoon (about) apple cider vinegar
- 1 teaspoon honey

In a large bowl, mix the almonds, oats, rose petals, kelp, and clay. Discard any large unground chunks of almonds. Store the dry mixture in a jar with a tight-fitting lid.

To use, combine 1 tablespoon of the dry mixture with apple cider vinegar until it is the consistency of sour cream. Stir in the honey. Spread the paste over your face and neck, avoiding the tender area around the eyes. Leave the mask on 10 to 30 minutes. (Less time is advisable for sensitive skin.) Rinse with warm water.

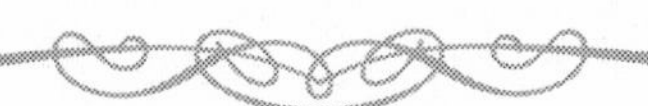

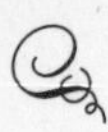

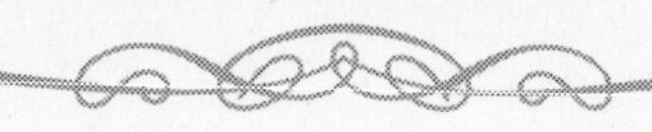

Rosemary

Rosmarinus officinalis

DEW OF THE SEA, GUARDROBE, INCENSIER, ROSMARINE, SEA DEW

Part Used: leaves

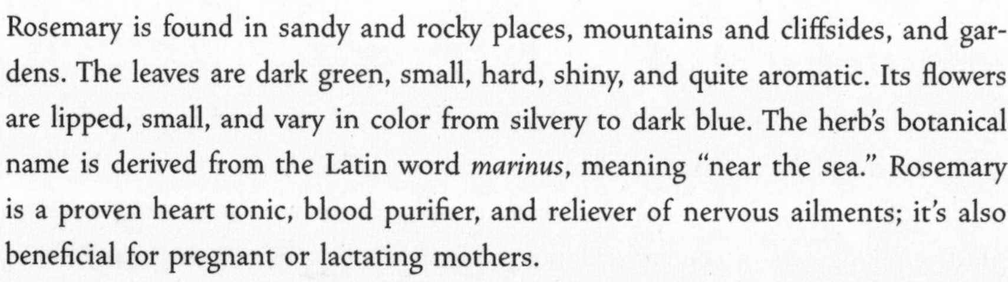

Rosemary is found in sandy and rocky places, mountains and cliffsides, and gardens. The leaves are dark green, small, hard, shiny, and quite aromatic. Its flowers are lipped, small, and vary in color from silvery to dark blue. The herb's botanical name is derived from the Latin word *marinus*, meaning "near the sea." Rosemary is a proven heart tonic, blood purifier, and reliever of nervous ailments; it's also beneficial for pregnant or lactating mothers.

In addition to helping stimulate memory, rosemary also restores energy. For an energizing foot bath, fill a wide, shallow bucket with warm water. Sprinkle two fistfuls of fresh rosemary sprigs in the water, and soak your feet for ten minutes.

Mix ten drops of rosemary essential oil with four ounces of base oil as a rub for arthritis or other joint pain or to stimulate capillary circulation. (Do not use this remedy on any person or animal with a seizure disorder.) In magick, rosemary is used for purification, love, protection, abundance, weather changes, grounding, and intellect.

Rosemary Remembrance Steak

SERVES 4

Long ago, according to old European legend, winter came rushing over the earth in cold frigid blasts. Many of the trees lost their leaves. When the sun did not reach high into the sky, most dryads (tree spirits) grew barren. Some dryads and plant devas wondered if the sun's warmth would ever return. As the winter raged on and the snowstorms blinded their sight, most of them forgot altogether about the sun's heat—most, that is, except for the evergreens. Rosemary was one of the evergreens. She kept the warmth of the sun close to her heart so that she would never forget the radiant glow upon her prickly leaves and purple flowers. Many moons passed this way.

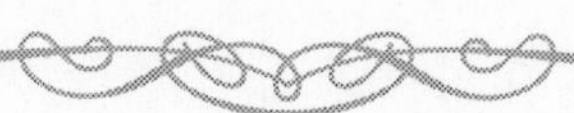

When the sun finally returned to the skies, growing stronger each day, he looked across the land at all the leafless trees and grew sad. *Has everyone forgotten me?* Then his sparkling rays caught sight of the glossy, dark leaves of the rosemary. *This one has not forgotten*, the sun thought. At that very moment, he blessed the little rosemary with the gift of remembrance. From that day forward, whenever anyone smells rosemary's aromatic scent, they will remember. When you make this dish, infuse your positive intent into it so that when you smell rosemary at a later date you will remember the good vibrations you created.

Rosemary loves the sun and dew. It does well with loose, permeable, well-drained soil. The flowers attract many bees. Plant near beans to enhance their growth. Rosemary is native to the Mediterranean.

1 cup warm water
½ ounce dried porcini mushrooms
4 boneless (8-ounce) top sirloin steaks, each 1 inch thick
3 teaspoons garlic cloves, minced
½ cup Marsala wine
½ cup thyme vegetable stock (see page 239)
3 tablespoons unsalted butter, cut into 6 pieces
3 teaspoons chopped fresh rosemary
Salt
Pepper

Bring 1 cup water to a boil; remove from heat. Soak the mushrooms in the water for 10 minutes. Heat a large skillet over high heat 3 minutes. Reduce the heat to medium and place the steaks in the pan. Cook 4 minutes. Flip the steaks and cook 4 more minutes for rare, 5 minutes for medium rare, 6 minutes for medium, or 7 to 8 minutes for well done. Transfer the steaks to a large plate and tent with foil. Do not discard the fat in the skillet.

Drain the mushrooms and chop, reserving the soaking water. Add the garlic to the skillet over low heat and sauté, stirring constantly, 15 to 20 seconds. Return the skillet to high heat. Add the Marsala, thyme broth, mushrooms, and reserved soaking water. Boil 3 minutes to reduce the liquid. Remove the skillet from the heat and add the butter, rosemary, salt, and pepper. Spoon the sauce over the steaks.

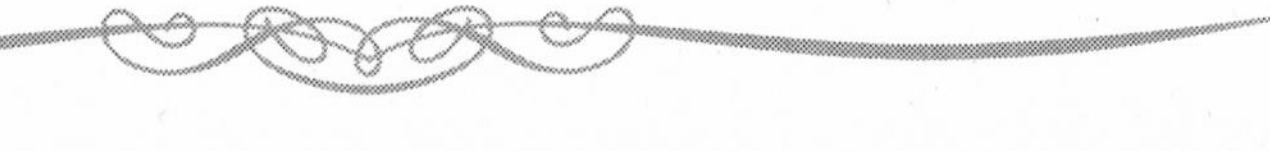

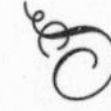

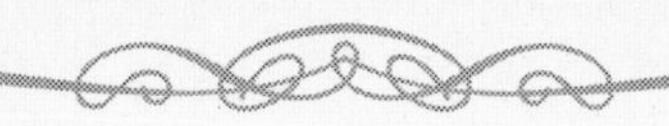

Rowan

Sorbus aucuparia

DELIGHT OF THE EYE, LUIS, MOUNTAIN ASH, QUICKBEAM, WICKEN TREE, WITCHBANE

Parts Used: branches, leaves, berries

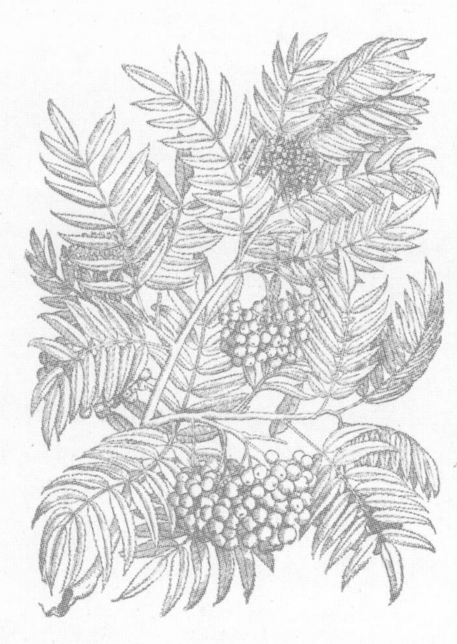

Rowan trees have deciduous compound leaves; red berries, which attract birds in autumn; and clusters of white, starry flowers. It is a tradition that before the Beltane fires are lit, boughs of rowan tied with a red cord should be hung to decorate the house. Walking sticks made from the rowan tree are believed to protect and to ensure that the owner does not get lost. Additionally, because this tree is known to increase intuitive powers, meditative walks will be especially enhanced by rowan walking sticks. Rowan is a healing agent and vibrates with a strong life force, helping to enhance intuitive abilities and to strengthen personal power. Rowan is associated with the Norse word *runa,* meaning "a charm," and the Sanskrit word *runa*, meaning "magician." In ancient Celtic, rowan is known as *luis*, the name for the second of the ogham letters. It provides the "quickening" of energy set in motion by birch, the first tree. The rune staves, sticks on which ogham characters were inscribed, were made of rowan wood. The Druids used rowan for dyeing the ceremonial black robes that they used for certain lunar ceremonies. Often, the leaves and berries are added to divination incenses, while the twigs are used for metal divining.

Rowan can assist meditation and promotes the development or uncovering of one's psychic abilities, so it helps us to tap into our limitless resources. Rowan is associated with Imbolc, the great fire festival of early February, held to mark the dawning or stirring of the light energy from out of the darkness of winter. This coincides with the rebirth of our divine inspiration, illumination, and intuition. It is a time for quiet reflection, crafting, divination, fire-gazing, scrying, meditation, drawing, and writing—all of which invite the intuitive process to unfold.

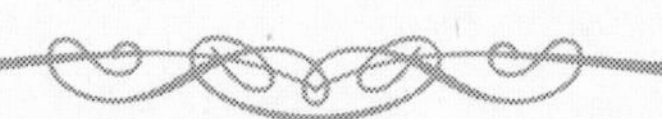

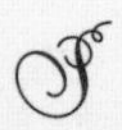

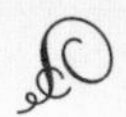

The juice from rowan berries is mildly laxative, high in vitamin C, works as an astringent, and soothes sore throats and hoarseness. To extract the juice from the dried berries, soak a teaspoonful of berries in a cup of cold water for ten hours, and then strain and use as a gargle. To make rowan jam, collect fresh berries in the autumn and trim off the stalks. Boil the berries, strain off the seeds and skins, and reboil the liquid until it sets. You may need to add some crab apples to provide pectin.

THERE ARE CONCERNS THAT ROWAN BERRIES CONTAIN A CARCINOGEN AND THAT THE RAW BERRIES ARE UNSAFE FOR CHILDREN, BUT COOKING THEM ELIMINATES THE POTENTIAL TOXINS.

ROWAN TREES DO WELL WITH SUN OR LIGHT SHADE AND MODERATE WATER. THEY NEED A CLIMATE WITH WINTER FROST. ROWAN TREES GROW THROUGHOUT THE NORTHERN HEMISPHERE.

Rowan Faery Sighting

Whenever you work with rowan, be attuned to the changes that occur as a result of communication with this tree. Its influence will bring about an acceleration of energy on many subtle levels. For this reason, it has always been treated with the greatest respect, used by the wise ones, and revered as a powerful influence. The following ceremony was gleaned from early pagan rituals.

Gather several small fallen rowan branches. (Never break branches off, especially for magickal purposes.) On Beltane Eve, at twilight, bless yourself and the rowan branches in the smoke from a smoldering bundle of dried sage. Cast a circle. Ground yourself by imagining a cord leaving your perineal floor (around the perineum) and extending downward to link with the subtle energy of Mother Earth permeating the soil. Wrap that cord around her fiery crystal center. Draw the energy back into the bottoms of your feet, and let it course up your legs and throughout your body. Imagine the sun above your head. Allow the warm energy to descend upon and through you.

Arrange the branches on the ground in a circle about eighteen inches in diameter. Use green cord to bind the branches together. As you do this, imagine the lightness of faeries. In your mind's eye, call to yourself the energy of being free and wild, able to ride with winds without a moment's hesitation. Make this faery ring with much intention and concentration. Sprinkle faery dust or powder over the ring. When it is completed, say,

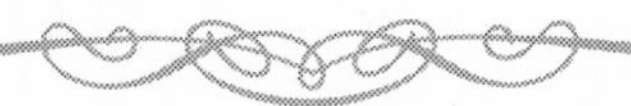

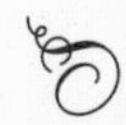

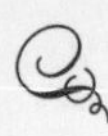

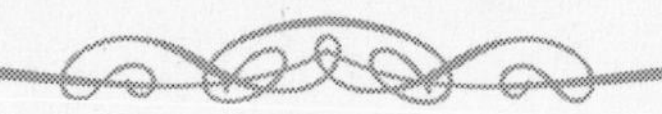

By the magick of this rowan wise
I ask the faeries to bless my eyes
With their wings and gift of flight
I beckon you this very night.

Hold up the ring and look through it. Remember, faeries appear to people in many different ways. You may see different shades of light, faded images, clear faeries, flashes in your peripheral vision, or small flying objects; or, you may sense their presence and just know that they are with you. You may choose to partake of a dessert and wine with your faery friends. When you have finished looking through the ring, place it on the ground again. Say good-bye to the faeries and close your circle. Continue to practice looking for faeries; they like regular visits.

Note: The incense used in this ritual can be anything that reminds you of faeries or an incense that was made specifically for visioning.

Angelic Well-Being

All the rituals, spells, and meditations in this book serve as a stimulus for your own creative powers. They are intended as catalysts to help you call on the energy needed for the diverse facets of your life. Spells are practice for perfecting manifestation. You use the elements of earth, air, water, and fire; colors; and other symbols to help you focus your intent. All humans are designed with the ability to manifest needs without these tools; all we need are intent and desire; the tools are props that eventually will not be used as often once you have learned to manifest and create the life of choosing with your heart, soul, and mind.

During this ritual, you will practice calling on the secure and health-giving powers to rise up within you and bless your environment with peace of mind and well-being. You will use rowan and the archangels Michael, Raphael, Gabriel, and Uriel as guides and representation.

Cut eight ½-inch strips of rowan bark from a fallen branch. Arrange two strips in a cross with arms of equal length for balance. Tie with natural twine, hemp, or raffia. Sprinkle with crushed or powdered angelica root and three drops of archangel oil. Make three additional crosses in the same way. Ground and center,

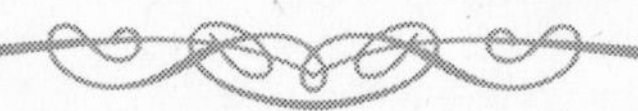

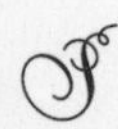

and then cast a circle, paying close attention to calling in the angels. Beginning in the east, place a rowan cross in the corner of your house or room, and say,

> Before me, Archangel Raphael
> Bless this home with divine tranquillity
> Let there be health, well-being, and serenity
> By my will, so mote it be.

Walk to the south, place a rowan cross in the corner of your house or room, and say,

> Before me, Archangel Michael
> Bless this home with your divine tranquillity
> Let there be health, well-being, and serenity
> By my will, so mote it be.

Walk to the west, place a rowan cross in the corner of your house or room, and say,

> Before me, Archangel Gabriel
> Bless this home with your divine tranquillity
> Let there be health, well-being, and serenity
> By my will, so mote it be.

Walk to the north, place a rowan cross in the corner of your house or room, and say,

> Before me, Archangel Uriel
> Bless this home with your divine tranquillity
> Let there be health, well-being, and serenity
> By my will, so mote it be.

Thank your guides and guardians and close the circle.

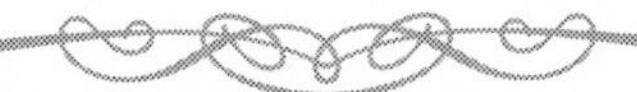

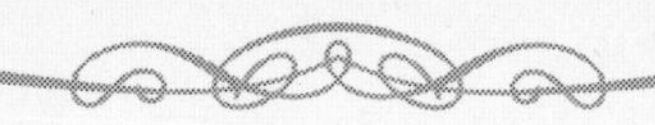

Rue

Ruta graveolens

BASHOUSH, HERB-OF-GRACE, HERBYGRASS, MOTHER OF THE HERBS, RUTA

Parts Used: leaves, flowers

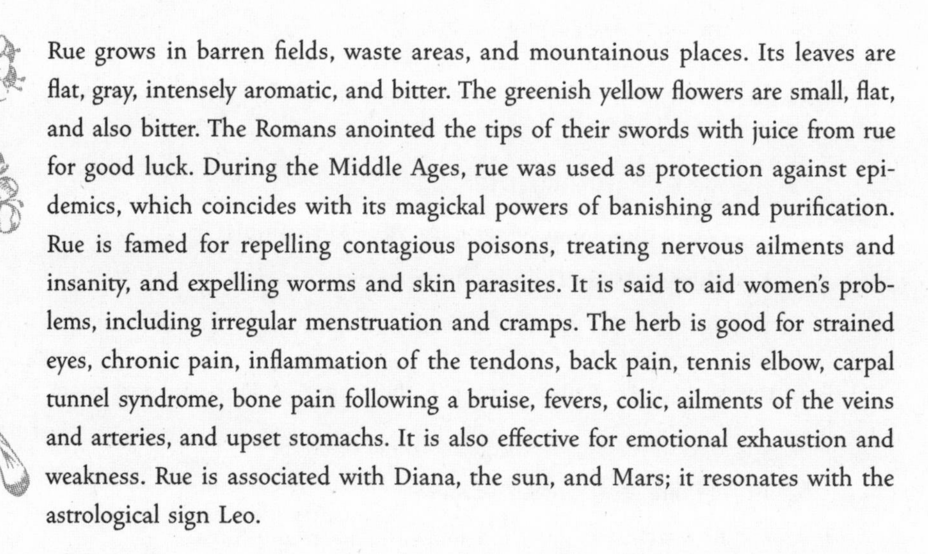

Rue grows in barren fields, waste areas, and mountainous places. Its leaves are flat, gray, intensely aromatic, and bitter. The greenish yellow flowers are small, flat, and also bitter. The Romans anointed the tips of their swords with juice from rue for good luck. During the Middle Ages, rue was used as protection against epidemics, which coincides with its magickal powers of banishing and purification. Rue is famed for repelling contagious poisons, treating nervous ailments and insanity, and expelling worms and skin parasites. It is said to aid women's problems, including irregular menstruation and cramps. The herb is good for strained eyes, chronic pain, inflammation of the tendons, back pain, tennis elbow, carpal tunnel syndrome, bone pain following a bruise, fevers, colic, ailments of the veins and arteries, and upset stomachs. It is also effective for emotional exhaustion and weakness. Rue is associated with Diana, the sun, and Mars; it resonates with the astrological sign Leo.

RUE IS NOT SAFE TO TAKE INTERNALLY. IT CONTAINS AN ACRONARCOTIC POISON THAT WHEN TAKEN INTERNALLY CAN CAUSE NERVE DERANGEMENT. RUE SHOULD NEVER BE USED BY PREGNANT WOMEN; IT HAS BEEN SAID TO CAUSE ABORTION. THE LEAVES ARE A SKIN IRRITANT TO SOME PEOPLE, SO HANDLE RUE WITH CARE.

Creative Air

Rue is a particularly effective herb for increasing mental clarity and intellect. Many people prefer seclusion, quiet, or inspirational background music or nature sounds, possibly a few candles, and no interruptions when they are trying to create. And yet usually the most successful approach is to fit the creative process into our everyday lives, where we are provided with loads of inspiration by our interactions with people, places, and things.

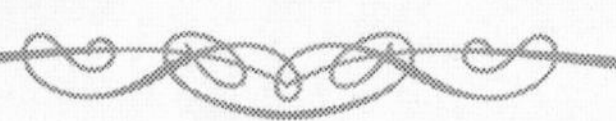

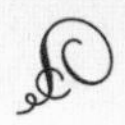

When you are feeling the urge to create but have only a short time and mindless worries are threatening to gobble all your precious time, burn some rue incense. Rue carries a powerful magickal intention or vibration of protection, exorcism, intellect, and purification. Its quickly banishes the chatter in your head, clearing a path for creative intellectual endeavors.

Light a charcoal and place in a fire-safe container such as a cauldron. Sprinkle about a tablespoon or a large pinch of dried rue leaves and flowers over the hot charcoal and blow on it gently. Allow the rich woodsy scent to waft over you. As you breathe in this magickal aroma, say,

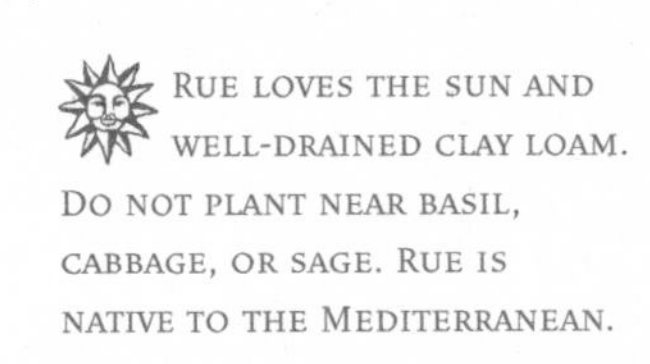

Rue loves the sun and well-drained clay loam. Do not plant near basil, cabbage, or sage. Rue is native to the Mediterranean.

I exorcise the worries, fears, and in their place
Seal and protect the boundaries of my space
I call upon creative and intellectual power
To come and bless me this very hour.

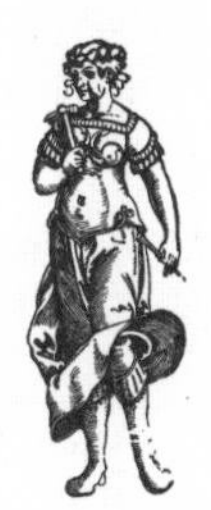

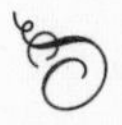

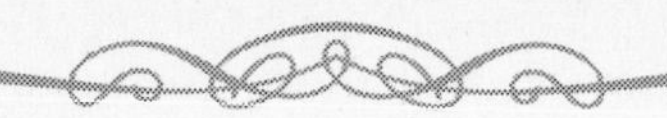

Saffron

Crocus sativus

AUTUMN CROCUS, SPANISH SAFFRON

Part Used: stigmas

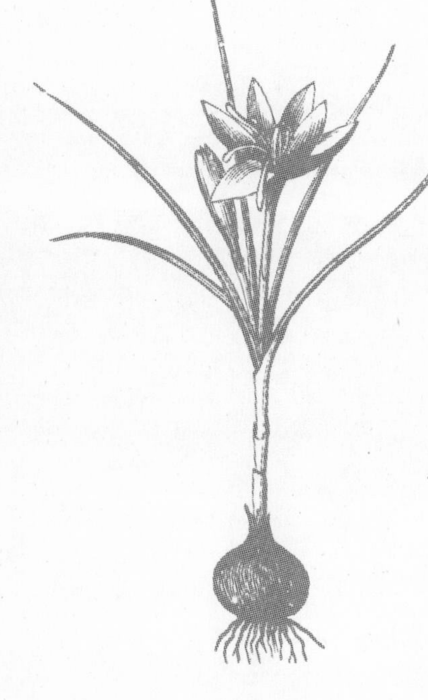

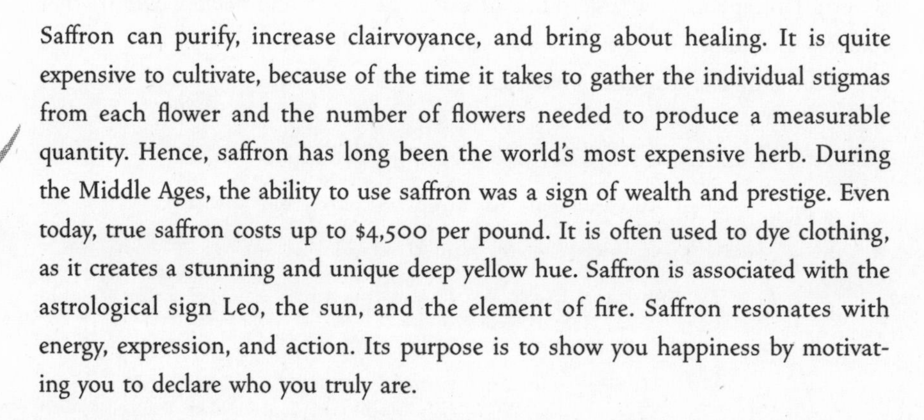

Saffron can purify, increase clairvoyance, and bring about healing. It is quite expensive to cultivate, because of the time it takes to gather the individual stigmas from each flower and the number of flowers needed to produce a measurable quantity. Hence, saffron has long been the world's most expensive herb. During the Middle Ages, the ability to use saffron was a sign of wealth and prestige. Even today, true saffron costs up to $4,500 per pound. It is often used to dye clothing, as it creates a stunning and unique deep yellow hue. Saffron is associated with the astrological sign Leo, the sun, and the element of fire. Saffron resonates with energy, expression, and action. Its purpose is to show you happiness by motivating you to declare who you truly are.

Saffron Rice with Shrimp

SERVES 4

The showiness and vibrancy of saffron implores you to honor yourself. If you have promised yourself to take a vacation, throw a party, or just relax after a difficult project, period of life, procedure, or other life experience, but still haven't done it, saffron will motivate you. Dive into life. Live lusciously. This is your day to shine.

¼ cup olive oil
2 cloves garlic
2 cups white rice
4 cups hot chicken or thyme vegetable stock (page 239)
2 teaspoons saffron threads
5 plum tomatoes, chopped
2 cups fresh peas
6 chopped marinated artichoke hearts

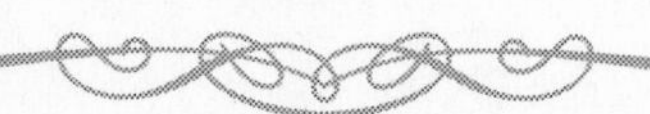

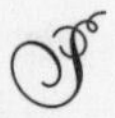

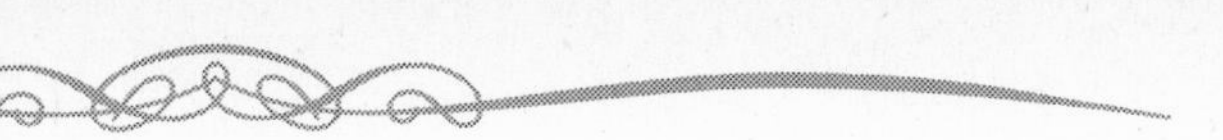

1 red bell pepper, chopped
1 orange or yellow bell pepper, chopped
8 uncooked large shrimp, peeled, deveined

In a large shallow pan, heat the oil over medium-high heat. Add the garlic and mash it with the back of a spoon. Remove the garlic when brown, about 2 minutes. Add the rice, and stir about 5 minutes. In a cup with a spout, mix the hot broth and saffron. Add the mixture to the pan. Cover and steam the rice until almost done, about 20 minutes. Stir in the tomatoes, peas, artichoke hearts, bell peppers, and shrimp. Replace cover and cook 10 minutes longer. Serve hot.

Saffron bulbs prefer light, well-drained soil and full sun to light shade. Saffron is native to India, the Balkans, and the eastern Mediterranean.

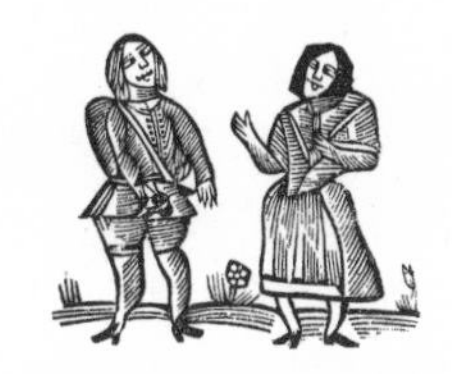

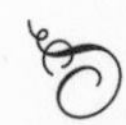

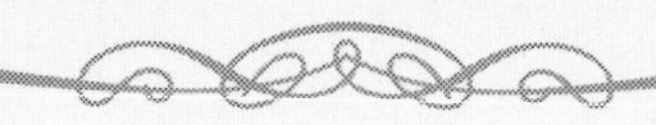

Sage

Salvia officinalis

GARDEN SAGE, COMMON SAGE

Part Used: leaves

Sage grows on sunny hillsides and rocky ground, and in gardens. The oval leaves are woolly and aromatic. The strongly scented flowers grow in whorls and range in color from silver to deep blue. There are many species originating in southwestern America, Asia, and the northern Mediterranean coast. The name is derived from the Latin *salvere,* meaning "to be well" or "to save." Sage is a valued fever treatment, heart tonic, and restorer of the human spirit. It is known to increase virility, relieve coughs, soothe wounds and ulcers, and support milk yield. Indigenous North Americans drank a tea made from the leaves of a related plant, hummingbird or pitcher sage (*Salvia spathacea*), as a treatment for colds, and to receive visions; they also used the concoction as a shampoo. Crushed leaves have been effectively used in eliminating body orders by cleansing the sweat glands.

Native Americans popularized the use of sage as a purifier of negative energy centuries ago. The leaves of white sage (*Salvia opiana*) were gathered under an auspicious moon, usually the full moon in the month of May. A song of thanksgiving was sung before reaping. Only one-third of the plant was harvested, leaving plenty for the plant to rejuvenate itself. Later, the leaves were bundled together and dried, and then used in all manner of prayer and protection rituals; the most popular is smudging. During a smudging ritual, dried sage leaves are set afire; the flames are extinguished, leaving the bundle to smolder. The sage smoke is directed all over the body, with special attention paid to areas vulnerable to negative energy, such as between the shoulder blades, the solar plexus, and the soles of the feet. (This ceremony is still revered and repeated today.) Another ritual utilizing sage calls for ten fresh sage leaves to be placed on a green cloth. Bind the cloth as a satchel with a gold ribbon for prosperity or a red ribbon for healing. Tie nine knots on

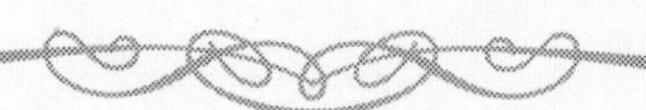

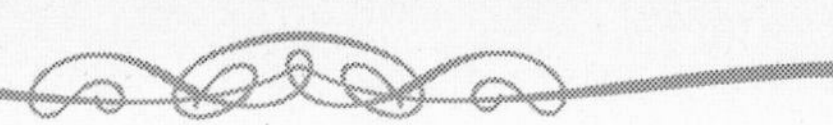

the ribbon and place on your altar. Sage's medicinal value has been connected with aiding night sweats, muscle tension, halitosis, coughs, stomachaches, sore throats, and mouth irritants.

Aromatic sage has been associated with immortality, longevity, health, prosperity, protection, purification, wisdom, and healing. Sage is associated with the planets and gods Jupiter and Venus. Artemis, Diana, and Hygeia are goddesses most often associated with this herb.

SAGE GROWS BEST IN ALKALINE SOIL WITH LITTLE MOISTURE AND FULL SUN TO LIGHT SHADE. PLANT NEAR CABBAGE, CARROT, STRAWBERRY, TOMATO, AND MARJORAM TO ENHANCE GROWTH. DO NOT PLANT NEAR ONIONS. SAGE IS NATIVE TO THE MEDITERRANEAN AND NORTH AMERICA.

Sage Tea

Sage is a powerful healing herb that has the ability to cleanse an area of all negative and stagnant energy. Sage lifts the feeling of lack of self worth, replacing it with the freedom to see yourself as a divine child of the universe. Many negative emotions boil down to a question of worth. As a holy being you deserve gentle, unconditional love. Sometimes we hold on to unhealthy attitudes because they are familiar and comfortable. Release them. As you prepare this tea, take the time to reflect on whether you are restricting joy from entering your life. Allow sage to remove these blocks.

Add 1 cup of dried sage leaves to 1 quart boiling water. Steep for 10 to 20 minutes. Strain out the herbs and allow the concoction to cool. Pour over your head to bring about a normal pH balance (this mixture also darkens hair, hiding gray).

Alternatively, you can make sage tea to eliminate night sweats. Add ½ cup of dried sage leaves to 1 cup of boiling water. Cover tightly and steep for 4 hours. Know that there is a sagacious Creator whose helpers can handle your problems if you let them do so. When you drink the tea, give your concerns to the ancient ones; hand the worries over to Spirit and realize that all will be well. (Avoid sage tea when pregnant.)

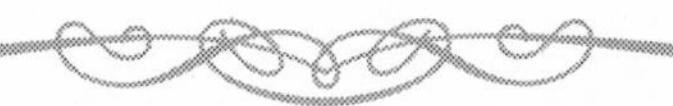

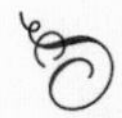

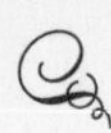

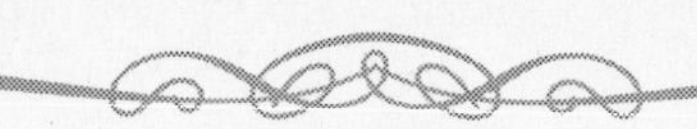

St. John's Wort

Hypericum perforatum

HERBA JON, HYPERICUM, KLAMATH WEED, RAISIN ROSE, ST. JOAN'S WORT, TOUCH-AND-HEAL

Parts Used: leaves, stems, flowers

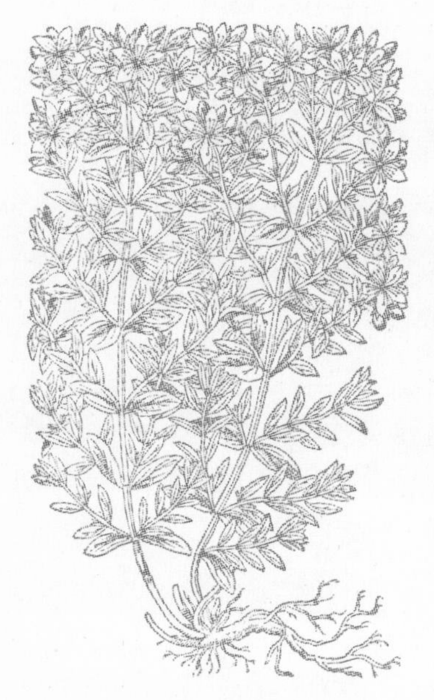

St. John's wort is found in woodlands and along waysides. The leaves are frail and multiform with bright specks of oil glands. The small, bright yellow flowers have prominent silky stamens and are poppy-shaped. The herb possesses medicinal gum, resins, and acids. St. John's wort is a soothing astringent. A medicinal oil can be taken internally to treat wounds, external and internal ulcers, hemorrhages, rheumatic joint inflammations, bronchitis, bruises, sprains, diarrhea, jaundice, earache, toothache, nervousness, fainting, and arthritis.

For a medicinal oil, finely chop a quarter-cup of fresh St. John's wort flowers. Combine with half a cup of virgin olive oil in a glass container. Allow to steep in a sunny location, uncovered or sealed, for two weeks. Shake the bottle occasionally. Using a coffee filter, strain out the red oil and discard the flowers. Decant the oil into a container with a tight-fitting lid.

ST. JOHN'S WORT SHOULD BE USED ONLY IN VERY SMALL DOSES AND AVOIDED BY FAIR-SKINNED PEOPLE, AS IT CAN CAUSE SKIN BURNING, SENSITIVITY TO LIGHT, AND OTHER PROBLEMS.

Protection Pomander

Since at least 500 B.C., St. John's wort has been used as a wound healer and an aid against melancholy, madness, and bodily pains. It was used in ancient love potions. European country folk burned the herb on St. John's Day, June 24, to ward off evil spirits. Its magickal vibrations work for protection, banishing, and to strengthen personal will. Make this pomander whenever you need courage to make a difficult change in your life. Consecrating this pomander as a symbol of

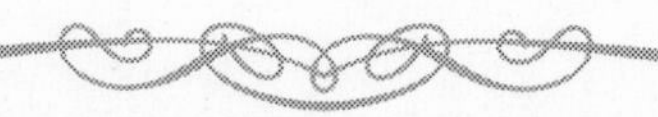

your strength, and using St. John's wort to invoke your will, gives your commitment to honor yourself a physical declaration.

1 Styrofoam ball, any size
3 cups dried St. John's wort flowers, enough for 3 coats
White carpenter's glue (will dry clear)

Paint the Styrofoam ball with carpenter's glue. Place a heap of St. John's wort on a sheet of waxed paper. Roll the glue-covered ball in the St. John's wort until it is fully coated. Place the ball on a sheet of waxed paper to dry, turning it periodically so that it won't have a flat side. As you make the pomander, say,

> I take a stand for my highest good today
> So that nothing now stands in my way.
> By my will, so mote it be
> Three times three times three.

Repeat 2 more times until the ball is covered in 3 layers of St. John's wort. Allow the pomander to dry overnight between coats. Hang in your house as a decoration and a proclamation of your will. (If the fragrance of the pomander diminishes with age, it can be renewed with a few drops of essential oil.)

This herb prefers partial to full sun and moderately moist, humusy, well-drained soil. It is propogated easily from cuttings or root divisions. Harvest the leaves, stems, and flowers when the flowers are in bloom, traditionally at the summer solstice. Plant next to onions. St. John's wort is found in temperate regions worldwide.

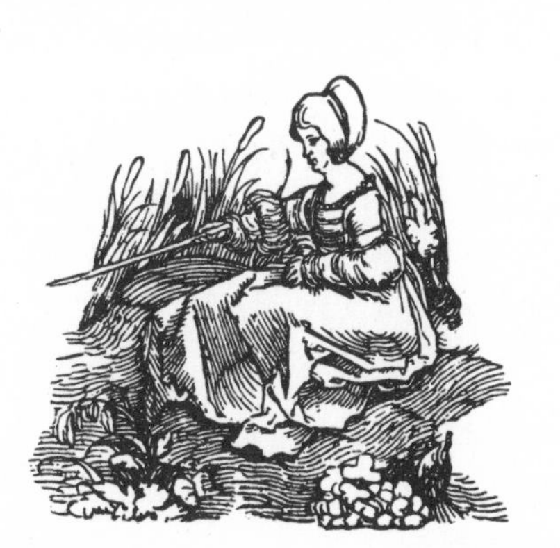

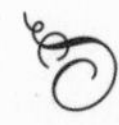

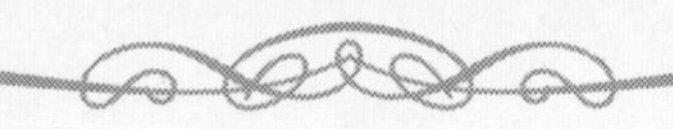

Sandalwood

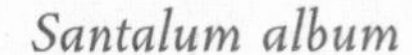

Santalum album

SANDAL, SANTAL, WHITE SAUNDERS, YELLOW SANDALWOOD

Parts Used: wood, inner part of root

Sandalwood is a semiparastic evergreen tree that can grow up to thirty feet. It has clusters of pale yellow or purple flowers; small, nearly black fruit; and lance-shaped leaves. It is widely cultivated in southeastern Asia. Its scent has been highly regarded in both China and India for centuries. In China, sandalwood has been used medicinally since at least 500 A.D. Sandalwood is burned in many Hindu rituals. Sandalwood confers protection, purification, and healing. It can be used as an aphrodisiac, appetite depressant, or stress reliever and sedative.

Purifying Deodorant

Our bodies are incredible: a conglomeration of interconnected systems, each relying on the others for a unified being. The lymphatic system cleanses our bodies of toxins. Its primary method for discharging these toxins is through sweat. The lymph nodes are located in the groin, underarms, colon, and elsewhere on the body. When released, these toxins often smell, resulting in what we call body odor.

In modern society, we have disrupted or ignored the natural processes of the body. In order to appear unconstrained by its physical limitations, we cover up our natural scents. But antiperspirants send the impurities directly back into the body. Natural deodorant can kill the odor-causing agents instead of keeping them in the body. Sandalwood is ideal because of its unisex scent. In addition, the oil from this fragrant tree is known to have a purifying element.

¼ cup vodka
2 tablespoons witch hazel astringent lotion
10 drops sandalwood essential oil
1 drop juniper essential oil
1 drop grapefruit essential oil

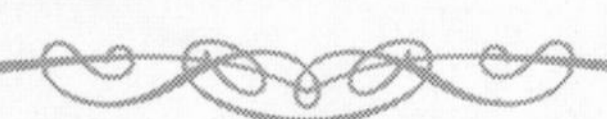

Combine all the ingredients in a sterilized bottle with a pump mechanism. Spray on clean armpits, preferably after showering. Shake well before each use. If the sprayer gets clogged, run it under warm water. Store in a cool, dry place and use within a year.

Sláinte

Sandalwood is cooling and sensual for both men and women, and is widely used in women's perfumes and men's colognes alike. This cologne might sound a bit flowery, but it's for men. It makes a great aftershave or body splash when mixed with some witch hazel. Aromatherapeutically antibiotic, I call this by the Irish term *sláinte*, meaning "to your health!" (Michael Riley, who has been a practicing Celtic pagan for more than twenty years and worked in herbal alchemy for almost ten, donated this recipe.)

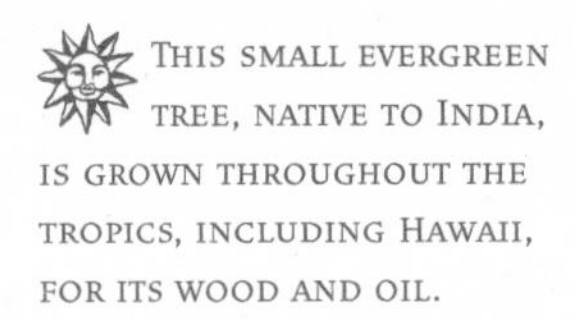

THIS SMALL EVERGREEN TREE, NATIVE TO INDIA, IS GROWN THROUGHOUT THE TROPICS, INCLUDING HAWAII, FOR ITS WOOD AND OIL.

3 drops rose essential oil
3 drops carnation essential oil
3 drops citron essential oil
3 drops gardenia essential oil
10 drops myrrh essential oil
20 drops sandalwood essential oil
5 drops clove essential oil
5 drops (or less) eucalyptus essential oil

Mix together all ingredients, cover, and let sit at least 7 days. Use alone, dabbed on as cologne; or mix with 2 to 3 ounces witch hazel astringent lotion as an aftershave or body splash; or add to bath salt base (page 141). You can also add it to the Saturn's potpourri (page 192) to enrich the scent and make it last longer.

Note: If you want to multiply or reduce this recipe the parts go as follows: 1 part each of rose, carnation, citron, and gardenia oil; 4 parts myrrh oil; 8 parts sandalwood oil; and 2 parts each of clove and eucalyptus oil. Store in an airtight glass container in a cool place. Use within 3 years.

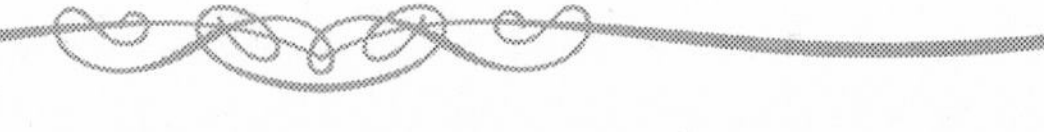

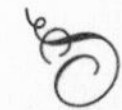

Skullcap

Scutellaria resinosa

BLUE PIMPERNEL, HELMET FLOWER, MAD-DOG WEED

Parts Used: leaves, flowers

THIS PERENNIAL LIKES PLENTY OF MOISTURE AND SUN, GROWING WILD IN DITCHES AND AROUND PONDS; BUT GIVE IT GOOD DRAINAGE FOR BEST RESULTS. IT IS NATIVE TO NORTH AMERICA.

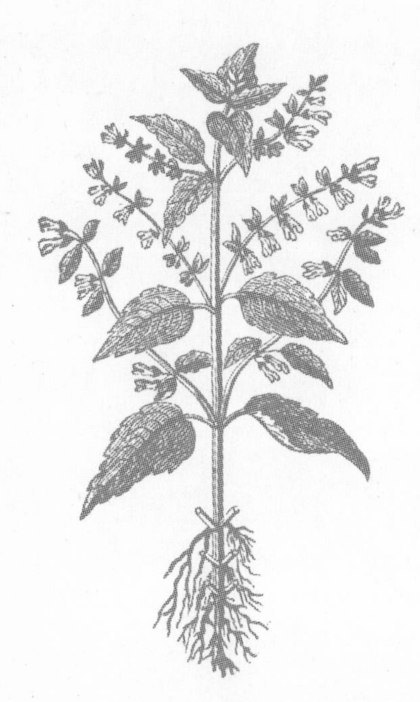

Skullcap is found by streams and low-lying meadows. The leaves are oblong; the bright blue flowers large and downy. The shieldlike form of the calyx, an outer whorl of protective leaves, gives it the nickname "helmet flower." Native Americans have long used skullcap to promote the menstrual cycle, relieve cramps, and ease breast pain. It relieves tension headaches, exhaustion, panic attacks, depression, and anxiety. Skullcap is used to treat wounds, soothe inflamed skin, repair a torn perineum after childbirth, and restore vaginal lubrication. Used as a relief for insomnia, skullcap will ease you to sleep and not leave you feeling groggy in the morning. This gentle quality also makes it an effective tool to help your body make the transition when you stop using chemical tranquilizers and antidepressants. Skullcap should be harvested while in flower and kept in a sealed container in a cool place. Skullcap is associated with the god and planet Saturn.

Success Satchel

Skullcap is used to ensure fidelity in handfasting (marriage) ceremonies. It carries with it a vibration of commitment. Ask yourself what are you committed to, and skullcap will help you manifest your desire here on earth. Combine the following herbs together on a waxing or full moon for virility, health, success, vitality, and strength. Light a red candle and pay close attention to the male energy, calling on God. Ask that his vibrant, vigorous force guide you toward achieving a set goal.

2 teaspoons dried skullcap
1 teaspoon dragon's blood powder
1 cinnamon stick

Grind the herbs in a mortar, moving the pestle clockwise (deosil). Visualize your goal and desire. Place the mixture in a small red pouch and wear it around your neck or carry it with you until your objective has manifested.

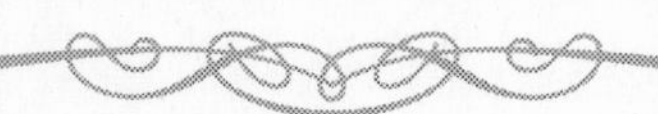

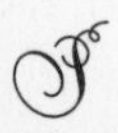

Slippery Elm

Ulmus rubra

INDIAN ELM, MOOSE ELM, RED ELM, SWEET ELM

Part Used: inner bark

Slippery elm is a large deciduous tree with rough, reddish brown bark, toothed oval leaves, and papery seedpods. Native Americans found that the inner bark produced a mucilage that makes a successful poultice for treating wounds and sore eyes. Infused as a tea or taken raw, slippery elm was used to ease childbirth and relieve diarrhea and ulcers. Slippery elm is rare or endangered in many parts of the United States, so its bark should not be harvested from wild plants. In magick, it is often used for meditation, communication, protection, and dreaming. It is associated with the god and planet Saturn.

SLIPPERY ELM TREES PREFER FULL SUN AND REGULAR WATERING; THEY CAN TOLERATE POOR SOIL.

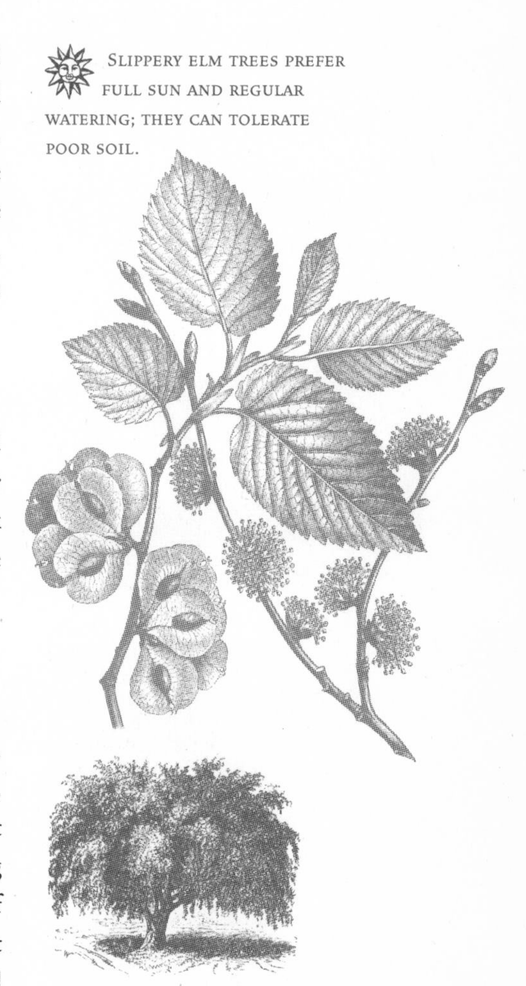

Throat Drops

Research has shown that the mucilage in slippery elm relieves inflammation and irritation of the reproductive, digestive, and respiratory systems. Bundle the inner bark and place in cool water for several hours; then strain out the bark and drink the liquid. Or make the drops here and keep them on hand for whenever you have a scratchy or sore throat.

- ½ cup slippery elm bark pieces
- 1 cup water
- ½ cup honey

Put the slippery elm bark in a tea bag, tea ball, or infuser, or place in a saucepan. Boil the water in a kettle. When the bubbles subside, pour the water over the bark, cover, and steep 10 to 20 minutes. Keep covered so that the essential oils don't escape. Strain out the bark. Add the honey. Simmer over low heat, stirring occasionally, about 25 to 30 minutes. Test for readiness by dropping ½ teaspoon of the mixture onto waxed paper; as it cools, it should harden and hold its form. Let cool completely; wrap the drops individually in waxed paper and store in a cool place. Drops will last for several weeks if kept in a cool place.

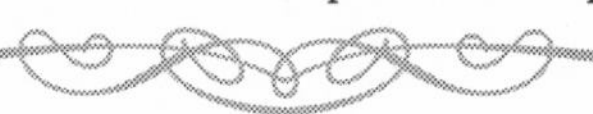

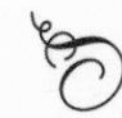

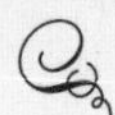

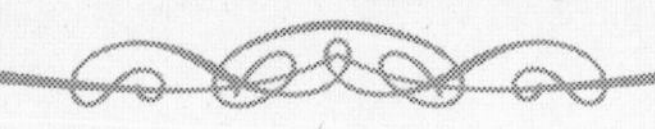

Star Anise

Illicium verum

Part Used: Seeds

Two related species are more commonly seen in the United States, but they do not produce the star-shaped fruit. Infused in oil, it has aromatherapy uses similar to those for regular anise. It also scents perfumes and soaps. Star anise is used magickally to increase clairvoyance, prophetic dreams, and luck. It is believed to protect holy sites and cleanse them of all negativity. Star Anise is associated with the moon, the astrological sign of Aquarius, and the god and planet Jupiter.

THE RELATED SPECIES *Illicium anisatum*, FOUND IN THE UNITED STATES, IS TOXIC IF EATEN.

Vietnamese Star-Anise Noodles

SERVES 4

Star anise's association with Aquarius is symbolic of personal independence and loyalty to one's true self. As you claim and bring forth your power, you need to feel safe to express your feelings; don't fall back on stoicism. Stoicism can separate you from your most intimate emotions. When you deny your inner feelings, you lose your sense of intuition. Jupiter serves to expand, so as you make these noodles, think of ways in which you can be powerful and human. Don't try to understand with your mind. You cannot theorize feelings. Allow your heart to lead.

1 (16-ounce) package rice noodles
4 cups chicken or vegetable broth
4 cloves garlic, smashed and peeled
1 (1½-inch) piece fresh ginger, peeled, cut into thin rounds, smashed
2 (3-inch-long) cinnamon sticks
2 pods star anise

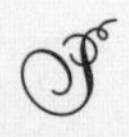

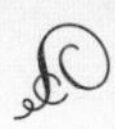

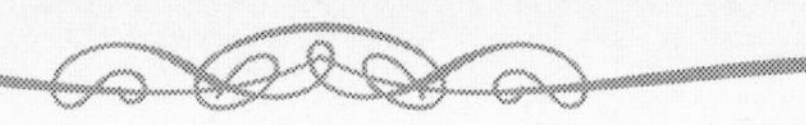

1 tablespoon soy sauce
1 tablespoon Thai fish sauce
1 tablespoon sugar
½ cup chopped Napa cabbage
¼ cup bean sprouts
2 tablespoons chopped fresh mint
2 tablespoons chopped fresh cilantro

Soak the noodles in hot water 20 minutes until tender. Meanwhile, mix together the broth, garlic, ginger, cinnamon, star anise, soy sauce, fish sauce, and sugar in a medium saucepan. Bring to a boil over medium-high heat. Decrease heat, cover, and simmer 20 minutes. Using a slotted spoon, remove and discard solids. Divide the noodles, cabbage, and sprouts evenly among 4 bowls. Ladle in the broth. Sprinkle the mint and cilantro on top and serve.

Star anise is a slow-growing tree native to Southeast Asia. Sow seeds in warm ground and grow in light soil with full sun. Star anise does not transplant easily.

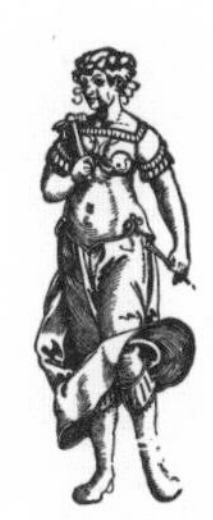

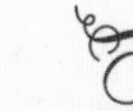

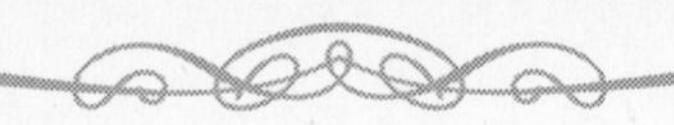

Thyme

Thymus vulgaris

COMMON THYME, GARDEN THYME

Parts Used: leaves, flowers

Thyme is found wild on heaths and sunny banks; it is widely cultivated in gardens. The small leaves are flat, dark, and highly aromatic. The name *thyme* is derived from a Greek word *thymon,* meaning "to make a burnt offering." The herb is used to treat whooping cough and digestive complaints. Thyme is used to dispel nightmares, refresh the spirit, increase clairvoyance, attract praise, and purify a room. The herb confers tranquillity, peace, and security. It is believed that if a bride wears thyme in her shoe, her groom will be forever true. Thyme yields thymol, an essential oil, which is used as a disinfectant and in hair lotions. Add dried and powdered thyme at a rate of one teaspoon per pound of food to a dog dish, or sprinkle on a cat's food, to help dispel parasites. Thyme is associated with the goddess and planet Venus.

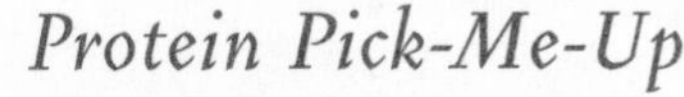

Protein Pick-Me-Up

SERVES 4 AS A SNACK OR APPETIZER

This is a great snack to make around the time the afternoon begins to drag. Kids can help make it; mine love to assist with whipping it up. It provides a great opportunity to teach them to ask Mother Earth's permission before taking from plants. You can alter the quantities of the fresh herbs, depending on which plant has more to offer. Add thyme flowers for a colorful touch. Cooking the chips takes some practice; expect to burn some. Also, your family members may have different preferences about how crispy they should be, but trial-and-error is part of the fun.

1 (6-ounce) can albacore tuna, packed in water
2 tablespoons chopped fresh thyme
1 tablespoon chopped fresh parsley

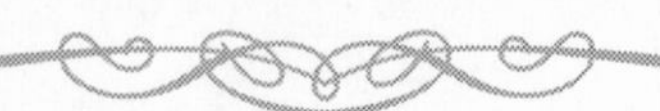

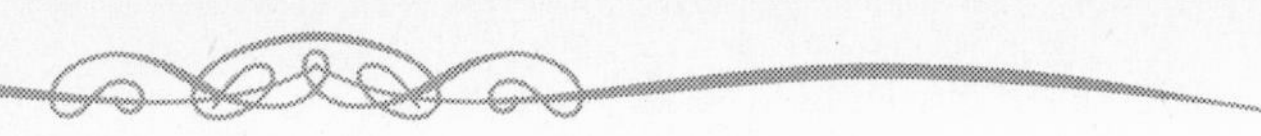

1 teaspoon chopped fresh chives
¼ cup chopped green onions
¼ cup finely chopped red bell pepper
2 tablespoons balsamic vinegar
1 heaping tablespoon mayonnaise
¼ teaspoon celery salt
6 corn tortillas
6 tablespoons vegetable oil

Drain the tuna and place in a small bowl. Break up the chunks with a fork. Add the thyme, parsley, chives, green onion, bell pepper, vinegar, and mayonnaise. Mix well. Sprinkle the dip with celery salt and stir to combine.

Cut the tortillas in half. Cut the halves vertically to make 4 strips from each half. Heat the oil in a frying pan over medium-high heat. Test the oil by adding a small drop of water. If it sparks, add 4 strips to the oil. After 3 to 5 minutes, the chips will curl slightly at the edges; turn over. Test for readiness by touching the chips with the tongs; if they feel crispy take them out of the pan and place on a paper towel to drain the oil. Season lightly with salt. Repeat with the remaining tortilla strips. Let the chips cool, then eat with the dip.

Thyme prefers light, dry, well-drained soil and full to partial sun. Plant in groups for a fuller look. Thyme does well in rock gardens and as edging for flower borders. It is a successful partner to eggplants, potatoes, and tomatoes and is known to repel whitefly. It is native to southern Europe.

Thyme Vegetable Stock

Makes 1½ quarts

This incredible stock can be used as a soup or gravy base, or whenever vegetable broth is called for. Lemongrass can be found in some grocery stores and most Asian markets. If you cannot find it, you can substitute half a teaspoon minced lemon zest, or leave out the lemon flavor altogether.

2 medium onions, peeled, coarsely chopped
1 head garlic, cloves peeled and smashed
8 shallots, thinly sliced
1 medium celery stalk, coarsely chopped
1 carrot, peeled, coarsely chopped
Nonstick vegetable oil spray

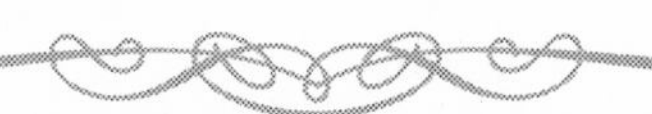

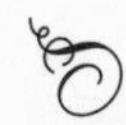

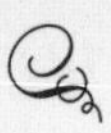
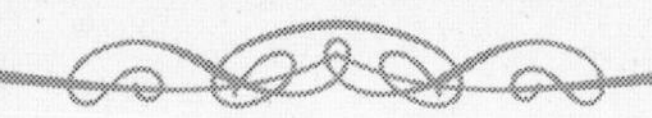

4 leeks (white part only), chopped
1½ cups plus 2 quarts water
½ cup chopped fresh parsley
3 small bay leaves
1 pound collard greens, rinsed, sliced crosswise into strips
¾ cup chopped fresh thyme
1 stalk lemongrass (bottom 6 inches only)
4 green onions (white and green parts), chopped
2 teaspoons rice vinegar

Combine the onions, garlic, shallots, celery, and carrot in a large stockpot. Spray the vegetables lightly with nonstick spray and toss to coat. Cover and cook over low heat, stirring occasionally, 20 to 30 minutes. Increase the heat to medium and add the leeks. Cook until the leeks are tender, about 10 minutes. Add 1½ cups of the water and cook, partially covered, until the water evaporates, about 30 minutes. Add the parsley, bay leaves, salt, pepper, and remaining 2 quarts water. Cover and cook 15 minutes. Add the collard greens, thyme, lemongrass, and green onions. Decrease the heat and simmer 15 minutes. Strain the stock through a large strainer into a 2-quart container. Do not press on the solids. Stir the vinegar into the stock. The stock will last in the refrigerator for 4 days, or in the freezer up to 2 months.

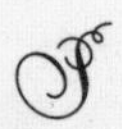

Tobacco

Nicotiana tabacum

TABACA, TABACI FOLIA

Part Used: leaves

Tobacco is a thin herbaceous shrub with long, narrow, pointed leaves and tubular greenish white flowers tipped in dark rose. Tobacco is burned magickally to dispel negativity, including sickness. Native Americans use it for blessings. The symptoms tobacco causes when used in excess—dizziness, nausea, trembling, headaches, and diarrhea—are the same it treats as a diluted homeopathic remedy. It can also relieve motion sickness, violent vomiting, heart palpitations, disturbed vision, and hiccups.

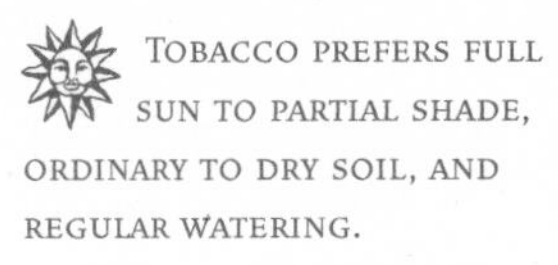

TOBACCO PREFERS FULL SUN TO PARTIAL SHADE, ORDINARY TO DRY SOIL, AND REGULAR WATERING.

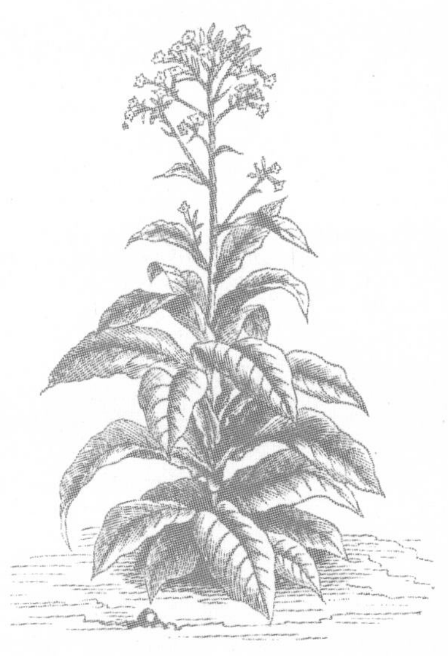

Tobacco Blessing

As children of this earth we would do well to remember that we are part of the cycle of give and take. By the gratitude we show, we give back to the Creator who has provided so lavishly for us. In this way we illustrate our willingness to be humble and appreciative of all our blessings, such as health, family, and love. This ceremony is designed for a gathering of people; children are necessary. Invite your guests to bring tobacco, any amount from a fistful to a bag. Flowers to smoke are welcome, including lobelia, mint, lavender, or any plant sacred to the Indian nations. This blessing ceremony was adapted from a Southern California Tongva Indian tobacco-blessing ritual, given to me by spiritual leader Jimi Castillo, also known as Walks with Bears; it was given to him by an Algonquin elder. Tobacco is not native to Southern California but the Tongva people are very active and celebrate Spirit in ceremonies that use the blessing qualities associated with tobacco.

Gather your friends in a circle. Traditionally, women who are in their moon time (menstrual period) will form a separate circle outside the main circle. They are considered already in ceremony and very powerful. Place a very large bowl or container (called the mother bowl) in the center. Light a bundle of dried sage or

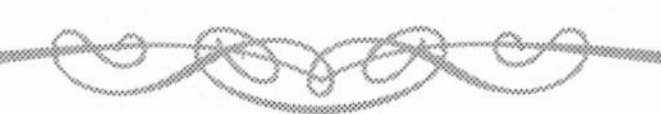

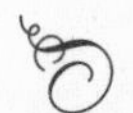

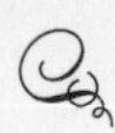

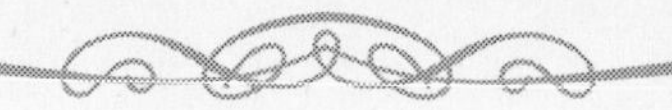

loose sage leaves in a fire-retardant container such as an abalone shell. Waft the smoke over every participant, when possible getting the bottoms of their feet. At this time, you can ask designated musicians to begin playing their instruments, such as flutes, rattles, clapsticks, or drums.

After everyone has been blessed with the smoke, ask the first person to come to the mother bowl, envision a wish, and place tobacco in it. One by one, or in groups of 3 to 5 if you have a large gathering, invite people to add their tobacco and make a silent wish. Select a boy and a girl to mix the tobacco. Offer a blessing over the tobacco.

Invite your guests back to the mother bowl to take whatever amount of tobacco they need. The women in the moon circle can have a friend or family member collect tobacco for them. If your guests need a lot of tobacco, it will be provided. If they are not experiencing pain or suffering, then they will know the proper amount to take is less. Tell your guests to use this tobacco as a gift when making a prayer, harvesting nature's herbs or fruits, or any time an offering is suggested.

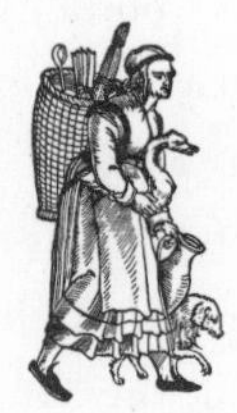

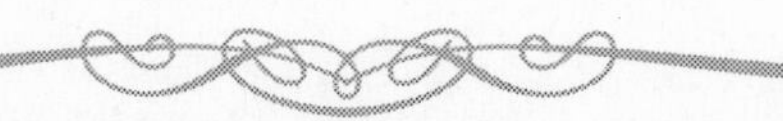

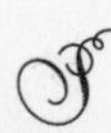

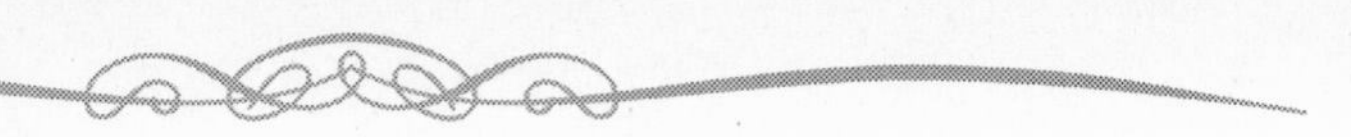

Valerian

Valeriana officinalis

AMATILLA, CAPON'S TAILOR, ENGLISH VALERIAN, GARDEN HELIOTROPE, MOON ROOT, SET WELL, ST. GEORGE'S HERB, VANDAL ROOT

Part Used: root

Valerian is a perennial herb that grows along walls and sunny riverbanks. The leaves are shiny and bright green; the flowers are white or rose-colored and carried on branching stems up to five feet tall. Its name is derived from the Latin *valere*, meaning "to be well." For more than a thousand years its stinky root has been used as an effective sleep aid, nerve remedy, and tranquilizer. Its mild approach helps you sleep without morning grogginess or dependency. It is used for cleansing, purification, protection, love, and harmony in magick. Valerian is associated with the astrological sign of Virgo and the purity that comes with this earth sign.

VALERIAN PREFERS MOIST, HUMUSY SOIL AND IS PARTIAL TO FULL SUN. IT CAN BE INVASIVE IN THE GARDEN BORDER. VALERIAN IS NATIVE TO EUROPE AND NORTHERN ASIA.

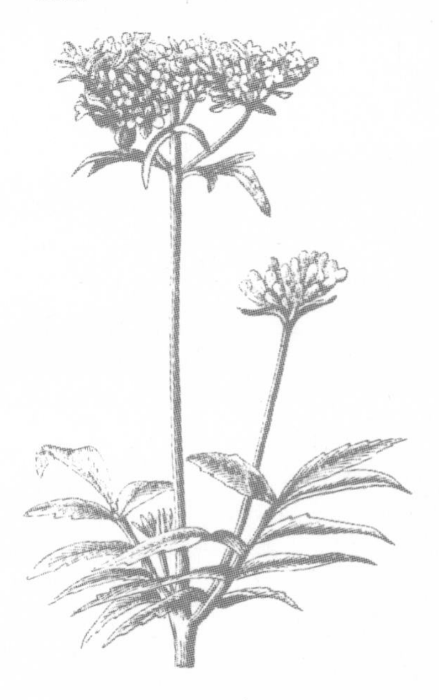

Peaceful Sleep and Dreams Sachet

Valerian cleanses through its association with Virgo's pure energy. Virgo and valerian combine to show you that the universe is unfolding according to a perfect plan. If a decision or other life experience has got you feeling out of control, incorporate valerian into the following resting spell. You will find a stillness that cannot be agitated by chaos in your mind or environment.

1 teaspoon dried valerian root
2 teaspoons dried chamomile buds
Pinch of dried lavender flowers

Grind all ingredients in a mortar with a pestle. As you do so, say,

Quiet mind, restful body
May peaceful dreams grace me tonight.

Place the mixture in a small muslin bag and put under your pillow or beside you on a nightstand.

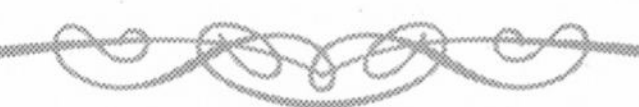

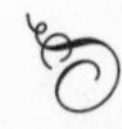

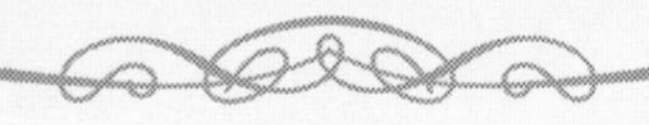

Vanilla

Vanilla planifolia

Part Used: seedpods

Vanilla is a parasitical, tropical vine with long, green, fleshy stems that cling to trees. Its bunching yellow or orange orchidaceous flowers attract bees. During vanilla's two-month blooming period, it opens a new flower each day. Many cultures consider vanilla's heady aroma to be an aphrodisiac. Vanilla invokes glamour, luxury, beauty, love, lust, attraction, sensuality, love, prosperity, bliss, inspiration, romance, and restoration. It is used to remove obstacles and instill vitality. Vanilla is associated with the gods Oxun, Kokopelli, and Shakti, and the planets Jupiter and the sun.

Van-Berry Bran Muffins

Makes 12 muffins

These delicious muffins are a great way of sneaking fiber into children; they'll never know! An added benefit is that if you make the muffins with intent and eat them in rituals for the purpose listed above, you will find they are very powerful indeed.

- 1 cup all-purpose flour
- 1 cup wheat bran
- 1 teaspoon baking soda
- ½ teaspoon salt
- 1 cup mashed hulled strawberries
- ½ cup (1 stick) unsalted butter
- ⅓ cup sugar
- 1 large egg
- 1 teaspoon vanilla extract

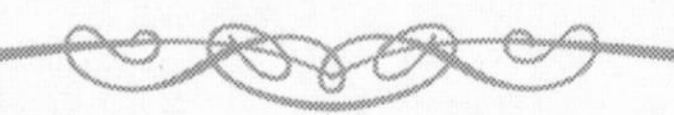

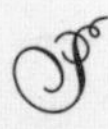

Preheat oven to 400°F. Grease a muffin tin with butter or nonstick cooking spray, or line it with cupcake holders. Mix all ingredients together in a medium bowl. Spoon into the muffin tin until ¾ full. Bake 13 minutes for a mini-muffin tin and 18 minutes for full-size muffins, or until golden brown.

Fruit Ice Cream

MAKES 1 QUART

The scent of vanilla can reduce anxiety. It is a sensual odor that carries you away from the worries and complications of the day and into the moment. It is associated with Venus. This planet's energy gives birth to harmony, aesthetic pleasures, and inner serenity. Venus is the goddess of beauty, peace, love, and trust. Let Venus help you birth balance and serenity in your life. This recipe uses strawberries, another Venusian ingredient, but you can substitute any fruit you like. (This recipe was donated by Jason Scheuner, a music junky who loves to make ice cream, especially for goddesses that he meets.)

VANILLA, A VINING PLANT IN THE ORCHID FAMILY, IS CULTIVATED IN THE TROPICAL REGIONS OF THE WESTERN HEMISPHERE. IT GROWS BEST IN A MOIST, SHADED ENVIRONMENT.

- 2 cups fresh sliced strawberries, or frozen, thawed
- 1¼ cups sugar
- 4 cups heavy whipping cream
- 1 tablespoon vanilla extract

Place the strawberries in a large bowl and sprinkle ¼ cup of sugar on top. Pour over 1 cup of the cream. Let stand 1 hour. Mash the strawberries, sugar, and cream into mush. Let stand 30 minutes. Add the vanilla and the remaining 1 cup sugar and 3 cups cream; stir until you get a nice pink soup. Place the mixture in the refrigerator at least 4 hours and up to 3 days. When you are ready to make your ice cream, put the bowl into the freezer to chill. Stir every 30 minutes, scraping down the sides each time. When the mixture starts to harden around the edges, it is ready to churn. Process according to your ice cream maker's instructions. If you do not have an ice cream maker, keep the mixture in the freezer and give it a good stir every 15 to 30 minutes until it hardens.

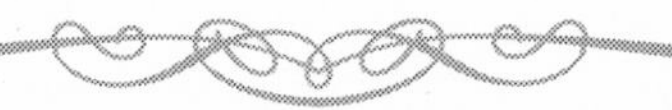

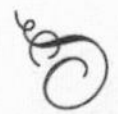

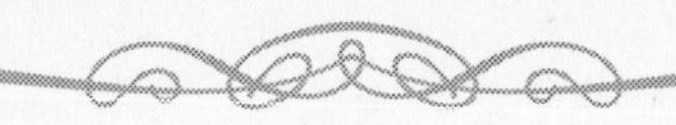

Vervain

Verbena officinalis

ENCHANTER'S PLANT, HERB OF GRACE, HERB-OF-THE-CROSS, JUNO'S TEARS, PIGEON'S GRASS, SIMPLER'S JOY

Parts Used: leaves, stems, flowers

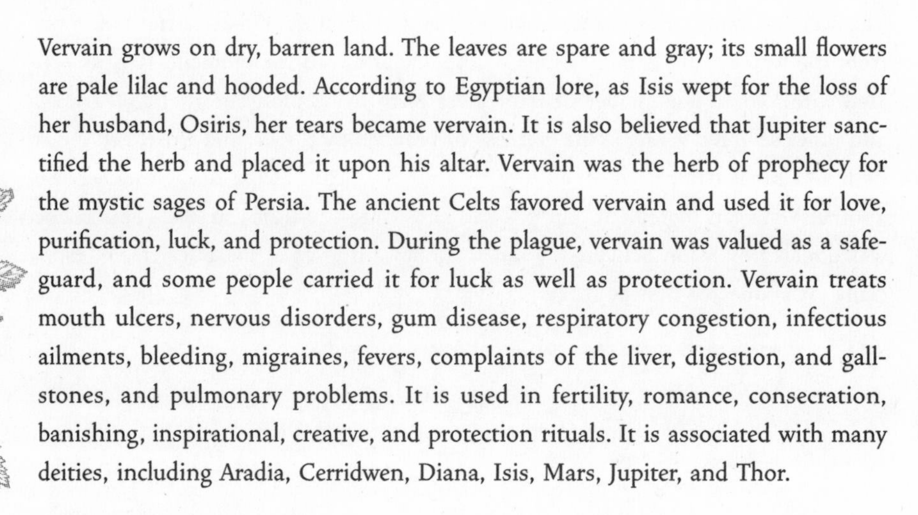

Vervain grows on dry, barren land. The leaves are spare and gray; its small flowers are pale lilac and hooded. According to Egyptian lore, as Isis wept for the loss of her husband, Osiris, her tears became vervain. It is also believed that Jupiter sanctified the herb and placed it upon his altar. Vervain was the herb of prophecy for the mystic sages of Persia. The ancient Celts favored vervain and used it for love, purification, luck, and protection. During the plague, vervain was valued as a safeguard, and some people carried it for luck as well as protection. Vervain treats mouth ulcers, nervous disorders, gum disease, respiratory congestion, infectious ailments, bleeding, migraines, fevers, complaints of the liver, digestion, and gallstones, and pulmonary problems. It is used in fertility, romance, consecration, banishing, inspirational, creative, and protection rituals. It is associated with many deities, including Aradia, Cerridwen, Diana, Isis, Mars, Jupiter, and Thor.

Forgiveness Incense

Hanging on to resentments blocks you from being able to give and receive love. This very powerful ceremony will help you release the past. You can get the powder for this incense at magickal shops, along with the forgiveness oil. (Robynn Zender—mother, writer, weaver, potter, and artist—donated this recipe and ritual.)

- 9 pinches dried vervain flowers
- 7 pinches sandalwood powder
- 7 pinches dragon's blood powder
- 5 pinches dried lavender flowers
- 3 pinches dried bergamot flowers
- 2 pinches dried rue flowers
- 2 pinches frankincense powder
- 2 pinches copal
- 4 whole peppercorns
- 4 drops patchouli essential oil
- 2 drops gardenia essential oil
- 1 drop ylang-ylang essential oil

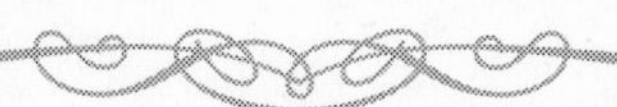

To make the incense, combine the vervain, sandalwood, dragon's blood, lavender, bergamot, rue, frankincense, copal, and peppercorns together in a mortar and grind with a pestle. Stir in the patchouli, gardenia, and ylang-ylang oils to form the incense.

Perform this ritual on the day before a new moon. Make a list of people whom you need to forgive in order to let go of the past. Write each name on a separate scrap of paper and place in a bag or pouch. Draw a warm bath and sip chamomile tea. When you have bathed, anoint your third eye (in the center of your forehead) with gold glitter and dab forgiveness oil on every chakra point (for more on the chakras, see page 73). Dress in lavender or purple clothing. Take your altar outside.

Bless your ritual area by wafting smoke from a smoldering bundle of dried sage all around it. Cast a circle. Light candles in all the colors of the spectrum, as well as white. Light the forgiveness incense you have made and walk widdershins (counterclockwise) around the circle. One at a time, pull the names of the people out of the pouch. Meditate on each name, and look at their life objectively. Put yourself in their place and understand why they might have wronged you. This will help you to feel compassion for their behavior and forgive them. As you ponder, you will feel many emotions. Consciously forgive each person. You may spend a lot of time reflecting on some names and less on others.

After you have gone through all the names, place the scraps of paper in a fire-retardant container. Put more forgiveness incense in with the names and burn the pieces of paper. Raise the energy by chanting whatever comes to your mind. Bend your knees and stand with your feet shoulder-width apart for a grounding stance. Wielding your athame with your arm held straight up (as if you were swinging a lasso), circle widdershins and shoot the energy out of your body and up to the sky until your feel unconditional love filling your body. Rest and focus on your gratitude for the loving space you have created. Close the circle. Ground yourself in the space of the mundane world and enjoy some cakes and ale.

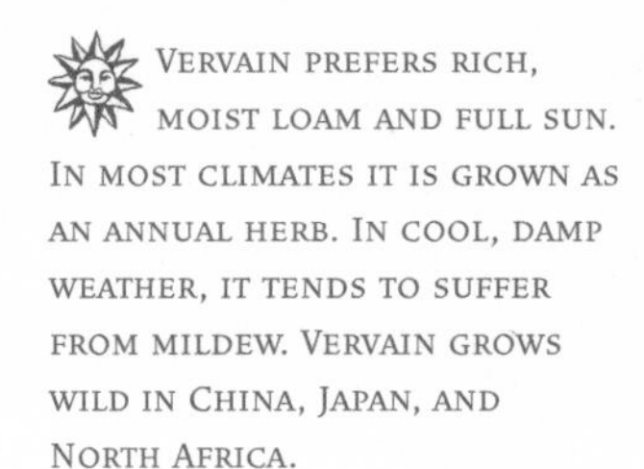

Vervain prefers rich, moist loam and full sun. In most climates it is grown as an annual herb. In cool, damp weather, it tends to suffer from mildew. Vervain grows wild in China, Japan, and North Africa.

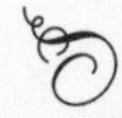

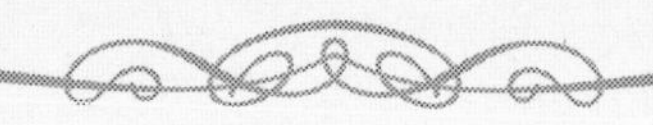

Walnut

Juglans regia

CAUCASIAN WALNUT, ENGLISH WALNUT, PERSIAN WALNUT, TREE OF EVIL

Part Used: nut

Walnuts are large, spreading, deciduous trees. Their leaves are divided into leaflets, and the nuts are round. Walnuts are used for healing, peaceful separation, and fertility. Walnut earned its reputation as the tree of evil because in olden times wary voyeurs spied on witches performing their work under the protection of its branches. We shall reclaim this tree in the name of the Goddess, among other names, as we once again walk together on our spiral path, reclaiming our birthright and title.

Pear-Walnut Salad

SERVES 4 TO 6

One of the most difficult things you may experience in life is becoming comfortable with what others think of you, especially if they discount what you value. Sometimes you may greatly desire to explain to them that what you believe has merit, history, and a solid foundation. What matters most is not convincing others, but rather holding on to your strong core of beliefs; do not let your values be undermined by your environment or by people who do not understand. My favorite affirmation for this topic is "What you think is none of my business." Walnut possesses the energy that will protect you from unwanted influences and help you maintain and strengthen your center. You cannot fight darkness. Judging others as unenlightened only binds you to them. Rest assured with the knowledge that spirituality is personal and can never be fully shared with another person but only with the Goddess. Know that you are a healer and a light-worker.

4 firm Anjou pears
1 tablespoon butter, melted
2 tablespoons sugar

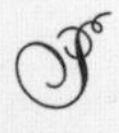

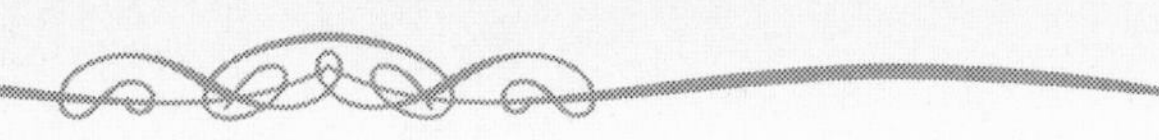

1 cup coarsely chopped walnuts

2 teaspoons white wine vinegar

1½ tablespoons extra virgin olive oil

½ teaspoon sea salt

¼ teaspoon freshly ground white peppercorns

7 cups arugula, torn into bite-size pieces (from about 2 bunches)

½ cup freshly grated Parmesan cheese

Position 1 rack in the bottom third of the oven, place a baking sheet on the rack, and preheat to 500°F. Halve each pear lengthwise and peel. Remove the core with a paring knife. Set each half on a working surface, cut side down, and slice into fifths. Coat the pear slices with butter and sugar. Lay out the slices in a single layer on preheated baking sheet. Roast until browned on the bottom, about 10 minutes. Flip each pear slice and continue roasting about 5 minutes. Let the pears cool. In a small skillet, toast the walnuts over medium heat 3 minutes. Set aside. In a small bowl, whisk together the vinegar, oil, salt, and pepper. In a large serving bowl, combine the arugula, pears, and Parmesan cheese. Add the dressing and toss. Sprinkle walnuts on top. Serve immediately.

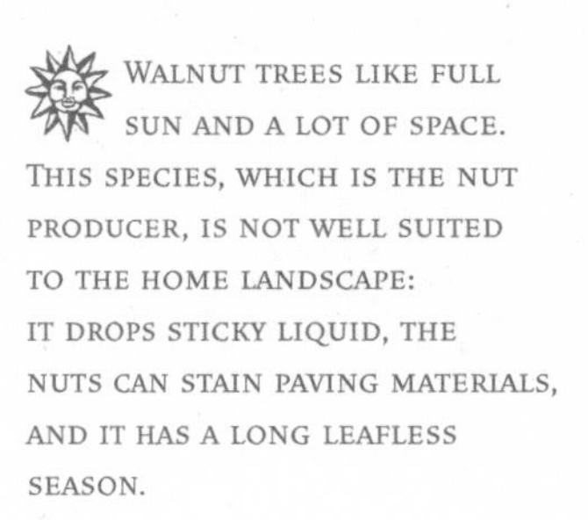

Walnut trees like full sun and a lot of space. This species, which is the nut producer, is not well suited to the home landscape: it drops sticky liquid, the nuts can stain paving materials, and it has a long leafless season.

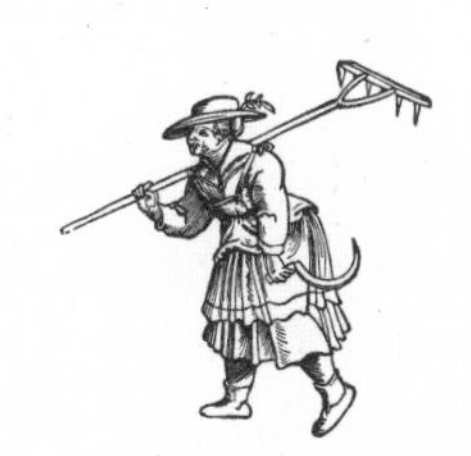

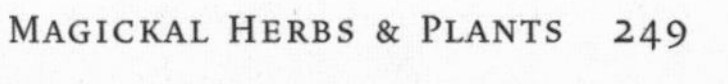

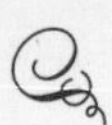

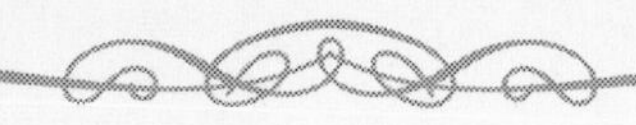

Willow

Salix alba

SAILLE, TREE OF ENCHANTMENT, WITCHES' ASPIRIN, WITHE, WITHY

Parts Used: branches, bark

There are about three hundred types of willows; the species we are most familiar with has thin, trailing branches and long, narrow leaves. Willow is often used for magick wands. On a waxing or full moon, attach a crystal to the end of a willow branch with wire to make a beautiful and powerful tool. As you do this, focus on a wish or on healing, as these are the two basic powers of the willow. Willow is associated with the moon, water, dreaming, intuition, deep emotions, the Goddess, all that is feminine, healing, separation, beginnings, binding, and wish making. Its moon energy puts us in touch with our feelings and deep emotions, and helps us be expressive, releasing pent-up feelings; it charges us with the energy to perform fantastical leaps of faith, inspiration, and understanding. You can make yourself a wand from a fallen willow branch and sleep with it under your pillow to increase intuitive dreaming. You will find your dreams will immediately become more vivid and meaningful. Willow is closely linked with Ostara, when nature stirs with new life and begins to burgeon. This connection reflects willow's ability to help us regenerate and rebirth. Willow's weeping shape has led to its symbolic association with grief. By its attunement to water, willow evokes movement on the emotional level, and dissolves blockages of deep emotional pain blocks by promoting expression. This graceful tree will stand guard while you move through the many levels of sadness and express your pain though tears and grief. Use the symbol of willow if you have experienced adversity or misfortune in life and remain embittered by it. Willow is associated with many deities, including Artemis, Belili, Ceres, Diana, Hecate, Hera, Mercury, and Persephone.

The Druids valued this tree so much that they named the letter *s* of their alphabet after it and called that letter *saille,* their name for willow.

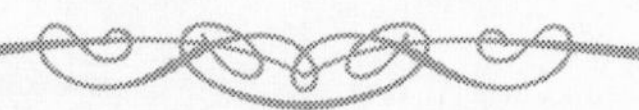

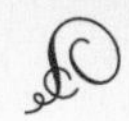

Sweet-Pea Trellis

Willow is pliable and has been used for various needs, including making baskets and wicker furniture. The Tongva and other Southern California Indian traditions use a species of willow native to their area as a support for their homes and sweat lodges. If you wish to make friends in your community, use the willow to form a trellis for the delicate twining sweet pea. Sweet peas are used in attraction spells.

Using hemp rope, tie three willow branches together to form three sides of a vertical rectangle; where the fourth side would be is where the trellis is inserted in the ground. An ideal height for your trellis is five feet; the crossbar is then three to five feet across, depending on your space. At the location where you wish to have your trellis, secure the vertical branches six to ten inches into the soil. Cut ten hemp ropes the width of the trellis, plus one foot. Just below the crossbar, tie a rope to the side and pull across the width of the trellis, securing it to the other side. Repeat this process, descending down the trellis, every six inches. Cut ten hemp ropes six feet long, or the height of your trellis, plus one foot. Six inches from the top corner, tie the rope to the crossbar branch. Wrap it around each horizontal line, tying it off on the bottom horizontal rope of the trellis. Repeat this process, moving along the trellis at six-inch intervals. When you are done, the trellis will resemble a grid.

WILLOW TREES DO WELL IN MOIST GARDENING SOIL WITH FULL SUN. WILLOW IS NATIVE TO NORTH AMERICA, EUROPE, ASIA, AND AFRICA.

One night before the full moon, set sweet pea seeds to soak, until they crack. By the light of the full moon, dig a one-foot trench for the seeds. Fill with a blend of compost, soil amendment, and all-purpose soil. Plant seeds one-inch deep in the trench, saying,

I now attract to me friends aplenty
To gather and build a community
Those of like mind I call you to me
By my will, so mote it be.

Water the seeds three times a day until they sprout. Share their sweet-smelling flowers with neighbors, friends, and family.

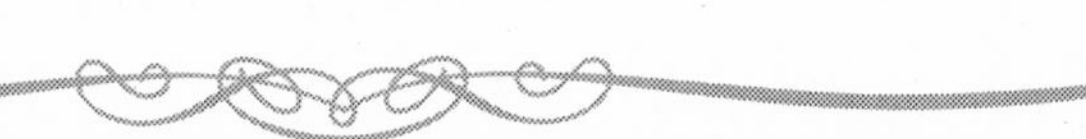

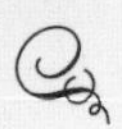

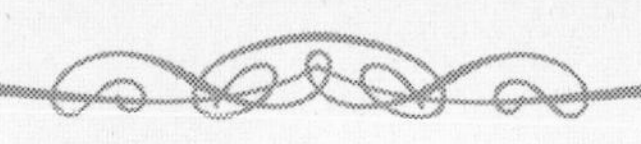

Woodruff

Galium odoratum

HERB WALTER, MASTER OF THE WOOD, WOODROVE, WUDEROVE

Parts Used: flowers, leaves

WOODRUFF PREFERS SHADE AND MOIST, HUMUSY, WELL-DRAINED SOIL. IN CLIMATES WITH SOME FROST, IT MAKES A PRETTY GROUND COVER FOR SHADY PLACES. IT IS NATIVE TO EUROPE.

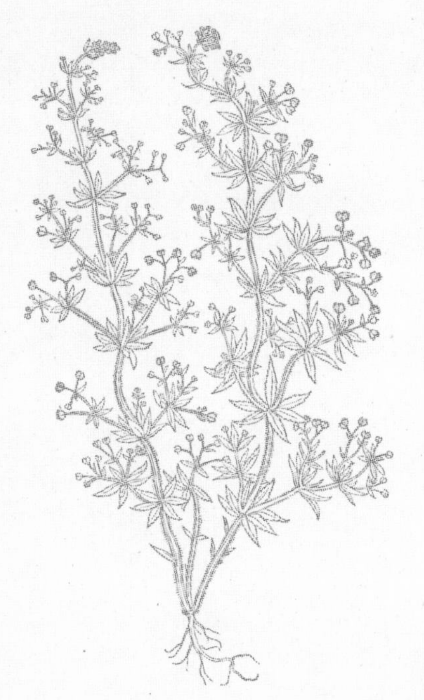

Woodruff grows wild in woodlands. Its leaves are tiny and dark and grow in whorls. The tiny flowers are fragrant, white, and frail. The perfume of the flower increases upon drying, so in the Middle Ages it was mixed with straw and scattered on the floor of the house to improve the odor. The herb is a tonic and nervine and increases milk production. It treats poor memory, depression, jaundice, constipation, children's fevers, and upset stomachs. Herbalists have applied the leaves as a dressing for cuts and as a tea to be drunk for these ailments. Magickally, woodruff is used for purification, balance, and rejuvenation. Woodruff is associated with the deities and planets Venus and Mars.

Spring Cleaning

Woodruff is an herb of spring—a time to celebrate new life, including paradigm shifts, belief repatternings, and all births. None of these transformations can come about if we do not cleanse and purify our minds of clutter.

Begin by sweeping your home with a broom of your choice. Follow by magickally sweeping out negative energy (instructions for making a magick broom appear on page 117). Sweep stale ideas or beliefs out of the door. (This spell was created by Constance DeMasters, also known as the Crimson Dragon.)

½ cup fresh woodruff flowers
1 gallon water
Juice of 1 lemon

Combine all the ingredients in either a sink or a large bucket. Dip your mop into the woodruff water. Bathe your floors in the sparkling freshness of spring. Imagine new possibilities filling the space, creating a foundation for them to grow and thrive. Anything is possible with an open, uncluttered mind.

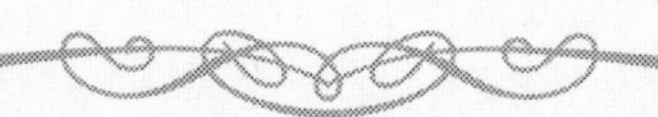

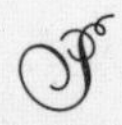

Wormwood

Artemisia absinthium

ABSINTHE, COMMON WORMWOOD, CROWN FOR A KING, OLD WOMAN, MADDERWORT

Part Used: leaves

Wormwood grows in dry regions and deserts, rocky places, and wastelands. The leaves are gray, downy, and fringed. The flowers are small and yellow-green. The plant is bitter, aromatic, and highly potent. Wormwood was once considered an effective tonic, antiseptic, nervine, vermifuge, and narcotic. It was used to treat women's issues, digestive ailments, fevers, jaundice, and balding.

WORMWOOD CONTAINS A NARCOTIC POISON THAT ACTS TO DEPRESS THE NERVOUS SYSTEM. LARGE DOSES CAUSE VERTIGO, HALLUCINATIONS, CONVULSIONS, PARALYSIS, AND EVEN DEATH. WORMWOOD CAN BE USED MAGICKALLY, BUT NOT MEDICINALLY.

WORMWOOD IS A MOUNDING SHRUB THAT PREFERS WELL-DRAINED CLAY LOAM AND FULL SUN TO PART SHADE. DO NOT PLANT NEAR MOST VEGETABLES OR THEY WILL BE HARMED. WORMWOOD IS NATIVE TO EUROPE. A LIQUEUR MADE FROM THIS HERB, ABSINTHE, HAS BEEN BANNED THROUGHOUT MOST OF THE WORLD.

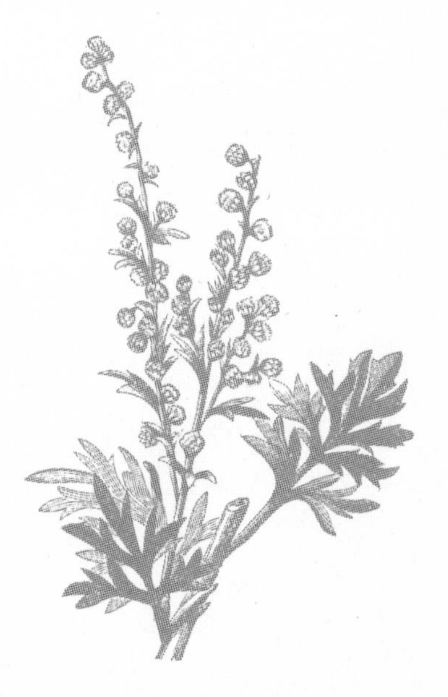

Samhain Candles

Wormwood is associated with clairvoyance, protection and the Samhain sabbat. Adorn your Samhain altar with these candles to represent the celebration of a new year. As you burn them, you can ask for clairvoyance from Diana or Iris, the herb's associated deities.

Samhain is known as Summer's End. It is the start of the Witches' New Year and the third and final harvest celebration. Our European ancestors timed their festivals in accordance with the movements of the stars as well as the seasons of the earth. The setting of the Pleiades marks Samhain. We become aware of the darkness and infertility of the land as produce shelves grow bare, or filled with fruits and vegetables imported from countries in the Southern Hemisphere. Samhain is a time of reflection, when the veil between the mundane world and the Otherworld is thin; it is the time to honor our ancestors and invite them to attend our ceremonies. Bonfires were traditionally part of the Samhain festivities, prepared during the day, preferably on a hilltop, and lit at dusk. Celebrations were

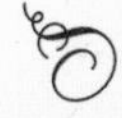

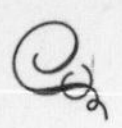

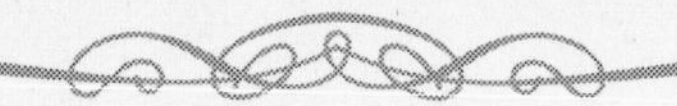

held round the fires, and apples and nuts were roasted. Samhain, when people felt close to the Otherworld, was seen as an appropriate time for divination of all sorts. The events of the coming year or the outcome of a wish could be foretold by tossing a nut into the fire and watching how it burned. If it burned brightly, the thrower's wish would come true.

2 Champagne flutes
10 ounces gold-colored candle gel wax
Candle glitter
4 to 6 drops Samhain oil
4 to 6 drops wormwood essential oil
2 candle wicks with tab
Purple and black wired ribbons

Wash and dry the flutes. Place the wax in a saucepan and warm over low heat until a candy thermometer registers 225°F. Do not allow the thermometer to touch the bottom of the pan, or you will receive an incorrect reading. Turn off the heat and allow the gel to cool slowly. When the temperature reads 190°F, stir in the glitter. When it cools to 180°F, add 3 to 5 drops each of the Samhain and wormwood oils. Using a metal spoon, stir well. Secure the wicks in the center of the flutes; make sure the wick is 1 inch taller than the flute. You can do this by resting a pencil on the top of the glass and winding the wick around the pencil. Pour the hot gel wax into each flute to a level ½ inch below the rim. Allow 1 hour to cool. Trim the wick to ¼ inch before lighting. Decorate the flute stems with purple and black wire ribbons.

Yarrow

Achillea millefolium

DEVIL'S PLAYTHING, HUNDRED-LEAVED GRASS, MILFOIL, SEVEN YEAR'S LOVE, SOLDIER'S WOUNDWORT, THOUSANDSEAL

Parts Used: flowers, leaves, stems

Yarrow grows in pastures and along waysides. The feathered leaves are grayish and fragrant. The disk-shaped flower heads are white or pink. This herb has been used to treat smallpox, typhoid fever, malaria, pneumonia, hysteria, and epilepsy. Chewing on the leaves will quell a toothache. It can also repel mosquitoes when infused in oil. The herb yields some of its healing potential to water and alcohol.

Yarrow is used to allay fears, induce love, increase clairvoyance, protect marriages or other committed relationships, and for banishing. A tea made from the leaves and flowers can be taken for a stomachache, sore throat, headache, colds, tired eyes, or as a laxative. Native Americans used yarrow to bring on their moon cycle, ease childbirth, treat breast abscesses, and expel the placenta after birth. Yarrow controls abnormal menstrual bleeding (taken in moderation), soothes menstrual cramps, and reduces a fever. A poultice prepared from the leaves or even a bunch of fresh herbs can stop bleeding, heal wounds, and draw out mild poisons. Yarrow is associated with the goddess and planet Venus.

YARROW IS A PERENNIAL GROUND COVER THAT LIKES MODERATELY RICH, WELL-DRAINED SOIL AND FULL SUN, BUT DOESN'T REQUIRE A LOT OF WATER. PLANT NEAR AROMATIC HERBS FOR MUTUAL GROWTH ENHANCEMENT. YARROW IS NATIVE TO EUROPE AND WESTERN ASIA.

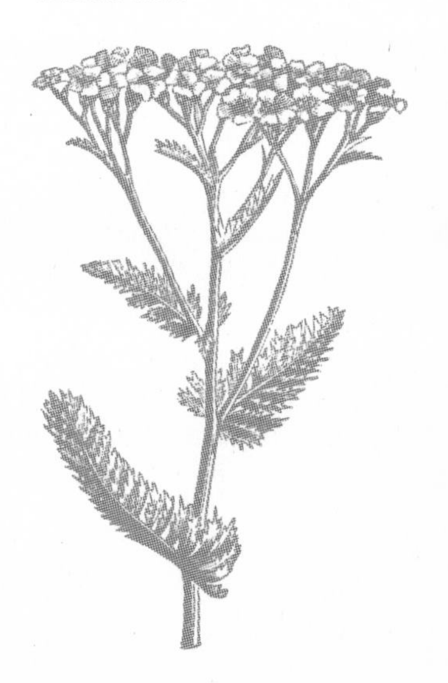

Stingless Bees

If you are stung by a bee, immediately scrape out the stinger using a credit card or similar firm, flat tool; if you pinch the skin around the stinger to extract it, it will squeeze out additional poison. Crush four to six yarrow leaves and rub them over the infected area for thirty seconds. If this remedy is applied quickly, before the poison has had a chance to seep deeper into the tissue, the yarrow will soothe the wound.

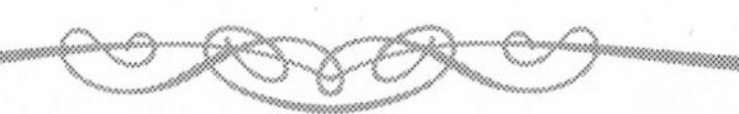

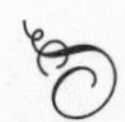

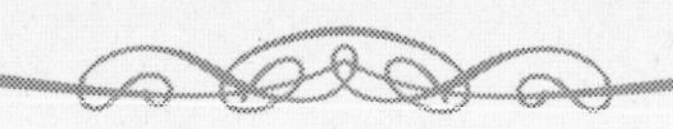

Ylang-Ylang

Cananga odorata

FLOWER OF FLOWERS, ILANG-ILANG

Part Used: flowers

Ylang-ylang is an evergreen tree that grows up to eighty feet tall. It has strongly scented yellow-green flowers and lance-shaped leaves. It is indigenous to Indonesia and the Philippines, and cultivated in tropical Asia and Africa. The flowers are a traditional adornment in the eastern Asia. Ylang-ylang's magickal associations include the ability to calm, attract, and make an impression; it is also an aphrodisiac. In aromatherapy, ylang-ylang is used to heighten the senses, increase sexuality, and relieve anxiety and jet lag.

Sensuous Bath Crystals

Falling in love with your sensuous self merely requires a little attention. Ylang-ylang carries with it the powers of seduction, love, and attraction.

10 to 12 drops ylang-ylang essential oil
6 to 8 drops vanilla essential oil
1 tablespoon freshly ground nutmeg
1 tablespoon freshly ground coriander
½ cup rock salt or sea salt
¼ cup baking soda
¼ cup Epsom salts

Combine all the ingredients in a medium bowl, cauldron, or large mortar. Grind with the pestle in a clockwise direction. As you do, think of a compliment you have received. Meditate on how it made you feel. Think of another word of praise or admiring comment about yourself, and then allow your emotions in response to the flattery to wash over you. Repeat this process, reviewing every kind word another has said about you, along with the fine attributes you admire about your-

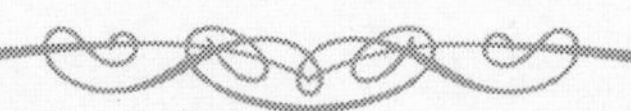

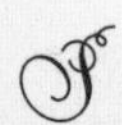

self. Pour your self-love into the mixture. When you are done, remove any large chunks from the mixture. Add 2 to 4 tablespoons to running bath water, or scatter them over the bottom of your shower. As you bathe, allow love and acceptance to themselves around you.

Ylang-Ylang Migraine Oil

The amalgamation of ylang-ylang, feverfew, and lavender works wonders on migraines. The two recipes that follow offer different ways to use this mixture: in a tea and in massage oil. In each case, equal parts of each herb are used, in order to draw on the powers of on the number three, which represents manifestation.

Ylang-ylang is a large tree that grows in the tropics of Asia, especially the Philippines. It can be cultivated as an ornamental in a tropical climate, and an extract made from the flowers is used in perfume.

4 to 6 drops ylang-ylang essential oil
4 to 6 drops feverfew essential oil (see Note)
4 to 6 lavender essential oil
4 ounces olive oil

Combine all the ingredients in a bottle with a squirt top. Massage it on your temples, the back of your neck, your occipital bulb, or any other place where you ache.

Note: If you cannot find feverfew oil, you can put 10 to 12 small feverfew leaves in the bottle.

Ylang-Ylang Migraine Tea

Dried ylang-ylang flowers can be purchased from bulk herbal companies (see page 263).

2 cups water
⅔ cup fresh or dried ylang-ylang flowers
⅔ cup fresh feverfew leaves
⅔ cup fresh lavender flowers

Bring the water to a boil. Add the ylang-ylang, feverfew, and lavender; remove from heat. Let steep 20 minutes. Strain out the herbs. Drink the tea warm.

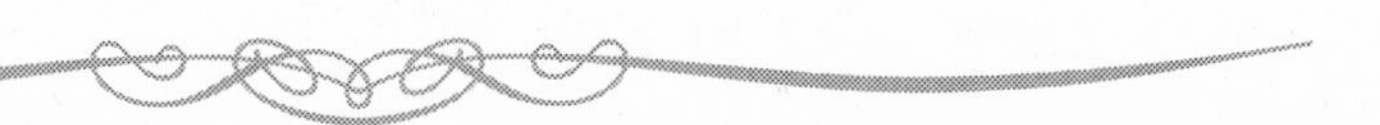

Glossary

Affirmation A positive, repetitive declaration about something you want to manifest in your life. It always needs to be in the positive and present form.

Amulet A consecrated piece of jewelry or coin, often worn or carried, which has been instilled with special desires, such as prosperity or inspiration, although it will often include protection.

Anoint To rub oil on something for ceremonial purposes.

Archetype An original, deep-seated image or model commonly believed to be the perfect example or representation of a group or type.

Astrology The art-science of identifying and clarifying the basic personality traits of a person through reference to planetary movement and position.

Athame A ritual knife used either to cut herbs or a doorway to the spiritual plane during ceremony.

Aura The magnetic force field surrounding a human being, which can be seen or photographed as pulsating and floating colors. The colors reveal one's state of mind.

Banishing To assertively drive energy away from a specific area or ourselves.

Book of Shadows Also known as grimiore, it is a diary or journal of rituals, spells, traditional lore, and journeys.

Censer A heat-proof container, usually a metal bowl or covered incense holder for burning herbs, incense, or resin used to smudge a circle or in performing magick.

Chakra Energy centers or vortexes located throughout body.

Charge To infuse an object with personal power.

Clairvoyant One who has the ability to foresee or intuit events.

Cone of Power A method of directing the energy of an individual or group for a singular purpose or to provide a connection to Spirit.

Consecrate The act of cleansing and blessing an item, most often for magickal or spiritual purposes. May also include infusing or filling a focused intent into the item.

Coven A group of magickal practitioners. The traditional number of members is thirteen.

Deosil Clockwise or going with the sun's direction. Used to gather, build, and strengthen positive energy.

Divination The art or practice of foretelling or predicting the future under the influence of Spirit.

Elements The four fundamental substances that constitute physical matter: air, earth, water, and fire. Also known as the four points of reference of consciousness.

Energy The celestial or primal force that is individually generated. It can be combined with others' energy for greater strength (as in a cone of power).

Esbat A Wiccan ritual, usually performed on a full or new moon.

Faeries A Celtic spelling of the word *fairies*. Faeries include everything from playful energy to the spiritual essence of nature, from an individual planet to a facet of one's being (and more).

Grounding The act of releasing unwanted energy and centering or aligning oneself with the balance of nature and Spirit.

Guardian A guardian represents a personal benefactor of the spiritual realm or caretakers and protectors of the energy represented in the four cardinal directions.

Image Candle A candle infused with your unmatched energy, personality, and power.

Incantation Chanting with the intention of bringing magick into your life.

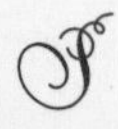

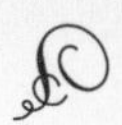

Incense Incense is an herb burned either in cone, stick, or loose dried form over an embering charcoal.

Intuition The truth within yourself. When you look in and sit peacefully, you will find it.

Invoking To call forth energy from your angels, guides, God, Goddess, and other spiritual beings.

Karma The universal law and order of cause and effect, which demonstrates that whatever you do will come back to you.

Macrocosm The spiritual realm of heaven where Spirit's collective consciousness, the heavens, and the deities exist.

Magick The art of getting desired results.

Meditation An exercise requiring the emphasis on breathing and relaxing the mind chatter for purposes of harmonizing and balancing oneself.

Metaphysical Events that occur beyond physical explanation.

Microcosm Your individual spiritual or physical existence.

Oracle A person of great knowledge who speaks the wisdom of Spirit.

Otherworld The world where spirits abide waiting to be reborn.

Pentacle A physical representation of a pentagram.

Pentagram A five-pointed star symbolizing the four elements in balance with Spirit.

Reincarnation The belief that life and death are a cycle. After you leave this life, you spend time with Spirit until you are reborn, learning lessons and having experiences.

Ritual A sacred system of ceremonial acts in observance and accordance of one's spirituality.

Runes An ancient alphabet inscribed on stones for the purpose of bringing in Spirit.

Sabbat One of eight festivals that celebrate the earth, God, Goddess, and the ever-changing cycle of the seasons.

Sacred Space A hallowed or blessed area that has been cleansed and prepared for magickal purposes.

Smudging A ritual used whenever or wherever you feel the need to cleanse, balance, protect, or purify yourself, others, a room, your crystals, or other special tools using the smoke from a smoldering bundle of sage.

Spell A means of helping one channel or direct wishes and desires from the spiritual realm to the material world.

Supernatural Events and experiences occurring "beyond the natural" order of things. Also unexplainable events and experiences attributed to the spiritual realm.

Talisman A consecrated item that brings good luck, averts evil, and embodies your personal magick.

Tarot A set of playing cards used to perceive the past, foretell the future, or divine current possible pathways.

Third-Dimensional Living Existing in the material or physical realm of earth and humans.

Totem An animal symbol or spirit that guides one throughout life.

Underworld The opposite side of the living. According to mythology the Underworld was formerly earth and then came under the rule of Hades, Greek god of the dead.

Visualization The act of using your mind to "see" events outside of your physically visual perception.

Wicca A nature-based religion derived from the Anglo-Saxon root word *wicce* meaning "to bend or shape" as well as "wise."

Widdershins Counterclockwise or going against the sun's direction. Used to banish, wither, or remove unwanted energy.

Wild-crafted A process of gathering herbs in their native habitat.

Wortcunning The art of growing and using herbs for magickal and healing purposes.

Zodiac The visible path of the planets, sun, and moon around the earth; the twelve signs.

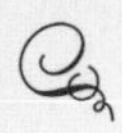

Resources

Ingredients

Base oils
Almond, sunflower, apricot, avocado, jojoba, grapeseed or coconut oil can be obtained at health food stores and whole food markets. The Herbal Products section, page 263, lists additional sources.

Beeswax
This salve base can be obtained at health food stores and whole food markets. The Herbal Products section, page 263, lists additional sources.

Cocoa butter
This salve can be obtained at health food stores and whole food markets. The Herbal Products section, page 263, lists additional sources.

Candles
Candles for imagery and in a variety of shapes and colors can be obtained from health food stores, whole food markets, and magickal supply shops.

Candle-making products
Wax, wicks, and other candle-making goods can be obtained at craft supply shops.

Deity oils
These oils, which have been made by a magickal practitioner with a specific intent—usually to invoke a particular God or Goddess—can be obtained at magickal supply shops.

Dried herbs
Herbs can be obtained at grocery stores, health food stores, whole food markets, and magickal supply shops. The Herbal Products section, page 263, lists additional sources.

Essential oils
Essential oils, which are extracted directly from the plant, can be obtained at health food stores, whole food markets, and magickal supply shops. The Herbal Products section, page 263, lists additional sources.

Evening primrose oil
Evening primrose oil can be obtained at health food stores and whole food markets. The Herbal Products section, page 263, lists additional sources.

Herbal product supplies
Supplies such as glass bottles, glass jars, lip balm tubes, and other containers can be obtained at magickal supply shops and craft stores. The Herbal Products section, page 263, lists additional sources.

Incense
Stick, cone, and herb incense can be obtained at health food stores, whole food markets, and magickal supply shops. The Herbal Products section, page 263, lists additional sources.

Ink
Ink prepared with a specific intent by a magickal practitioner can be purchased at magickal supply shops.

Intent oils
Oils with a specific intent, such as prosperity or blessing, prepared by a magickal practitioner are available at magickal supply shops.

Perfume oils
Perfume oils (made of essential oil that has been diluted) can be purchased at health food stores, whole food markets, and magickal supply shops. The Herbal Products section, page 263, lists additional sources.

Shea butter
This salve base is available at health food stores and whole food markets. The Herbal Products section, page 263, lists additional sources.

Soap-making products
Glycerin melt-and-pour soap base, gels, and colorants are for sale at craft supply shops.

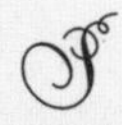

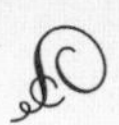

Tea tree oil

Tea tree oil is sold at health food stores and whole food markets. The Herbal Products section, page 263, lists additional sources.

Tinctures

Tinctures (herbal extracts mixed with water and alcohol) are available at health food stores and whole food markets. The Herbal Products section, page 263, lists additional sources.

Vitamin E oil

Vitamin E oil can be obtained at health food stores and whole food markets. The Herbal Products section, page 263, lists additional sources.

Herbal and Natural Medicine Associations

American Association of Naturopathic Physicians

3201 New Mexico Avenue, N.W., Suite 350
Washington, DC 20016
Toll-free: 866-538-2267
Local: 202-895-1392
Fax: 202-274-1992
www.naturopathic.org

This organization empowers its members with the knowledge, tools, skills, and guidance to help them succeed in educating and guiding their communities and patients toward greater health and well-being. This organization is useful for locating naturopathic practitioners and finding treatments for ailments.

American Botanical Council

6200 Manor Rd.
Austin, TX 78714-4345
Phone: 512-926-4900
Fax: 512-926-2345
www.herbalgram.org

The American Botanical Council offers nonprofit education by disseminating science-based information intended to promote the safe and effective use of medicinal plants and phytomedicines. On their website, you will find up-to-date information on beneficial herbs with an emphasis on a clinical approach.

American Herbal Products Association

4733 Bethesda Avenue
Bethesda, MD 20814
www.ahpa.org

The American Herbal Products Association serves its members and the public by promoting and regulating the responsible commerce of herbal products. Their website will keep you abreast of the latest regulatory and scientific issues related to herbal products.

American Herbalists Guild

1931 Gaddis Road Canton, GA 30115
Phone: 770-751-6021
Fax: 770-751-7472
www.americanherbalistsguild.com

The American Herbalists Guild seeks to create harmony between indigenous models of herbalism and modern clinical approaches. It is the only peer-review organization in the United States for professional herbalists specializing in the medicinal use of plants. It is a strong network for herbal practitioners.

American Holistic Health Association

P.O. Box 17400
Anaheim, CA 92817-7400
714-779-6152
www.ahha.org

The American Holistic Health Association promotes holistic principles: honoring the mind, body, and spirit of each person and encouraging people to participate actively in their own health and health care. Their website contains many useful, downloadable articles that can truly empower the healer within you.

Herb Research Foundation

1007 Pearl Street, Suite 200
Boulder, CO 80304
Phone: 800-748-2617, 303-449-2265
Fax: 303-449-7849
www.herbs.org

This foundation offers a resource for seeds and herbs for growers. Their website is full of scientific information about herbs. This organization also holds the media responsible for accurate reporting about herbs and their usage.

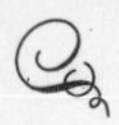

Herb Society of America
9019 Kirtland Chardon Road
Kirtland, OH 44094
Phone: 440-256-0514
Fax: 440-256-0541
www.herbsociety.org

The Herb Society of America offers new information about and shares its members' experiences with horticulture, science, literature, history, the arts, and economics. There is a refreshing angle to the gardening they promote.

Herbal Publications

Herbal Essences
LBHerbSociety@aol.com

The Long Beach Herb Society online newsletter is a free monthly publication of recipes, gardening and craft tips, and opinions. Though targeted to the Southern California region, it has relevance to a much broader area. The Society also holds regular meetings.

Herbal Gram
1007 Pearl Street, Suite 200
Boulder, CO 80304
Phone: 800-748-2617, 303-449-2265
Fax: 303-449-7849
www.herbs.org

A peer-reviewed quarterly journal with a scientific focus on medicinal herbs, copublished by the Herb Research Foundation and the American Botanical Council. Their articles are very detailed, covering government and scientific issues related to herbs.

Herb Research News
1007 Pearl Street, Suite 200
Boulder, CO 80304
Phone: 800-748-2617, 303-449-2265
Fax: 303-449-7849
www.herbs.org

Herb Research Foundation's quarterly newsletter covers herbs in the news, new herb research, current dietary supplement legislative and regulatory issues, and international activities of the foundation in sustainable herb-cultivation projects. It also covers outreach programs in the local community as well as national campaigns.

Herbs for Health
1007 Pearl Street, Suite 200
Boulder, CO 80304
Phone: 800-748-2617, 303-449-2265
Fax: 303-449-7849
www.herbs.org

This bi-monthly magazine by the Herb Research Foundation includes information on herbs' benefits and healing capabilities. It covers topics ranging from recent scientific research to consumer guides, medicinal recipes to legislative updates; they also provide handy information about herb usage.

The Herb Companion
www.discoverherbs.com

The Herb Companion provides the latest research on medicinal herbs, recipes, projects, and ideas for incorporating herbs into your life. It also contains beautiful photographs and artwork.

The Herb Quarterly
223 San Anselmo Avenue, Suite 7
San Anselmo, CA 94960
www.herbquarterly.com

This quarterly magazine offers down-to-earth tips on hard-to-grow herbs, new herbs, recipes, seasonal herbs, and herbal lore in a user-friendly format.

The Herbarist
9019 Kirtland Chardon Road
Kirtland, OH 44094
Phone: 440-256-0514
Fax: 440-256-0541
www.herbsociety.org

This annual publication of the Herb Society of America reports the latest writings, research, and information on herbs. It blends both scholarly and popular techniques in articles by experts on current herbal topics.

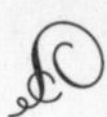

Organic Gardening
www.organicgardening.com

Each issue offers expert advice on making organic gardening easy and successful; there are also tips for growing vegetables and flowers naturally. They offer excellent resources for buying herb, vegetable, and flower seeds and information on getting involved with maintaining organic standards.

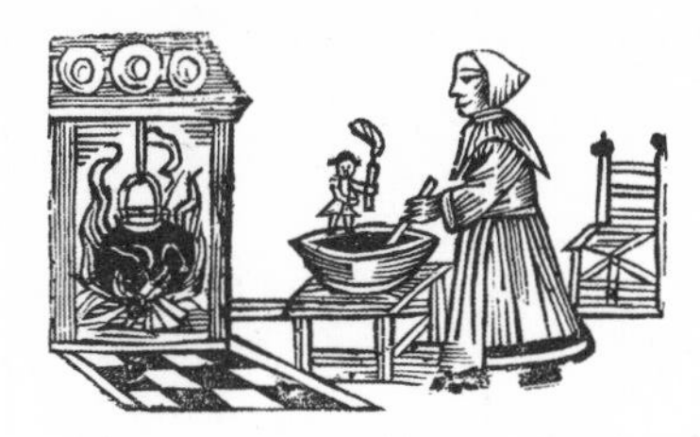

Herbal Products

Avena Botanicals

219 Mill Street
Rockport, ME 04856
Phone: 207-594-0694
Fax: 207-594-2975
www.avenaherbs.com

This company offers herbal education and products that carry on an herbal tradition kept alive by women with a nurturing, biodynamic approach. They have a catalog and their garden is open to the public.

Cheryl's Herbs

836 Hanley Industrial Court
St. Louis, MO 63144
Phone: 800-231-5971, 314-963-4449
Fax: 314-963-4454
www.cherylsherbs.com

This informative site offers therapeutic-quality pure essential oils and hydrosols, dried herbs, and a wide variety of aromatherapy and herbal products, supplies, and books. The site includes articles, an encyclopedia, newsletter, and answers to questions frequently asked about herbs.

Frontier Herb Co-op

P.O. Box 299
Norway, IA 53218
800-669-3275
www.frontiercoop.com

Offers organic foods, candles, fragrance oils, natural personal care products, baking and cooking products, and aromatherapy products. This is a great website for those who do not have access to health food stores or whole food markets in town.

Gaia Herbs

108 Island Ford Road
Brevard, NC 28712
Phone: 800-831-7780, 828-884-4242
Fax: 828-884-8967
www.gaiaherbs.com

This site offers liquid herbal extracts of guaranteed quality and certified organic purity. Gaia Herbs' products are located in health food stores and whole food stores nationwide, including herbal solutions for children. Their products are wild-crafted.

Herb Pharm

P.O. Box 116
Williams, OR 97544
Phone: 800-348-4372, 541-846-6262
Fax: 800-545-7392
www.herb-pharm.com

Offers more than 240 herbal products, including single liquid extracts, liquid extract compounds, alcohol-free glycerites, oils, a salve, and tablets and capsules. This website offers news, events, and answers to questions about herbal products. Some of their herbs are wild-crafted.

Herbalist & Alchemist

51 South Wandling Ave.
Washington, NJ 07882
800-611-8235
www.herbalist-alchemist.com

This resource for herbs is steeped in respect for tradition and dedicated to education; they offer high-quality organic and wild-crafted herbs, oils, tea blends, and books.

Horizon Herbs
P.O. Box 69
Williams, OR 97544
Phone: 541-846-6704
Fax: 541-846-6233
http://www.chatlink.com/~herbseed

Purveyors of strictly medicinal seeds and live roots. Their products are organically grown or wild-crafted.

Jean's Greens
119 Sulphur Spring Road
Newport, NY 13416
Phone: 888-845-8327, 315-845-6500
www.jeansgreens.com

This company sells herbal teas, herbal essences, dried bulk herbs, herbal beauty products, healthy edibles, and more. They have an online store and a catalog.

Mountain Rose Herbs
85472 Dilley Lane
Eugene, OR 97405
Phone: 800-879-3337
Fax: 510-217-4012
Outside USA phone: 541-741-7341
www.mountainroseherbs.com

Mountain Rose Herbs offers the finest organic botanical products and the freshest as well. They supply organic herbs, essential oils, natural body-care products, vials, tea bags, and other packaging goods.

Nichols Garden Nursery
1190 Old Salem Road N.E.
Albany, OR 97321-4580
Phone: 800-422-3985
Fax: 800-231-5306
www.nicholsgardennurserey.com

This family-run business has over fifty years' experience as purveyors of herb seeds, plants, some dried herb products, oils, extracts, and books. They offer rare and unusual seeds and plants, recipes, and answers to questions.

Pacific Botanicals
4350 Fish Hatchery Road
Grants Pass, OR 97527
Phone: 541-479-7777
Fax: 541-479-5271
www.pacificbotanicals.com

Pacific Botanicals' product line includes more than 175 organically grown medicinal herbs and spices in whole, cut, tea-bag cut, or powder forms.

Richters Herbs
Goodwood, Ontario
LoC 1AO, Canada
Phone: 905-640-6677
Fax: 905-640-6641
www.richters.com

The Richters are fine purveyors of herb seeds, plants, some dried herb products, and books. They offer answers to questions, workshops for herb lovers new at growing herbs, and information for commercial growers and buyers. They also have a catalog.

San Francisco Herb & Natural Food Co.
47444 Kato Road
Fremont, CA 94538
Phone: 510-770-1215
www.herbspicetea.com

Bulk herbs and botanicals, teas, spice blends, extracts, and tinctures—wholesale and retail—of excellent quality are available from this website. They offer excellent tools for making and containers for storing herbal products.

Simpler's Botanicals
P.O. Box 2534
Sebastopol, CA 95476
Phone: 800-652-7646, 707-887-2012
Fax: 707-887-7570
http://simplers.com

Simpler's intention is to supply high-quality plant extracts, aromatherapy, and essential oils. Information on the benefits of herbs and aromatherapy is available on their website.

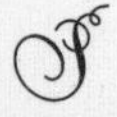

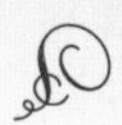

Vitality Works
5821-D Midway Park Boulevard N.E.
Albuquerque, NM 87109
Phone: 800-403-4372
www.vitalityworks.com

Organically grown and ethically wild-harvested herbs are used in extracts and formulas to bring you high-quality herbal preparations. This company will create unique herbal formulas just for you.

Young Living Essential Oils
250 South Main Street
Payson, UT 84651
Phone: 800-371-2928
Fax: 866-203-5666
www.youngliving.us

Young Living Essential Oils is world-renowned for exceptionally high-quality essential oils, dietary supplements, personal care products, and other unique products. Their formulas unite ancient traditions and modern science to promote health and longevity. Their oils are considered among the best available.

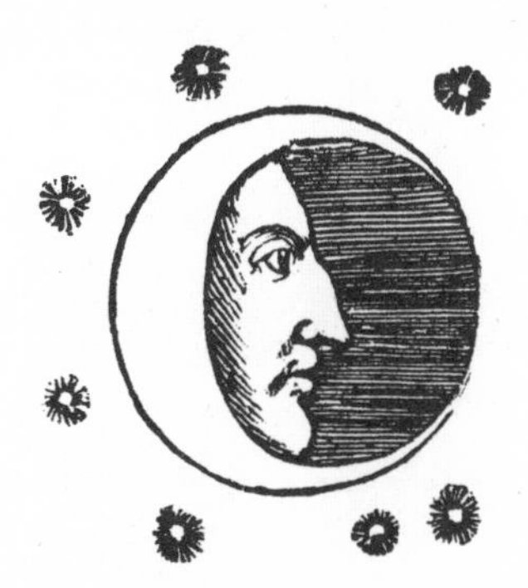

Wise Women Products

Country Spun Soaps and Scents
www.countryspunsoapsandscents.com

Handmade, all-natural soaps (including soaps for men and pets), bubble bath, bath salts, lotions, and creams.

Of the Goddess, Ltd.
www.aromatherapygoddess.com

Aromatherapy, bath, and body products, as well as gifts created with love and devotion. All products are created from old European and indigenous Native American recipes and infused with magickal intent. This company's focus is activating the healer within you.

Kelly's Magical Garden
43 Essex Road
Camp Hill, PA 17011
Phone: 717-737-7623
www.kellysmagicalgarden.com

Bath and body products, oils, herbs, and charms are made with a combination of magical energy and knowledge of aromatherapy to enhance your spiritual journey. They offer intent oils for magick practitioners.

Medieval Bath Products
818-771-5537
www.medievalinc.com

Bath and body products handcrafted in the wise woman tradition. All of their beautifully packaged products are made with all-natural ingredients, a little fantasy, love, simple natural wisdom, and a whole lot of old wives' tales.

Monk's Garden
949-369-5378
www.monksgarden.com

A line of herbal preparations for everyday living. Products include magickal botanicals, flower essences, herbal tea blends, Faeries for the Pot, pure weeds, incenses for your good intentions. Everything the proprietor, Jacquie, makes is handmade and enchanted with love and magick.

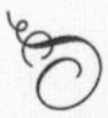

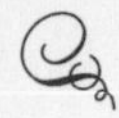

Bibliography

Alshul O'Donnell, Sara, and Sara Harrar. *The Woman's Book of Healing Herbs*. Emmaus, Penn.: Rodale Press, 1999.

Bach, Richard. *Illusions: The Adventures of a Reluctant Messiah*. New York: Dell, 1994.

______. *Jonathan Livingston Seagull.* New York: Avon, 1973.

Balch, Phyllis. *Prescriptions for Herbal Healing*. New York: Penguin, 2002.

Beyerl, Paul. *The Master Book of Herbalism*. Custer, Wash: Phoenix, 1984.

Bremness, Lesley. *Herbs.* Pleasantville, N.Y.: The Reader's Digest Association, 1990.

Carlton, Hanna. *The Complete Guide to Natural Healing*. Pittsburgh, Penn.: International Masters, 2001.

Chevallier, Andrew. *Encyclopedia of Herbal Medicine*. New York: Dorling Kindersley, 2000.

Coney, Norma. *The Complete Soapmaker*. New York: Sterling, 1996.

Cornell, Joseph. *Sharing Nature with Children.* Nevada City, Calif: DAWN Publications, 1998.

Cunningham, Scott. *Encyclopedia of Magical Herbs.* St. Paul, Minn.: Llewellyn, 1985.

______. *Magical Herbalism.* St. Paul, Minn.: Llewellyn, 1982.

De Bairacli Levy, Juliette. *Common Herbs for Natural Health.* Woodstock, N.Y.: Ash Tree, 1997.

Dunwich, Gerina. *Witch Craft.* Secaucus, N.J.: Citadel, 1997.

Eason, Cassandra. *A Complete Guide to Faeries and Magical Beings.* Boston, Mass.: Weiser Books, 2002.

Fairley, Josephine. *Organic Beauty.* New York: Dorling Kindersley, 2001.

Findhorn Community, The. *The Findhorn Garden.* New York: Harper & Row, 1975.

Forrest, Steven. *The Inner Sky.* San Diego, Calif.: ACS Publications, 1988.

Foy, Nicky, and Roger Philips. *The Random House Book of Herbs.* New York: Random House, 1990.

Gladstar, Rosemary. *Herbal Healing for Women.* New York: Fireside/Simon and Schuster, 1993.

Green, James. *The Herbal Medicine-Maker's Handbook.* Freedom, Calif.: The Crossing Press, 2000.

Kruger, Anna. *An Illustrated Guide to Herbs, Their Medicine and Magic.* Surrey, Eng.: Dragon's World, 1993.

Matthews, John. *The Winter Solstice.* Wheaton, Ill.: Quest Books, 1998.

McCoy, Edain. *Celtic Women's Spirituality.* St. Paul, Minn.: Llewellyn, 2001.

______. *Sabbats.* St. Paul, Minn.: Llewellyn, 2002.

Morrison, Dorothy. *Everyday Magic.* St. Paul, Minn.: Llewellyn, 1998.

Murray, Michael T. *The Healing Power of Herbs.* Rocklin, Calif.: Prima, 1992.

Patton, Mary Lee. *Mary Lee's Natural Health and Beauty.* New York: Jeremy Tarcher/Putnam, 2001.

Rodale's Illustrated Encyclopedia of Herbs, edited by Claire Kowalchik and William H. Hylton. Emmaus, Penn.: Rodale Press, 1987.

Schiffer, Mechthild. *The Encyclopedia of Bach Flower Therapy.* Rochester, Verm.: Healing Arts, 1999.

Starhawk. *The Spiral Dance.* San Francisco, Calif.: HarperCollins, 1999.

Stewart, R. J. *Earth Light.* Lake Toxaway, N.C.: Mercury, 1992.

Stout, Ruth. *The Ruth Stout No-Work Garden Book.* Emmaus, Penn.: Rodale, 1971.

Sunset Western Garden Book, edited by Kathleen Norris Brenzel. Menlo Park, Calif.: Sunset, 2001.

Tenney, Louise. *Today's Herbal Health.* Pleasant Grove, Utah: Woodland, 2000.

Thurston, Leslie Temple, and Brad Laughlin. *Returning to Oneness: The Seven Keys of Ascension.* Santa Fe, N.M.: CoreLight, 2002.

Tolle, Eckhart. *The Power of Now.* Novato, Calif.: New World Library, 1999.

Weed, Susan, and Durga Bernhard. *Healing Wise.* Woodstock, N.Y.: Ash Tree, 1995.

______. *Herbal for the Childbearing Year.* Woodstock, N.Y.: Ash Tree, 1995.

Weiss, Gaea, and Shandor Weiss. *Growing and Using the Healing Herbs.* New York: Wings Books, 1985.

Wildfeuer, Sherry. *Stella Natura 1998.* San Francisco, Calif.: Biodynamic Farming and Gardening Association, 1998.

Wood, Jamie, and Tara Seefeldt. *The Wicca Cookbook.* Berkeley, Calif.: Celestial Arts, 2000.

Index

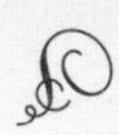

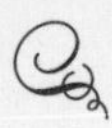

H

I

J

K

L

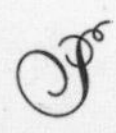

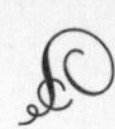

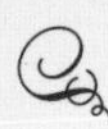

Q

R

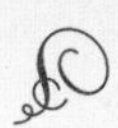

S

T

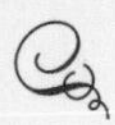

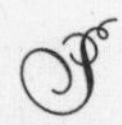